Pharmaceuticals: Clinical Studies

Pharmaceuticals: Clinical Studies

Editor: Meredith Morton

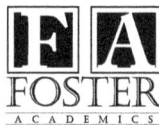

FA FOSTER
ACADEMICS

www.fosteracademics.com

www.fosteracademics.com

FA
FOSTER
ACADEMICS

Cataloging-in-Publication Data

Pharmaceuticals : clinical studies / edited by Meredith Morton.
   p. cm.
Includes bibliographical references and index.
ISBN 978-1-63242-909-4
1. Drugs. 2. Clinical pharmacology. 3. Pharmacy. 4. Materia medica. I. Morton, Meredith.
RM300 .P43 2020
615.1--dc23

© Foster Academics, 2020

Foster Academics,
118-35 Queens Blvd., Suite 400,
Forest Hills, NY 11375, USA

ISBN 978-1-63242-909-4 (Hardback)

Contents

Permissions

List of Contributors

Index

Preface

A pharmaceutical drug is a drug that is used to diagnose, treat or prevent disease. Pharmaceuticals are classified based on the level of control, mode of action, therapeutic effects, biological system affected or route of administration. Some classes of drugs are analgesics, antipyretics, antibiotics, antiseptics, oral contraceptives, tranquilizers, hormone replacements, etc. Drugs can be administered in various dosages in the form of pills, capsules or tablets, and their administration can be parenteral, enteral, topical, intranasal, rectal, etc. Drug discovery, drug development and drug delivery are important areas of research in pharmaceutical science. Biotechnology is a major driver in the discovery of biopharmaceuticals. There has been constant research around the development of novel antibiotics and antibacterials as well as on the use of biological agents for antibacterial therapy. This facilitates better drug design and development. This book is a compilation of chapters that discuss the most vital concepts and emerging trends in the field of pharmacology. From theories to research to practical applications, case studies related to all contemporary topics of relevance to pharmaceuticals have been included in this book. It will help the readers in keeping pace with the rapid changes in this field.

This book unites the global concepts and researches in an organized manner for a comprehensive understanding of the subject. It is a ripe text for all researchers, students, scientists or anyone else who is interested in acquiring a better knowledge of this dynamic field.

I extend my sincere thanks to the contributors for such eloquent research chapters. Finally, I thank my family for being a source of support and help.

Editor

Antimicrobial and Antibiofilm Activity of UP-5, an Ultrashort Antimicrobial Peptide Designed using only Arginine and Biphenylalanine

Ammar Almaaytah [1,*] 🆔, Mohammed T. Qaoud [1], Gubran Khalil Mohammed [1], Ahmad Abualhaijaa [2], Daniel Knappe [3], Ralf Hoffmann [3] and Qosay Al-Balas [4] 🆔

[1] Department of Pharmaceutical Technology, Faculty of Pharmacy, Jordan University of Science and Technology, Irbid 22110, Jordan; mqaud@daad-alumni.de (M.T.Q.); gubrankhalil@daad-alumni.de (G.K.M.)

[2] Department of Applied Biological Sciences, Faculty of Science and Arts, Jordan University of Science and Technology, Irbid 22110, Jordan; ahkhaled18@yahoo.com

[3] Institute of Bioanalytical Chemistry, Faculty of Chemistry and Mineralogy and Center for Biotechnology and Biomedicine, Universität Leipzig, Deutscher Platz 5, 04103 Leipzig, Germany; daniel.knappe@bbz.uni-leipzig.de (D.K.); ralf.hoffmann@bbz.uni-leipzig.de (R.H.)

[4] Department of Medicinal Chemistry, Faculty of Pharmacy, Jordan University of Science and Technology, Irbid 22110, Jordan; qabalas@just.edu.jo

* Correspondence: amalmaaytah@just.edu.jo

Abstract: The recent upsurge of multidrug resistant bacteria (MDRB) among global communities has become one of the most serious challenges facing health professionals and the human population worldwide. Cationic ultrashort antimicrobial peptides (USAMPs) are a promising group of molecules that meet the required criteria of novel antimicrobial drug development. UP-5, a novel penta-peptide, displayed significant antimicrobial activities against various standard and clinical isolates of MDRB. UP-5 displayed MICs values within the range of (10–15 µM) and (55–65 µM) against Gram-positive and Gram-negative bacteria, respectively. Furthermore, UP-5 displayed antibiofilm activity with minimum biofilm eradication concentration (MBEC) value as equal to twofold higher than MIC value. At the same inhibitory concentrations, UP-5 exhibited very low or negligible toxicity toward human erythrocytes and mammalian cells. Combining UP-5 with conventional antibiotics led to a synergistic or additive mode of action that resulted in the reduction of the MIC values for some of the antibiotics by 99.7% along a significant drop in MIC values of the peptide. The stability profile of UP-5 was evaluated in full mouse plasma and serum with results indicating a more stable pattern in plasma. The present study indicates that USAMPs are promising antimicrobial agents that can avoid the negative characteristics of conventional antimicrobial peptides. Additionally, USAMPs exhibit good to moderate activity against MDRB, negligible toxicity, and synergistic outcomes in combination with conventional antimicrobial agents.

Keywords: antimicrobial peptide; biofilms; ultrashort peptide; resistant bacteria

1. Introduction

The uncontrolled, outspread and extended use of antibiotics in recent decades has led to an unbounded resistance development by bacteria against most conventional antibiotics. Antimicrobial resistance develops when microorganisms (such as bacteria, fungi, viruses, and parasites) start to combat the effectiveness of antimicrobial agents. As a result, these agents gradually become ineffective. The multidrug resistance (MDR) phenomenon has become one of the most serious challenges in the clinical management of human infections [1].

From an economic point of view, the patients with resistant infections increase the cost of health care due to the longer duration of illness and hospitalization. The requirement for additional tests and the use of more expensive drugs contributes further in increasing the cost of health care for those patients than patients with non-resistant infections [2]. This issue has turned into a main concern worldwide, as there is no clear medication strategy to handle these types of serious infections. Therefore, massive efforts have been applied in order to develop new antimicrobial agents with unique modes of actions and low potential of bacterial resistance development to manage multidrug-resistant related infections and the post-antibiotic era.

All species of living organisms produce antimicrobial peptides (AMPs), which play a vital function within the organism by acting as fast weapons in the innate immune system against infecting pathogens, such as bacteria, fungi, and yeast [3–6]. These peptides are usually less than 50 amino acid residues long, display net positive charges, and exhibit an amphipathic nature [7].

The mode of action of AMPs is significantly different when compared to conventional antibiotics that act by targeting specific sites within the microbial cell, such as enzymes, ribosomes, or bacterial DNA. On the other hand, the mode of action of AMPs is related to causing irreversible damage to the cell membrane, thus allowing the AMPs to permeate the cell membrane physically and rapidly. Due to this unique mechanism of action, the probability of bacterial cells developing microbial resistance is very low compared to the available conventional antibiotics [8]. Furthermore, many models were proposed in order to explain AMPs' modes of action, these models are matched by the diversity of AMPs in sequences, structures, and lengths [4,9–11].

In general, the antimicrobial activity of AMPs is governed by two substantial merits: positive net charge and hydrophobic residues. Based on the previous structure-activity related studies [12–14], the cationic and hydrophobic residues should be in a properly balanced state in order to avoid eukaryotic toxicity. There is a strong belief that the initial binding of cationic AMPs with the lipopolysaccharide (LPS) layer or lipoteichoic acids that hold a negative charge in Gram-negative and Gram-positive bacteria, respectively, is an essential step. It is the first substantial step to govern the antimicrobial activity of cationic AMPs. After that, AMPs navigate into and permeate the inner phospholipid membrane. Furthermore, it is suggested that DNA is another potential target for AMPs where binding to DNA leads to inhibition of DNA replication and transcription without damaging the cell membrane of bacteria [15–18]. It is believed that the bacterial membrane is broken down through the "carpet" mechanism which results in piling up of these peptides on the microbial surface till reaching a sensitive threshold concentration that eventually leads to the devastation of the bacterial membrane in a detergent-like a manner [19,20].

Regrettably, several factors limit the use of native peptides as therapeutics, including mammalian cell toxicity which is considered as a major disadvantage for AMPs, very poor bioavailability due to poor absorption and low metabolic stability towards proteolytic enzymes in the gastrointestinal tract after oral ingestion, in addition to the rapid excretion through the kidneys and liver [21]. Furthermore, complex structure and relatively large size are important factors that limit the chemical synthesis of the natural antimicrobial peptides, so accordingly significant efforts and high costs are needed to synthesize them. The defensins group is an example of AMPs of such criteria that consists of 18–45 amino acids including six disulphide linked cysteines [3,22].

Despite of all these drawbacks, development of new therapeutics based on proteins and peptides has attracted interests and therefore efforts are oriented toward the development of peptidomimetics, a new concept that have shown great promise both in medicinal and organic chemistry. This approach is based on enhancing the bioavailability and activity of native peptides and proteins, which are considered as tools to develop drug candidates and new therapeutic classes, by introducing both functional and structural specific modifications while maintaining main features responsible for biological activity [21]. Apart from displaying greater oral bioavailability and biological activity, peptidomimetics may also show high cell selectivity than native peptides [23,24]. Peptidomimetics are divided into three classes depending on their functional and structural characteristics and these include [25]:

- Class I (structural mimetics): show a structural analogy with the native substrate in a well-defined spatial orientation, they carry all the functionalities responsible for the interaction with a receptor or an enzyme.
- Class II (functional mimetics): the analogy of this type is based on the interaction with the target enzyme or receptor regardless of their apparent structural similarity with the native compound.
- Class III (functional-structural mimetics): all the functional groups required for biological activity are mounted in a scaffoldwith a structure different from that of the starting compound.

Thyrotropin-releasing hormone (TRH) mimetic represents an elegant example of a peptidomimetic scaffold. This mimetic is based on a cyclohexane scaffold that replaces the peptide backbone. The pharmacophore represented by three functional groups are placed on the scaffold with maintaining spatial orientation of the amino acid side chains found in TRH hormone [26].

Current efforts for developing AMPs and enhancing their development towards the clinic are being focused on the design of a new sub-family called ultrashort antimicrobial peptides (USAMPs) which consist of three to eight amino acids. Several environmental and economic advantages are associated with the development of these new promising peptides. Chemically, they can be synthesized easily and purified simply. The amount of solvent and time required for synthesis is limited [27–38].

It was observed that according to previous studies aimed to design ultrashort peptides that using only two lysine or two ornithine amino acids to represent charged residues has led to loss of activity [28]. Further investigations showed that the antimicrobial and antibiofilm activity was significantly reduced as a result of replacing arginine with lysine residues due to favoring particular binding characteristics to bacterial membrane and DNA [39,40]. These results prove that membrane disruption is cation residue specific and furthermore cationic charges must arise from arginine and not lysine or ornithine, especially when the peptide is ultrashort in length. On the other hand, the hydrophobic moieties were represented by tryptophan which has a significant preference for the membrane interface compared to other hydrophobic amino acids. Also, biphenylalanine was used to represent hydrophobic moieties in order to enhance membrane insertion properties and using it led to reinforce peptide activity against methicillin-resistant *staphylococcus aureus* (MRSA) [28,41]. Furthermore, incorporation of non-natural amino acids was used as a main strategy to enhance peptide stability [42,43]. The biphenylalanine motif was reported as the shortest antimicrobial peptide-based agent. A severe damage to bacterial morphology and bacterial cell death were observed as a result of biphenylalanine interaction with bacterial cell membrane [44]. Besides that, the substitution of H by phenyl group in biphenylalanine is expected to incorporate a superior biological protection against enzymatic degradation compared to other non-natural motifs used alkyl substitution. This stability enhancement is secured via increasing basicity and decreasing polarity in addition to eliminate the predominance of *trans* versus *cis* peptide bond confirmation and some inter- and intramolecular hydrogen bonds [42,45].

Taking this into consideration, biphenylalanine (an unnatural amino acid) and arginine were used rationally in the present study to design a novel penta-peptide named UP-5. The peptide displayed potent antimicrobial activities against various standard and clinical isolates of MDRB. Additionally, UP-5 displayed potent antibiofilm activity with MBEC values as equal to MIC values. At the same inhibitory concentrations, UP-5 exhibited very low or negligible toxicity toward human erythrocytes and mammalian cells (Vero cells).

2. Materials and Methods

2.1. Peptide Design, Synthesis and Purification

The pentapeptide UP-5 (NH_2-RBRBR-COOH, where B represents biphenylalanine and R represents arginine), was synthesized by G.L. Biochem (Shanghai, China), employing solid-phase methods and Fmoc chemistry. The purity and the identity (>98%) of the synthetic peptide were confirmed by reversed-phase high performance liquid chromatography (RP-HPLC) and electrospray Ionization (ESI-MS) mass spectrometry, respectively (supplementary material).

2.2. Antibiotics

Conventional antibiotics levofloxacin, chloramphenicol, rifampicin, and ampicillin were obtained from Sigma-Aldrich (Shanghai, China) and erythromycin from Sigma-Aldrich (St. Louis, MO, USA). According to the manufacture's recommendations, the antibiotic powders and stock solution preparations were stored at the optimum temperature for each antibiotic.

2.3. Bacterial Strains

All bacterial susceptibility, biofilm, and synergistic assays of peptides, antibiotics, and peptides-antibiotics combinations used bacterial strains obtained from the American Type Tissue Culture Collection (ATCC, Manassas, VA, USA) that states the mechanism of resistance for each strain according to ATCC number. Gram-positive bacteria were represented by five strains, the wild type strain *Staphylococcus aureus* (ATCC 29213) and methicillin-resistant *S. aureus* (MRSA) (ATCC 33591) in addition to clinically isolated strains *S. aureus* (ATCC BAA-41& 43300) and *Enterococcus faecalis* (ATCC BAA-2316). The Gram-negative bacteria strains were represented by wild type strains of *Escherichia coli* (ATCC 25922 & 35218) and *Pseudomonas aeruginosa* (ATCC 27853) as well as the clinically isolated multidrug-resistant strain *P. aeruginosa* (ATCC BAA-2114). The bacteria were cultured onto Muller Hinton Agar (Scharlab, S.L, Barcelona, Spain). Mueller Hinton Broth (Oxoid Ltd., Basingstoke, UK) was used to prepare all bacterial suspensions and to dissolve the peptides and the antibiotics. The assay was performed in sterile 96-well polypropylene microtiter plates.

2.4. Bacterial Susceptibility Assays

All bacterial susceptibility assays were conducted according to the microbroth dilution method outlined by the Clinical and Laboratory Standards Institute (CLSI) guidelines [46,47].

2.4.1. MIC and MBC Values of UP-5

Briefly, pre-sterilized MHB was used as a growth medium for organisms obtained from stock media with glycerol. Bacterial cells were grown overnight in MHB and diluted to 10^6 CFU/mL in the same medium prior to use. For peptide, serial concentrations in the range of 0.5–100 μM were prepared. Then, 50 μL of each peptide concentration and 50 μL of diluted bacterial suspension were added to each well of a 96-well microtiter plate. Peptide solutions were prepared by dissolving the peptide in sterile MHB. Then, the plates were incubated overnight in a humidified atmosphere, and at 37 °C. Bacterial growth was determined by measuring the optical density (OD) at $\lambda = 600$ nm using an ELISA plate reader (Epoch, BioTek, Winooski, VT, USA) and the minimum inhibitory concentration (MIC) was determined. For the minimum bactericidal concentration (MBC), 10 μL was withdrawn from wells having various concentrations of the peptide, clear negative wells, and turbid positive control wells, and were allowed to grow after sub-culturing on pre-sterilized labeled agar plated for 24 h at 37 °C. The lowest concentration that led to having <0.1% viable cells (killing 99.9%) of the subcultures refers to the MBC value.

2.4.2. MICs and MBC Determination of Individual Antibiotics

As described in the previous section, the MIC and MBC values of antibiotics employed in this study were determined against subjected bacterial strains via preparing different concentrations of each antibiotic.

2.4.3. MIC and MBC Determination for Peptide and Antibiotics in Combinations

According to the broth microdilution checkerboard technique [48], the MIC and MBC values of peptide-antibiotics combinations against wild type and multidrug resistant bacterial strains were determined. Serial concentrations of peptide and each antibiotic were prepared in the range of 0.005–100 μM. In each well of a 96-well microtiter plate, 25 μL of each peptide concentration were added to 25 μL of each antibiotic concentration which is followed by adding 50 μL of diluted bacterial suspension (10^6 CFU/mL) to each well. The prepared concentrations of peptide and each antibiotic were arranged into rows and columns, respectively, in a 96-well microtiter plate according the checkerboard technique. Then as described previously (see Section 2.4.1), the procedure was followed. All MIC and MBC determinations of all assays were made in triplicate.

2.4.4. FIC Determination

The fractional inhibitory concentration (FIC) is defined as the inhibitory concentration of the antimicrobial combination divided by that of the single antimicrobial component. To calculate FIC index for peptide-antibiotic combinations, the following equation was used:

$$\text{FIC index} = \frac{\text{MIC of drug X in combination}}{\text{MIC of drug X alone}} + \frac{\text{MIC of drug Y in combination}}{\text{MIC of drug Y alone}} \tag{1}$$

The FIC indices were interpreted as follows: ≤0.5: synergistic activity, 0.5–1: additive activity, 1–4 indifferent, >4: antagonism. Interpretation and assessment of the FIC indices were performed according to the broth microdilution checkerboard technique [48].

2.5. Antibiofilm Assay

Biofilm formation relied on a published protocol employing the Calgary biofilm device (Innovotech, Edmonton, AB, Canada) [49,50]. Briefly, *S. aureus* (ATCC 33591) bacterial strain was incubated in MHB and cultures were diluted in the same medium to achieve a concentration of 10^5 CFU/mL. Next, diluted bacterial suspension (150 μL) was added to the sterile 96 peg-lids on which biofilm cells can build up. Negative control lanes were prepared by adding 150 μL MHB to six wells. And then the pegs were incubated for 14–16 h under rotation of 125 rpm at 37 °C to allow biofilm formation on the purpose designed pegs. The pegs were rinsed twice with phosphate-buffered saline (PBS) to remove planktonic cells as a washing step. Each peg-lid was then transferred into a "challenge 96-well microtiter plate" containing 200 μL of different peptides concentrations and the peg-lids containing the biofilms were incubated for four hours at 37 °C under rotation at 125 rpm. After biofilm treatment with the challenge plate, the biofilms were re-washed twice with PBS then transferred into the recovery plate for eight hours. The minimum biofilm eradication concentration MBEC value is defined as the minimum concentration needed to inhibit the re-growth of biofilms after four hours of peptide treatment, washing twice with PBS and incubating in pre-sterilized MHB (recovery plate) for 8 h, using an ELISA plate reader λ = 600 nm. Additionally, the biofilms were assessed for their minimum bactericidal concentration (MBECb), this assay was conducted similar to MBC assay (see Section 2.4.1). MBECb parameter is defined as the lowest concentration able to eradicate $3\log^{10}$ of the viable microorganisms in a biofilm (99.9% killing) after 8 h of incubation in recovery plates using the colony count method.

2.6. MTT Cell Proliferation Assay

Vero cells were seeded at 5×10^3 cells per well in flat-bottomed 96-well plates, and the plate was incubated for 18–24 h at 37 °C under 5% CO_2 to allow cell attachment on the bottom of the plates. Next day, different concentrations of the peptide were prepared as a gradient using growth medium as the diluent (150, 200, 250, 300, 400, 500, and 600 μM). The plates were incubated for 24 h at 37 °C under 5% CO_2. Next, 30 μL (2.5 g/L) MTT solutions were added to all wells and the plates were incubated for 4–6 h. After incubation, the MTT-Peptide solution was removed and a 100 μL of DMSO was added to each well and mixed thoroughly by pipetting to dissolve the Formazan crystals at the bottom of the wells until a clear purple color was achieved. The plates were then placed on an ELx808™ Absorbance Microplate Reader (BioTek, Winooski, VT, USA) and the absorbance was measured at $\lambda = 540$ nm.

2.7. Erythrocyte Hemolytic Assay

Two milliliters of human blood were placed into a 50 mL centrifuge tube and centrifuged ($3000 \times g$). The supernatant was discarded, the cell pellet re-suspended in 48 mL of PBS, and centrifuged as above; this step was repeated twice. Finally, 2 mL of cell pellet were re-suspended in a sterile tube containing 48 mL PBS to reach a final concentration of 4% RBC. Different concentrations of the peptide were prepared (40, 60, 80, 100, 125, 150, 175, and 200 μM), and then 1 mL of each peptide concentration was added to 1 mL of erythrocyte suspension. Positive controls were prepared by adding 5 μL of 0.1% (Triton 100X) to 2 mL of 4% RBC suspension and negative controls were prepared by adding 2 mL of 4% RBC suspension only. All preparations were incubated for 60 min at 37 °C. Next, the tubes were gently vortexed and 1 mL of each sample were removed and placed into sterilized eppendorf tubes and then centrifuged ($3000 \times g$). Then, 200 μL of each supernatant was placed into a 96 well-plate. Absorbance was measured at $\lambda = 450$ nm with the aid of an ELISA reader [51]. The percentage hemolysis was calculated according to the following equation:

$$\% \text{ Hemolysis} = \frac{A - AO}{AX - AO} \times 100 \tag{2}$$

where A is the optical density at 450 nm (OD_{450}) of the peptide solution, AO is the OD_{450} of the negative control (0.9% NaCl) and AX is the OD_{450} of the positive control (0.1% Triton 10X).

2.8. Stability Assays

The stability assay of UP-5 relied on a previously reported stability test procedure [52] employing mouse plasma or mouse serum (PAA Laboratories, Pasching, Austria). Briefly, a stock solution of the peptide was prepared in 5% aqueous DMSO. The highest DMSO concentration was less than 0.5% after dilution in order to have a final concentration of peptide equal to 1 g/L. Each peptide was dissolved in plasma or serum at a final concentration corresponding to 75 μg/mL and incubated at 37 °C (750 rpm, Eppendorf, Hamburg, Germany). After different time periods, aliquots (47.5 μL) were taken and proteins were precipitated by addition of 150 μL of a mixture composed acetonitrile, water, and formic acid (89:10:1 by volume). The samples were incubated on ice for 45 min and centrifuged for 10 min at $13,000 \times g$ (Eppendorf, Hamburg, Germany). After transfer to a new reaction tube, the supernatant (170 μL) showed partial precipitation and was therefore centrifuged a second time. The second supernatant (155 μL) was collected and dried under vacuum. The samples were dissolved in 3% aqueous acetonitrile containing, 0.1% formic acid, and were analyzed using an Agilent 1100 HPLC system (Agilent Technologies, Santa Clara, CA, USA), coupled online to an Esquire HCT mass spectrometer (Bruker Daltonik GmbH, Bremen, Germany) equipped with an analytical Jupiter C_{18}-reversed phase column (2 mm inner diameter, 150 mm length, 5 μm particle size, 125 nm pore size). Eluent A contained 0.1% formic acid in water and Eluent B was 60% aqueous acetonitrile containing 0.1% formic acid.

2.9. Statistical Analysis

All statistical analyses were performed using the GraphPad Prism 7 software (La Jolla, CA, USA) program and Microsoft Office excel 2016.

3. Results

3.1. Design of UP-5

UP-5 was designed rationally with the balance between the hydrophobic and charged moieties taken into account. Arginine (R) was chosen to represent the charged moieties, while biphenylalanine (B) was incorporated in between to represent the hydrophobic residues. Five amino acids residues represents the overall sequence of UP-5 (Mw = 932.15 g/mol) which exhibited a charge of +3. The structure of UP-5 is displayed in Figure 1.

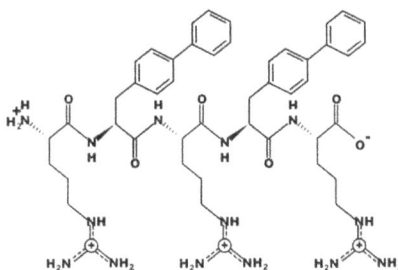

Figure 1. Chemical structure of UP-5.

3.2. In Vitro Antimicrobial Activity of UP-5

The in vitro antimicrobial activity of UP-5 was assessed against representative wild type and multidrug resistant bacterial strains of Gram positive and Gram negative bacteria (Table 1). UP-5 managed to inhibit the growth of wild type and methicillin resistant G+ bacterial strains of *S. aureus* (ATCC 29213 & 33591, respectively) with a MIC value of 10 μM. The other G+ bacterial strains including the two clinically isolated methicillin resistant strains *S. aureus* (ATCC 43300 & BAA-41) were less susceptible with MIC values of 15 μM. The vancomycin resistant bacterial strain *E. faecalis* (ATCC BAA-2316) was inhibited at a significantly higher MIC value of 70 μM. UP-5 was less potent against G− bacteria, *E. coli, P. aeruginosa,* with MIC values ranging from 55 to 65 μM.

Table 1. Minimum inhibitory concentrations (MIC) and minimum bactericidal concentrations (MBC) of UP-5 against the subjected bacterial species.

Bacterial Species	ATCC #	MIC Value (μM)	MBC Value (μM)
Staphylococcus aureus	29231	10	10
Staphylococcus aureus	43300	15	15
Staphylococcus aureus	BAA-41	15	15
Staphylococcus aureus	33591	10	10
Enterococcus faecalis	BAA-2316	70	70
Escherichia coli	25922	55	55
Escherichia coli	35218	60	60
Pseudomonas aeruginosa	27853	65	65
Pseudomonas aeruginosa	BAA-2114	55	55

Additionally, the bactericidal activity of UP-5 against all the subjected bacteria strains was evaluated by quantifying the minimum bactericidal concentration (MBC) (Table 1). All measured MBC values of UP-5 were equal to MIC values of the tested G+ and G− bacterial strains indicating that UP-5 is a bactericidal peptide.

3.3. Antimicrobial Synergistic Assays

The antimicrobial activity of UP-5 in combination with five conventional antibiotics (levofloxacin, chloramphenicol, rifampicin, ampicillin, and erythromycin) was assessed against *S. aureus* (ATCC 29213), *S. aureus* (ATCC 33591), *S. aureus* (ATCC 43300), *S. aureus* (ATCC BAA-41), and *P. aeruginosa* (ATCC BAA-2114).

3.3.1. Determination of the MIC and MBC of the Individual Antibiotics

The five studied antibiotics were tested against wild type and multidrug-resistant bacterial strains in order to determine the antimicrobial activity of each antibiotic against the employed bacterial strains. In addition to the MIC values, the bactericidal activity of the applied antibiotics was evaluated by determining the minimum bactericidal concentrations (MBCs). All reported data of MIC and MBC values of antibiotics are summarized in (Table 2). As reported, the MIC values of levofloxacin, rifampicin and ampicillin were on a par with the MBC values. This is an indication of the bactericidal activity of these antibiotics. On the contrary, a bacteriostatic activity was reported for chloramphenicol and erythromycin due to having higher MBC values when compared to their MIC values.

Table 2. Minimum inhibitory concentrations (MICs) and minimum bactericidal concentration (MBCs) of the individual antibiotics; MICs of UP-5 and the antibiotics in combination; Percentage reduction of antibiotic MIC values in combination with UP-5 compared to the individual MICs; the fractional Inhibitory concentrations (FIC) indices for the antimicrobial combinations against tested bacterial species.

Bacterial Species	Antibiotics				UP-5	
		MIC/MBC Alone (μM)	MIC in Combination (μM)	Reduction in MIC (%)	MIC in Combination (μM)	FIC Index
S. aureus ATCC 29213	Levofloxacin	0.5/0.5	0.05	90	0.125	0.11
	Chloramphenicol	20/30	10	<50	2.5	0.75
	Rifampicin	0.025/0.025	0.025	<50	10	2
	Ampicillin	2.5/2.5	2.5	<50	0.25	1.025
	Erythromycin	0.5/1.5	0.5	<50	10	2
S. aureus ATCC 33591	Levofloxacin	10/10	1.25	87.5	0.125	0.13
	Chloramphenicol	130/150	65	50	5	1
	Rifampicin	0.04/0.04	0.005	87.5	0.125	0.13
	Ampicillin	85/85	12.5	85.3	1.25	0.27
	Erythromycin	8/10	8	<50	0.125	1
S. aureus ATCC 43300	Levofloxacin	20/20	5	<50	0.025	0.25
	Chloramphenicol	15/20	7.5	<50	7.5	1
	Rifampicin	1/1	0.125	87.5	5	0.45
	Ampicillin	20/20	2.5	<50	7.5	0.62
	Erythromycin	100/150	100	<50	7.5	1.5
S. aureus ATCC BAA-41	Levofloxacin	10/10	10	<50	15	2
	Chloramphenicol	25/30	7.5	70	7.5	0.8
	Rifampicin	0.005/0.005	0.002	60	15	1.4
	Ampicillin	40/40	20	<50	7.5	1
	Erythromycin	350/400	125	64.3	15	1.35
P. auroginosa ATCC BAA-2114	Levofloxacin	12/12	5	58.3	20	0.78
	Chloramphenicol	200/325	12.5	93.7	10	0.24
	Rifampicin	50/50	0.25	99.5	25	0.46
	Ampicillin	>500/>500	250	>50	20	0.86
	Erythromycin	125/150	50	60	27.5	0.9

3.3.2. Checkerboard Assay Results

As shown in (Table 2), the MIC values of peptide decreased dramatically, while calculating the percentage of dropping of MIC values of antibiotics in combination with UP-5 compared to MIC alone displayed a significant reduction (p value $p \leq 0.05$). A reduction equal to 99.5% to rifampicin MIC value compared to MIC alone was reported when tested against the MDR strain *P. aeruginosa* (ATCC 2114), displaying the most synergistic behavior (FIC value = 0.46). Additionally, this combination led to an 87.5% reduction of rifampicin MIC value when tested against the *S. aureus* (ATCC 43300 and 33591) strains and displayed synergistic effects with FIC values equal to 0.45 and 0.13, respectively. On the other hand, according to FIC values, this combination led to indifferent effects when tested against the clinical isolate of *S. aureus* (ATCC BAA-41) strain, despite showing a 60% reduction of antibiotic MIC value compared to MIC alone, and *S. aureus* (ATCC 29213). The chloramphenicol-UP-5 combination led to a 93.7% and 70% reduction of antibiotic MIC values compared to the MIC alone when tested against *P. aeruginosa* (ATCC 2114) and *S. aureus* (ATCC BAA-41), respectively. Based on FIC values, this combination displayed only one synergistic effect against *P. aeruginosa* (ATCC 2114) with FIC value equal to 0.24, otherwise, it displayed additive effects. Combining levofloxacin with UP-5 against *S. aureus* (ATCC 29213 & 33591) strains led to a percentage of reduction of levofloxacin MIC value equal to 87.5% and 90%, respectively, compared to MIC alone. Levofloxacine-UP-5 combination exhibited synergistic effects against *S. aureus* (ATCC 29213, 43300 and 33591), additive effect against *P. aeruginosa* (ATCC 2114) and indifferent outcome when tested against *S. aureus* (ATCC BAA-41). A reduction of MIC value equal to 85.3% of ampicillin compared to MIC alone was obtained when tested against *S. aureus* (ATCC 33591) with FIC value equal to 0.27 that showed a synergistic effect. The ampicillin-UP-5 combination also displayed additive effects when tested against *P. aeruginosa* (ATCC 2114) and *S. aureus* (ATCC 43300) with FIC values equal to 0.86 and 0.62, respectively. The last combination (erythromycin-UP-5) displayed an additive effect with a 60% reduction of erythromycin MIC value compared to MI alone, FIC value was equal to 0.9. Other combinations displayed a reduction of 50% or less of antibiotics' MIC values when combined with UP-5 against subjected bacterial species. In summary, out of the overall twenty-five antimicrobial combinations of UP-5 and the antibiotics, 32% were synergistic and 44% were additive against the tested bacterial strains while the other combinations did not show any antagonism effect according to the FIC index.

3.3.3. Determination of MBCs of UP-5 and Antibiotics in Combinations

Determining the MIC values of UP-5 and antibiotics in combinations was followed by evaluating the bactericidal activity of those combinations. This issue was evaluated by measuring the minimum bactericidal concentration (MBC) against the subjected bacterial species included in this study. Both chloramphenicol and erythromycin, which exhibit bacteriostatic antimicrobial activity, displayed bactericidal activity in combination with UP-5. Thus, the MBC values of all antibiotics were equal to the MIC values in all combinations (see Table 2).

3.4. Antibiofilm Activity of UP-5

The antibiofilm activity of UP-5 against biofilm structures formed by the multidrug resistant strain *S. aureus* (ATCC 33591) was evaluated by two distinct techniques using the Calgary device: measuring the minimum biofilm eradication concentration (MBEC) and counting viable bacterial cell (MBCb) after treatment in accordance to the colony count method. As summarized in (Table 3), treatment of bacterial biofilm cells with peptide concentration equal 10 µM caused a reduction of viable biofilm cells to about 0.35% (99.65% killing) compared to negative control (untreated formed biofilm). The reported UP-5 concentration required to eradicate biofilm formation after 4 h of exposure at 37 °C was equal to 20 µM, a concentration that is twofold higher than the MIC value. This is a clear indication that UP-5 has a potent antibiofilm activity at relatively a low concentration. Additionally, the minimum UP-5 concentration needed to reduce the number of viable biofilm cells to almost zero (99.9% killing) (MBECb) against biofilm cells was also found equal to the MBEC value (20 µM) (Table 3). These results clearly display the antibiofilm potential of UP-5 and the innate antimicrobial resistance of biofilms towards ultrashort peptides.

Table 3. The antibiofilm activity of UP-5 against a standard resistant *S. aureus* (ATCC 33591) strain.

Peptide Concentration (μM)	Viable Biofilm Cells (%)	±SD
100	0	0.0002
80	0	0.0005
60	0	0.0006
40	0	0.002
30	0.054	0.005
20	0.108	0.03
10	0.35	0.09
MBEC value	20	
MBCb	20	

3.5. Hemolytic Assay

The hemolytic activity of UP-5 peptide was assessed against human erythrocytes. All the results are summarized in (Table 4). The obtained results indicate that only 1% hemolysis was reported after 1h of incubation with human erythrocytes at 100 μM concentration, which is equal to about a sevenfold higher concentration than UP-5 MICs (10–15 μM) against G+ and G− bacteria. Additionally, UP-5 didn't cause a hemolytic effect over 4% even at 200 μM concentration.

Table 4. Hemolytic activity of UP-5 against human erythrocytes. The results were recorded at $\lambda = 450$ nm.

Hemolysis (%)	Concentration (μM)	±SD
0.09	40	0.0005
1.01	60	0.004
1.04	80	0.001
1.04	100	0.0005
2.06	125	0.002
3.0	150	0.001
3.04	175	0.001
3.09	200	0.01

3.6. Cell Cytotoxicity

The cytotoxicity and selectivity of UP-5 against eukaryotic mammalian cells was also assessed using MTT cell proliferation assay and employing Vero mammalian cells. Different peptide concentrations (150, 200, 250, 300, 400, 500 and 600 μM) were subjected against the employed cell line and the proliferation activity was studied. Cell viability (%) equal to 79% (killing 21%) of Vero cells was obtained at concentration of 150 μM concentration of peptide treatment. Reaching a concentration of 600 μM led to a killing of 79% of Vero cells. The relationship between cell viability (%) and the UP-5 concentrations was also determined (Figure 2), the $IC_{50\%}$ value of UP-5 against Vero mammalian cells was more than 250 μM, which is equal to about seventeen fold higher than UP-5 MICs (10–15) against G+ and G− bacteria. The results obtained from the hemolytic assay and cell toxicity assay indicate that UP-5 is exerting negligible toxicity against eukaryotic cells at the antimicrobial concentrations needed to inhibit bacterial growth.

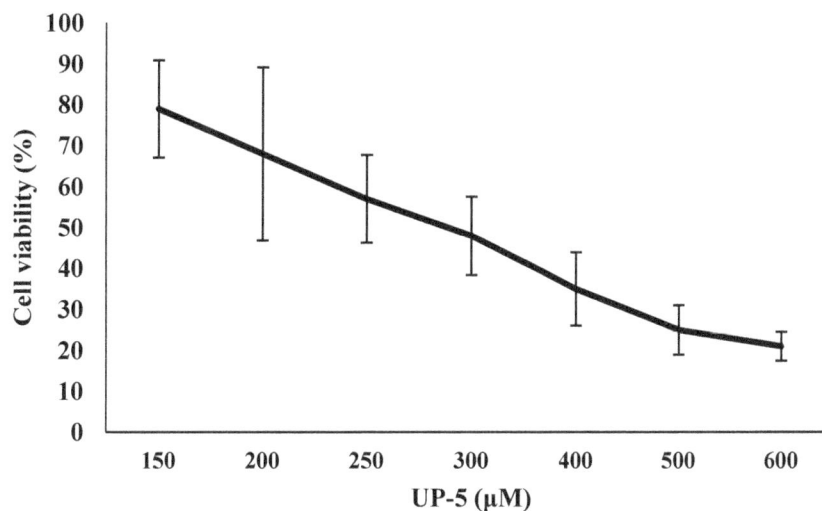

Figure 2. Cell viability (%) of Vero mammalian cells as a response to different UP-5 concentrations exposure. Bars represent the standard deviation ($\pm$SD). Values represent means of three different experiments.

3.7. Stability Assay

The stability assay was used to provide preliminary information about the in vivo profiles of UP-5. To what extent the peptide has the ability to resist proteolytic degradation by blood enzymes was determined in the assay. As summarized in Figure 3, the stability of UP-5 in full mouse plasma was studied at different time points. The peptide amount was determined based on the peak areas relative to the initial peptide quantity at 0 min (set to 100%). It was reported that: after 1-h incubation in plasma, only 27% of initial amount was degraded (73% intact peptide) and at 4 h of incubation the peptide was degraded by 66% (34% intact peptide).

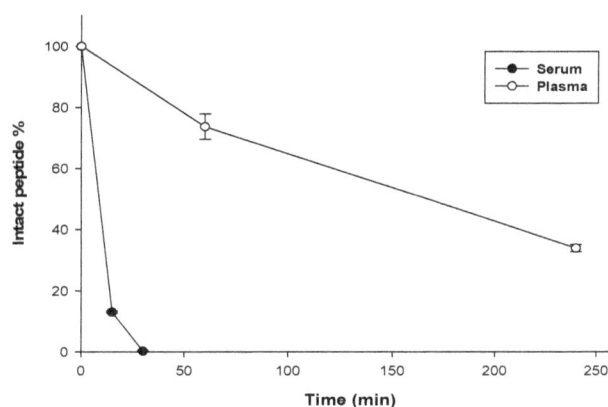

Figure 3. The serum and plasma stability profiles of UP-5. Samples were incubated at 37 °C with full mouse serum and plasma. Aliquots were taken at different time points. Results are the mean values $\pm$ SEM of three independent experiments.

On the other hand, regarding the serum stability test, UP-5 was studied in full mouse serum at different time points (Figure 3). As reported, more than 80% of the initial peptide amount was degraded after 15 min and after 30 min, the peptide was totally degraded. These results indicate that UP-5 is more stable in plasma ($t_{1/2}$ = 173 min = 2.9 h) than in serum ($t_{1/2}$ < 15 min). This data indicates that the peptide suffers from high in vivo degradation and poor stability which would consequently limit the application of this peptide for topical antimicrobial therapy.

4. Discussion

"Fight the resistance", has become one of the most famous slogans launched by all the human health-care communities worldwide in view of the alarming emergence of infectious diseases as well as the increase in bacterial multi-resistance. In order to manage this issue, new antimicrobial agents using new modes of action have been in development to meet this imminent challenge [53]. AMPs represent a promising class of antimicrobial agents providing a lot of advantages compared to conventional antibiotics including the lower likelihood of resistance development, accompanied with high potency against multi-drug resistant strains. In the literature, over 600 AMPs have been reported as potent agents against multi-drug resistant bacteria (MDRB) and biofilm forming strains [54]. The last research efforts were directed to the introduction of novel or modified amino acids displaying several features which have represented a promising approach to develop valuable and effective peptidomimetics. For instance: replacing proteinogenic amino acids with their corresponding D-variants resulted in enhanced in vivo biological activity, introduction of a stereocenter at the β-position using β-methylamino acids has been reported to result in a conformational restriction of bioactive peptides and substitution of proline with 5,5-dimethylthiazolidine-4-carboxylic acid (an unnatural amino acid) resulted in 39% greater agonist activity toward angiotensin II, a key peptide in blood pressure regulation [21]. The current efforts are aimed at developing AMPs with ultrashort sequences (ultrashort peptides) based on a selection of specific amino acids that exhibit specific and unique characteristics suitable for antimicrobial activity. Those ultrashort sequences represent new alternative antimicrobial agents designed to mitigate and avoid the negative shortcomings of the long and short peptides that are reflected by the occurrence of high mammalian toxicity as well as high cost issues. The ultrashort peptides are cost effective as they can be chemically synthesized via simpler and less complex procedures [55].

The antimicrobial activity of AMPs is mainly governed through targeting the bacterial cell membranes. Targeting is facilitated by the notable hydrophilic positively charged residues of AMPs and the microbial negatively charged surfaces leading to pore formation and hence cell membrane lysis and death. As UP-5 displays a net cationic charge of +3, which carries a sufficient positive charge in order to create sufficient electrostatic attraction and hence achieves complete interaction with the negative head groups of phospholipids in the bacterial cell membrane and cationic residues of the peptide [28].

The charged moieties of UP-5 were represented by arginine since the side chain can interact through the formation of hydrogen bonds and also through electrostatic interactions with the negatively charged surface of bacteria. The arginine's guanidine moiety as well as arginine side chain play a vital role for anchoring cationic AMP to the membrane surface via formation of a complex with the phosphate groups of the phospholipid bilayer [28,56].

The hydrophobic moieties of UP-5 were represented by the unnatural amino acid biphenylalanine, as well as the C5-chain of arginine amino acid. Insertion of two lipophilic residues created a sufficient 'grip' to these residues for the peptide, thus allowing the peptide to disrupt the bacterial membrane integrity after membrane insertion. The existence of at least two lipophilic residues will ensure a maximal thinning of the membrane at a certain radius around the peptide followed by membrane disruption [28].

As demonstrated in the present study, the MIC values of Gram-negative bacteria were significantly higher than the MICs of the Gram-positive bacteria; these differences could be explained due to differences in their respective cell wall compositions. Gram-negative bacteria contain a thin peptidoglycan lipid bilayer (~7–8 nm) which is a three-dimensional rigid structure consisting of a linear polysaccharide chains cross-linked by short peptides. and is also surrounded by an additional outer membrane of a lipopolysaccharide (LPS) layer while Gram-positive bacteria possess a thick peptidoglycan lipid bilayer (~20–80 nm) but lacks an outer layer of LPS [20,57,58]. The MBC values reported for UP-5 against subjected bacterial species were equal to the MIC values, which indicate that the peptides are bactericidal in nature.

The antimicrobial activities of UP-5 in different combinations with antibiotics were also evaluated. The results of the targeted MIC assay of five conventional antibiotics and UP-5 differed according to the bacterial strain; furthermore, the MIC values of the same antibiotics were significantly different from the MICs of the ultrashort peptide on the same strains. These differences can be explained due to differences in the mechanism of action that is suggested for the ultrashort peptides and the known mechanisms of action of the antibiotics used in the study. The antibiotics used in our study have different mechanisms of action such as inhibiting protein synthesis, interfering with nucleic acid synthesis, and blocking cell wall synthesis while, the antimicrobial activity of AMPs is mainly governed by cell membrane disruption and destabilization that leads to increasing membrane permeability through pore formation, which ultimately causes cell lysis and death [59–61].

As many of the tested combinations displayed synergistic activities or at least additive effects, this behavior suggests that the possible membrane targeting of UP-5 might have potentiated the effects of antibiotics. However, the mechanisms of the synergistic effects of the peptide- antibiotic combinations are still unclear. One of the proposed mechanisms for the synergistic effect was the destruction, permeabilization, and pores formation effects of AMPs against bacterial membranes which facilitates and enhances the intracellular entry of antibiotics. Additionally, it is suggested that the peripheral membrane proteins essential for cell wall biosynthesis and respiration are mainly delocalized, cellular energy is limited and cell wall integrity is undermined by the small cationic antimicrobial peptides. All antibiotics used act intracellularly except ampicillin, which functions via inhibiting bacterial cell wall synthesis. Therefore, combining antimicrobial agents with different mechanisms of action usually leads to the enhancement of the performance of each combination's constituent, and causes bacterial cell disruption rapidly and efficiently [62–64]. Based on these studies data, we propose that these proposed mechanisms are the most probable mechanisms for peptide-antibiotic combinations.

In regards to the results of combining UP-5 with five different types of antibiotics, the MIC values for both antibiotics and peptides in combination decreased dramatically (Table 2) in most groups. It is reported in general that 10 to 1000-folds higher concentrations of conventional antibiotics are required to restrain biofilm growth effectively, when compared with planktonic cells due to the presence of the extracellular lipopolysaccharide matrix surrounding the biofilms [65]. The development of antibiofilm therapeutics has generally been based on enhancing the dispersion of biofilm pioneer cells, inhibition of adhesion and interfering with the quorum sensing system. In the present study, the antibiofilm activity was determined and UP-5 displayed potent antibiofilm activity Compared to previous rare studies that investigated the antibiofilm activities of different ultrashort peptides. For instance: the MBEC values of OOWW-NH2 and C6-OOWW-NH2, two ultrashort peptides previously designed by Bisht et al., were sometimes 128-fold higher than the MIC values [30,65]. This is a clear indication that UP-5 is a potent antibiofilm agent that displays significant antibiofilm activity at relatively low concentrations.

Based on previous studies, some AMPs such as melittin and newly synthesized antimicrobial peptides (long and short sequences) displayed hemolytic and cytotoxicity activity ranging from moderate to high rates toward eukaryotic cells [66–68] while, very low or negligible toxicity was reported for UP-5. The low toxicity of the ultra-short peptide is thought to be due to its low hydrophobicity and short size. Furthermore, the high cationic charges of UP-5 (+3 net charges) mainly participated in minimizing the toxicity towards eukaryotic cells. Thus, mass charge plays a major role in creating sufficient electrostatic attraction and hence targeting the negative head groups of the bacterial cell membrane and consequently increasing the peptide's selectivity. This higher selectivity towards bacterial cell membrane is thought to be due to having a higher proportion of anionic phospholipids compared to the zwitterionic phospholipids in eukaryotic cells [12,69–71]. Additionally, it is suggested that erythrocytes are protected against the peptides lysis via neutralization of the cationic peptides with the negatively-charged sialic acid that is available abundantly and is located about 80 Å above the cells' surface.

The stability of UP-5 was studied in full mouse plasma and serum at different time points. The results indicated that UP-5 has a better stability profiles in plasma ($t_{1/2}$ = 173 min = 2.9 h) than in serum (<15 min). The mechanism of this enhanced stability profiles in plasma than in serum is unclear but, it's proposed that the presence of clotting factors and fibrinogens in blood plasma is playing a major rule for maintaining peptide intact and protecting cleavage sites.

In a previous study in accordance to our results, Nguyen et al., investigated the stability profiles of short AMPs that are rich in arginine and tryptophan residues. It is reported that short peptide sequences usually display low stability profiles ($h_{1/2}$ < 2 h) and they are considered susceptible agents for proteolytic enzymes especially that they exhibit a linear conformation [72]. In the present study, UP-5 displayed a better stability profile in plasma ($h_{1/2}$ > 2 h) compared to the other short peptides reported in literature. This enhancement proves that incorporation of non-natural amino acids have a positive effect against enzymatic degradation. However, that degradation pattern is not yet optimal for systemic delivery and places restrictions on the peptide to be applied in topical antimicrobial applications only.

5. Conclusions

Herein, we report the design of a novel pentapeptide named UP-5, which displayed significant antibacterial activity against wild type and clinical isolates of multidrug resistant strains, including MRSA, with a bactericidal mode of action. Additionally, UP-5 displayed potent antibiofilm activity with negligible hemolytic activity and cytotoxicity towards human erythrocytes and mammalian Vero cells. The UP-5 combinations with conventional antibiotics led to a remarkable reduction of the peptide and antibiotics' MIC values that usually were represented by a synergistic or additive outcome. The ultrashort peptide displayed better stability profiles in plasma than in serum. All these results indicate that UP-5 is a promising antimicrobial agent against both planktonic and biofilm forming MDR G+ and G− bacterial species and could have potential for developing topical antimicrobial applications.

Acknowledgments: This study was funded by the Deanship of Research at the Jordan University of Science and Technology. The authors also express their gratitude to the generous financial support provided by the German Academic Exchange Service (DAAD) for supporting Mohammed T. Qaoud's master studies at Jordan University of Science and Technology. The authors are extremely grateful and sincerely acknowledge the guidance, encouragement, and help of Nid"a Alshraiedeh at the Faculty of Pharmacy, Jordan University of Science and Technology, during the course of this study.

Author Contributions: Ammar Almaaytah, Mohammed T. Qaoud, Daniel Knappe, Ahmad Abualhaijaa and Ralf Hoffmann conceived and designed the experiments; Gubran Khalil Mohammed and Daniel Knappe performed the stability assay. Mohammed T. Qaoud, Ammar Almaaytah, Gubran Khalil Mohammed, Daniel Knappe, and Qosay Al-Balas analyzed the data; Ralf Hoffmann and Qosay Al-Balas revised the manuscript; Ammar Almaaytah, Mohammed T. Qaoud, and Qosay Al-Balas, wrote the paper.

References

1. World Health Organization (WHO). Antimicrobial Resistance. Available online: http://www.who.int/mediacentre/factsheets/fs194/en/ (accessed on 13 November 2017).
2. Laxminarayan, R.; Duse, A.; Wattal, C.; Zaidi, A.K.; Wertheim, H.F.; Sumpradit, N.; Vlieghe, E.; Hara, G.L.; Gould, I.M.; Goossens, H.; et al. Antibiotic resistance—The need for global solutions. *Lancet Infect. Dis.* **2013**, *13*, 1057–1098. [CrossRef]
3. Selsted, M.E.; Ouellette, A.J. Mammalian defensins in the antimicrobial immune response. *Nat. Immunol.* **2005**, *6*, 551–557. [CrossRef] [PubMed]

4. Otero-González, A.J.; Magalhães, B.S.; Garcia-Villarino, M.; López-Abarrategui, C.; Sousa, D.A.; Dias, S.C.; Franco, O.L. Antimicrobial peptides from marine invertebrates as a new frontier for microbial infection control. *FASEB J.* **2010**, *24*, 1320–1334.

5. Wang, G.; Li, X.; Wang, Z. APD3: The antimicrobial peptide database as a tool for research and education. *Nucleic Acids Res.* **2016**, *44*, D1087–D1093. [CrossRef] [PubMed]

6. Lai, Y.; Gallo, R.L. AMPed up immunity: How antimicrobial peptides have multiple roles in immune defense. *Trends Immunol.* **2009**, *30*, 131–141. [CrossRef] [PubMed]

7. Yeung, A.T.; Gellatly, S.L.; Hancock, R.E. Multifunctional cationic host defence peptides and their clinical applications. *Cell. Mol. Life Sci.* **2011**, *68*, 2161. [CrossRef] [PubMed]

8. Yin, L.M.; Edwards, M.A.; Li, J.; Yip, C.M.; Deber, C.M. Roles of hydrophobicity and charge distribution of cationic antimicrobial peptides in peptide-membrane interactions. *J. Biol. Chem.* **2012**, *287*, 7738–7745. [CrossRef] [PubMed]

9. Chen, L.; Li, X.; Gao, L.; Fang, W. Theoretical insight into the relationship between the structures of antimicrobial peptides and their actions on bacterial membranes. *J. Phys. Chem. B* **2014**, *119*, 850–860. [CrossRef] [PubMed]

10. Wimley, W.C.; Hristova, K. Antimicrobial Peptides: Successes, Challenges and Unanswered Questions. *J. Membr. Biol.* **2011**, *239*, 27–34. [CrossRef] [PubMed]

11. Porto, W.F.; Silva, O.N.; Franco, O.L. Prediction and rational design of antimicrobial peptides. *InProtein Struct.* **2012**. [CrossRef]

12. Albada, H.B.; Prochnow, P.; Bobersky, S.; Langklotz, S.; Bandow, J.E.; Metzler-Nolte, N. Short Antibacterial Peptides with Significantly Reduced Hemolytic Activity can be Identified by a Systematic l-to-d Exchange Scan of their Amino Acid Residues. *ACS Comb. Sci.* **2013**, *15*, 585–592. [CrossRef] [PubMed]

13. Ong, Z.Y.; Wiradharma, N.; Yang, Y.Y. Strategies employed in the design and optimization of synthetic antimicrobial peptide amphiphiles with enhanced therapeutic potentials. *Adv. Drug Deliv. Rev.* **2014**, *78*, 28–45. [CrossRef] [PubMed]

14. Jacob, B.; Park, I.S.; Bang, J.K.; Shin, S.Y. Short KR-12 analogs designed from human cathelicidin LL-37 possessing both antimicrobial and antiendotoxic activities without mammalian cell toxicity. *J. Pept. Sci.* **2013**, *19*, 700–707. [CrossRef] [PubMed]

15. Mardirossian, M.; Grzela, R.; Giglione, C.; Meinnel, T.; Gennaro, R.; Mergaert, P.; Scocchi, M. The host antimicrobial peptide Bac7 1-35 binds to bacterial ribosomal proteins and inhibits protein synthesis. *Chem. Biol.* **2014**, *21*, 1639–1647. [CrossRef] [PubMed]

16. Li, Y.; Xiang, Q.; Zhang, Q.; Huang, Y.; Su, Z. Overview on the recent study of antimicrobial peptides: Origins, functions, relative mechanisms and application. *Peptides* **2012**, *37*, 207–215. [CrossRef] [PubMed]

17. Nguyen, L.T.; Haney, E.F.; Vogel, H.J. The expanding scope of antimicrobial peptide structures and their modes of action. *Trends Biotechnol.* **2011**, *29*, 464–472. [CrossRef] [PubMed]

18. Haney, E.F.; Petersen, A.P.; Lau, C.K.; Jing, W.; Storey, D.G.; Vogel, H.J. Mechanism of action of puroindoline derived tryptophan-rich antimicrobial peptides. *Biochim. Biophys. Acta (BBA)-Biomembr.* **2013**, *1828*, 1802–1813. [CrossRef] [PubMed]

19. Balhara, V.; Schmidt, R.; Gorr, S.U.; DeWolf, C. Membrane selectivity and biophysical studies of the antimicrobial peptide GL13K. *Biochim. Biophys. Acta (BBA)-Biomembr.* **2013**, *1828*, 2193–2203. [CrossRef] [PubMed]

20. Lee, T.H.N.; Hall, K.; Aguilar, M.I. Antimicrobial peptide structure and mechanism of action: A focus on the role of membrane structure. *Curr. Top. Med. Chem.* **2016**, *16*, 25–39. [CrossRef] [PubMed]

21. Trabocchi, A.; Guarna, A. The basics of peptidomimetics. In *Peptidomimetics in Organic and Medicinal Chemistry: The Art of Transforming Peptides in Drugs*; John Wiley & Sons: New York, NY, USA, 2014; pp. 1–7.

22. Rekha, R.S. Role of Antimicrobial Peptides in Tuberculosis and Respiratory Tract Infections: Clinical and Mechanistic Studies. Ph.D. Thesis, Inst för laboratoriemedicin/Dept of Laboratory Medicine, Karolinska Institute, Stockholm, Sweden, 14 October 2015.

23. Liskamp, R.M. Conformationally restricted amino acids and dipeptides, (non) peptidomimetics and secondary structure mimetics. *Recl. Trav. Chim. Pays-Bas* **1994**, *113*, 1–9. [CrossRef]

24. Olson, G.L.; Bolin, D.R.; Bonner, M.P.; Bos, M.; Cook, C.M.; Fry, D.C.; Graves, B.J.; Hatada, M.; Hill, D.E. Concepts and progress in the development of peptide mimetics. *J. Med. Chem.* **1993**, *36*, 3039–3049. [CrossRef] [PubMed]

25. Ripka, A.S.; Rich, D.H. Peptidomimetic design. *Curr. Opin. Chem. Biol.* **1998**, *2*, 441–452. [CrossRef]

26. Daily, A.E.; Greathouse, D.V.; van der Wel, P.C.; Koeppe, R.E., 2nd. Helical Distortion in Tryptophan- and Lysine-Anchored Membrane-Spanning α-Helices as a Function of Hydrophobic Mismatch: A Solid-State Deuterium NMR Investigation Using the Geometric Analysis of Labeled Alanines Method. *Biophys. J.* **2008**, *94*, 480–491. [CrossRef] [PubMed]

27. Chu, H.L.; Yu, H.Y.; Yip, B.S.; Chih, Y.H.; Liang, C.W.; Cheng, H.T.; Cheng, J.W. Boosting salt resistance of short antimicrobial peptides. *Antimicrob. Agents Chemother.* **2013**, *57*, 4050–4052. [CrossRef] [PubMed]

28. Lau, Q.Y.; Ng, F.M.; Cheong, J.W.D.; Yap, Y.Y.A.; Tan, Y.Y.F.; Jureen, R.; Hill, J.; Chia, C.S.B. Discovery of an ultra-short linear antibacterial tetrapeptide with anti-MRSA activity from a structure-activity relationship study. *Eur. J. Med. Chem.* **2015**, *105*, 138–144. [CrossRef] [PubMed]

29. Arnusch, C.J.; Ulm, H.; Josten, M.; Shadkchan, Y.; Osherov, N.; Sahl, H.G.; Shai, Y. Ultrashort peptide bioconjugates are exclusively antifungal agents and synergize with cyclodextrin and amphotericin B. *Antimicrob. Agents Chemother.* **2012**, *56*, 1–9. [CrossRef] [PubMed]

30. Bisht, G.S.; Rawat, D.S.; Kumar, A.; Kumar, R.; Pasha, S. Antimicrobial activity of rationally designed amino terminal modified peptides. *Bioorg. Med. Chem. Lett.* **2007**, *17*, 4343–4346. [CrossRef] [PubMed]

31. Mangoni, M.L.; Shai, Y. Short native antimicrobial peptides and engineered ultrashort lipopeptides: Similarities and differences in cell specificities and modes of action. *Cell. Mol. Life Sci.* **2011**, *68*, 2267. [CrossRef] [PubMed]

32. Fjell, C.D.; Hiss, J.A.; Hancock, R.E.W.; Schneider, G. Designing antimicrobial peptides: Form follows function. *Nat. Rev. Drug Discov.* **2012**, *11*, 37–51. [CrossRef]

33. Seo, M.D.; Won, H.S.; Kim, J.H.; Mishig-Ochir, T.; Lee, B.J. Antimicrobial peptides for therapeutic applications: A review. *Molecules* **2012**, *17*, 12276–12286. [CrossRef] [PubMed]

34. Makovitzki, A.; Baram, J.; Shai, Y. Antimicrobial lipopolypeptides composed of palmitoyl di- and tricationic peptides: In vitro and in vivo activities, self-assembly to nanostructures, and a plausible mode of action. *Biochemistry* **2008**, *47*, 10630–10636. [CrossRef] [PubMed]

35. Serrano, G.N.; Zhanel, G.G.; Schweizer, F. Antibacterial activity of ultrashort cationic lipo-β-peptides. *Antimicrob. Agents Chemother.* **2009**, *53*, 2215–2217.

36. Chen, X.; Zhang, M.; Zhou, C.; Kallenbach, N.R.; Ren, D. Control of bacterial persister cells by Trp/Arg-containing antimicrobial peptides. *Appl. Environ. Microbiol.* **2011**, *77*, 4878–4885. [CrossRef] [PubMed]

37. Mensa, B.; Howell, G.L.; Scott, R.; DeGrado, W.F. Comparative mechanistic studies of brilacidin, daptomycin, and the antimicrobial peptide LL16. *Antimicrob. Agents Chemother.* **2014**, *58*, 5136–5145. [CrossRef] [PubMed]

38. Hansen, T.; Alst, T.; Havelkova, M.; Strøm, M.B. Antimicrobial Activity of Small β-Peptidomimetics Based on the Pharmacophore Model of Short Cationic Antimicrobial Peptides. *J. Med. Chem.* **2010**, *53*, 595–606. [CrossRef] [PubMed]

39. Wang, G.; Mishra, B.; Epand, R.F.; Epand, R.M. High-quality 3D structures shine light on antibacterial, anti-biofilm and antiviral activities of human cathelicidin LL-37 and its fragments. *Biochi. Biophys. Acta (BBA)-Biomembr.* **2014**, *1838*, 2160–2172. [CrossRef] [PubMed]

40. Zarena, D.; Mishra, B.; Lushnikova, T.; Wang, F.; Wang, G. The π Configuration of the WWW Motif of a Short Trp-Rich Peptide Is Critical for Targeting Bacterial Membranes, Disrupting Preformed Biofilms, and Killing Methicillin-Resistant Staphylococcus aureus. *Biochemistry* **2017**, *56*, 4039–4043. [CrossRef] [PubMed]

41. Wang, G.; Hanke, M.L.; Mishra, B.; Lushnikova, T.; Heim, C.E.; Chittezham Thomas, V.; Bayles, K.W.; Kielian, T. Transformation of human cathelicidin LL-37 into selective, stable, and potent antimicrobial compounds. *ACS Chem. Biol.* **2014**, *9*, 1997–2002. [CrossRef] [PubMed]

42. Gentilucci, L.; De Marco, R.; Cerisoli, L. Chemical modifications designed to improve peptide stability: Incorporation of non-natural amino acids, pseudo-peptide bonds, and cyclization. *Curr. Pharm. Des.* **2010**, *16*, 3185–3203. [CrossRef] [PubMed]

43. Deepankumar, K.; Prabhu, N.S.; Kim, J.H.; Yun, H. Protein engineering for covalent immobilization and enhanced stability through incorporation of multiple noncanonical amino acids. *Biotechnol. Bioprocess Eng.* **2017**, *22*, 248–255. [CrossRef]

44. Schnaider, L.; Brahmachari, S.; Schmidt, N.W.; Mensa, B.; Shaham-Niv, S.; Bychenko, D.; Adler-Abramovich, L.; Shimon, L.J.W.; Kolusheva, S.; DeGrado, W.F.; et al. Self-assembling dipeptide antibacterial nanostructures with membrane disrupting activity. *Nat. Commun.* **2017**, *8*, 1365. [CrossRef] [PubMed]

45. De Marco, R. Synthesis of Modified Amino Acids and Insertion in Peptides and Mimetics. Structural Aspects and Impact on Biological Activity. ph.D. Thesis, University of Bologna, Bologna, Italy, 2012.

46. Brown, D.F.J.; Edwards, D.I.; Hawkey, P.M.; Morrison, D.; Ridgway, G.L.; Towner, K.J.; Wren, M.W. Guidelines for the laboratory diagnosis and susceptibility testing of methicillin-resistant Staphylococcus aureus (MRSA). *J. Antimicrob. Chemother.* **2005**, *56*, 1000–1018. [CrossRef] [PubMed]

47. Pereira, E.M.; Gomes, R.T.; Freire, N.R.; Aguiar, E.G.; Brandão, M.D.; Santos, V.R. In vitro antimicrobial activity of Brazilian medicinal plant extracts against pathogenic microorganisms of interest to dentistry. *Planta Medica* **2011**, *77*, 401–404. [CrossRef] [PubMed]

48. Sueke, H.; Kaye, S.B.; Neal, T.; Hall, A.; Tuft, S.; Parry, C.M. An in vitro investigation of synergy or antagonism between antimicrobial combinations against isolates from bacterial keratitis. *Invest. Ophthalmol. Vis. Sci.* **2010**, *51*, 4151–4155. [CrossRef] [PubMed]

49. Schwering, M.; Song, J.; Louie, M.; Turner, R.J.; Ceri, H. Multi-species biofilms defined from drinking water microorganisms provide increased protection against chlorine disinfection. *Biofouling* **2013**, *29*, 917–928. [CrossRef] [PubMed]

50. Feng, X.; Sambanthamoorthy, K.; Palys, T.; Paranavitana, C. The human antimicrobial peptide LL-37 and its fragments possess both antimicrobial and antibiofilm activities against multidrug-resistant Acinetobacter baumannii. *Peptides* **2013**, *49*, 131–137. [CrossRef] [PubMed]

51. Almaaytah, A.; Zhou, M.; Wang, L.; Chen, T.; Walker, B.; Shaw, C. Antimicrobial/cytolytic peptides from the venom of the North African scorpion, Androctonus amoreuxi: Biochemical and functional characterization of natural peptides and a single site-substituted analog. *Peptides* **2012**, *35*, 291–299. [CrossRef] [PubMed]

52. Knappe, D.; Henklein, P.; Hoffmann, R.; Hilpert, K. Easy strategy to protect antimicrobial peptides from fast degradation in serum. *Antimicrob. Agents Chemother.* **2010**, *54*, 4003–4005. [CrossRef] [PubMed]

53. Rolain, J.M.; Canton, R.; Cornaglia, G. Emergence of antibiotic resistance: Need for a new paradigm. *Clin. Microbiol. Infect.* **2012**, *18*, 615–616. [CrossRef] [PubMed]

54. Mataraci, E.; Dosler, S. In vitro activities of antibiotics and antimicrobial cationic peptides alone and in combination against methicillin-resistant Staphylococcus aureus biofilms. *Antimicrob. Agents Chemother.* **2012**, *56*, 6366–6371. [CrossRef] [PubMed]

55. Strøm, M.B.; Haug, B.E.; Skar, M.L.; Stensen, W.; Stiberg, T.; Svendsen, J.S. The Pharmacophore of Short Cationic Antibacterial Peptides. *J. Med. Chem.* **2003**, *46*, 1567–1570.

56. Wang, G. Determination of solution structure and lipid micelle location of an engineered membrane peptide by using one NMR experiment and one sample. *Biochim. Biophys. Acta (BBA)-Biomembr.* **2007**, *1768*, 3271–3281. [CrossRef] [PubMed]

57. Silhavy, T.J.; Kahne, D.; Walker, S. The Bacterial Cell Envelope. *Cold Spring Harb. Perspect. Biol.* **2010**, *2*, a000414. [CrossRef] [PubMed]

58. Fayaz, A.M.; Balaji, K.; Girilal, M.; Yadav, R.; Kalaichelvan, P.T.; Venketesan, R. Biogenic synthesis of silver nanoparticles and their synergistic effect with antibiotics: A study against gram-positive and gram-negative bacteria. *Nanomed. Nanotechnol. Biol. Med.* **2010**, *6*, 103–109. [CrossRef] [PubMed]

59. Ruden, S.; Hilpert, K.; Berditsch, M.; Wadhwani, P.; Ulrich, A.S. Synergistic interaction between silver nanoparticles and membrane-permeabilizing antimicrobial peptides. *Antimicrob. Agents Chemother.* **2009**, *53*, 3538–3540. [CrossRef] [PubMed]

60. Maróti, G.; Kereszt, A.; Kondorosi, E.; Mergaert, P. Natural roles of antimicrobial peptides in microbes, plants and animals. *Res. Microbiol.* **2011**, *162*, 363–374. [CrossRef] [PubMed]

61. Yang, P.; Ramamoorthy, A.; Chen, Z. Membrane orientation of MSI-78 measured by sum frequency generation vibrational spectroscopy. *Langmuir* **2011**, *27*, 7760–7767. [CrossRef] [PubMed]

62. Zhang, Y.; Liu, Y.; Sun, Y.; Liu, Q.; Wang, X.; Li, Z.; Hao, J. In vitro synergistic activities of antimicrobial peptide brevinin-2CE with five kinds of antibiotics against multidrug-resistant clinical isolates. *Curr. Microbiol.* **2014**, *68*, 685–692. [CrossRef] [PubMed]

63. Hirt, H.; Gorr, S.-U. Antimicrobial peptide GL13K is effective in reducing biofilms of Pseudomonas aeruginosa. *Antimicrob. Agents Chemother.* **2013**, *57*, 4903–4910. [CrossRef] [PubMed]

64. Mishra, B.; Wang, G. Individual and combined effects of engineered peptides and antibiotics on Pseudomonas aeruginosa biofilms. *Pharmaceuticals* **2017**, *10*, 58. [CrossRef] [PubMed]

65. Laverty, G.; McLaughlin, M.; Shaw, C.; Gorman, S.P.; Gilmore, B.F. Antimicrobial Activity of Short, Synthetic Cationic Lipopeptides. *Chem. Biol. Drug Des.* **2010**, *75*, 563–569. [CrossRef] [PubMed]

66. Corzo, G.; Escoubas, P.; Villegas, E.; Barnham, K.J.; He, W.; Norton, R.S.; Nakajima, T. Characterization of unique amphipathic antimicrobial peptides from venom of the scorpion Pandinus imperator. *Biochem. J.* **2001**, *359 Pt 1*, 35–45. [CrossRef] [PubMed]

67. Shin, S.Y.; Kang, J.H.; Lee, M.K.; Kim, S.Y.; Kim, Y.; Hahm, K.S. Cecropin A - magainin 2 hybrid peptides having potent antimicrobial activity with low hemolytic effect. *Biochem. Mol. Biol. Int.* **1998**, *44*, 1119–1126. [CrossRef] [PubMed]

68. Almaaytah, A.; Tarazi, S.; Alsheyab, F.; Al-Balas, Q.; Mukattash, T. Antimicrobial and Antibiofilm Activity of Mauriporin, a Multifunctional Scorpion Venom Peptide. *Int. J. Pept. Res. Ther.* **2014**, *20*, 397–408. [CrossRef]

69. Mohandas, N.; Gallagher, P.G. Red cell membrane: Past, present, and future. *Blood* **2008**, *112*, 3939–3948. [CrossRef] [PubMed]

70. Glukhov, E.; Stark, M.; Burrows, L.L.; Deber, C.M. Basis for selectivity of cationic antimicrobial peptides for bacterial versus mammalian membranes. *J. Biol. Chem.* **2005**, *280*, 33960–33967. [CrossRef] [PubMed]

71. Guilhelmelli, F.; Vilela, N.; Albuquerque, P.; Derengowski, L.D.; Silva-Pereira, I.; Kyaw, C.M. Antibiotic development challenges: The various mechanisms of action of antimicrobial peptides and of bacterial resistance. *Front. Microbiol.* **2013**, *4*, 353. [CrossRef] [PubMed]

72. Nguyen, L.T.; Chau, J.K.; Perry, N.A.; De Boer, L.; Zaat, S.A.; Vogel, H.J. Serum stabilities of short tryptophan-and arginine-rich antimicrobial peptide analogs. *PLoS ONE* **2010**, *5*, e12684. [CrossRef] [PubMed]

2

The Potential Protective Effect of Oligoribonucleotides-D-Mannitol Complexes against Thioacetamide-Induced Hepatotoxicity in Mice

Tetiana Marchyshak [1], Tetiana Yakovenko [1], Igor Shmarakov [2] and Zenoviy Tkachuk [1,*]

[1]   Institute of Molecular Biology and Genetics, National Academy of Sciences of Ukraine, 03680 Kyiv, Ukraine; biochem.imbg@gmail.com (T.M.); tetianayakovenko46@gmail.com (T.Y.)

[2]   Department of Biochemistry and Biotechnology, Yurii Fedkovych Chernivtsi National University, 58012 Chernivtsi, Ukraine; igor.shmarakov@gmail.com

*   Correspondence: ztkachuk47@gmail.com

Abstract: This study investigated the potential hepatoprotective effect of oligoribonucleotides-D-mannitol complexes (ORNs-D-M) against thioacetamide (TAA)-induced hepatotoxicity in mice. The hepatoprotective activity of ORNs-D-M was evaluated in thioacetamide (TAA)-treated C57BL/6J. Results indicate that treatment with ORNs-D-M displayed a protective effect at the TAA-induced liver injury. Treatment with ORNs-D-M, starting at 0 h after the administration of TAA, decreased TAA-elevated serum alanine aminotransferase (ALT) and γ-glutamyl transpeptidase (GGT). Activities of glutathione S-transferase (GST) and glutathione peroxidase (GPx), and levels of glutathione (GSH), were enhanced with ORNs-D-M administration, while the hepatic oxidative biomarkers (TBA-reactive substances, protein carbonyl derivatives, protein-SH group) and myeloperoxidase (MPO) activity were reduced. Furthermore, genetic analysis has shown that the ORNs-D-M decreases the expression of mRNA pro-inflammatory cytokines, such as tumor necrosis factor α (TNF-α) and interleukin-6 (IL-6), profibrogenic cytokine-transforming growth factor β1 (TGF-β1), as well as the principal protein of the extracellular matrix—collagen I. The present study demonstrates that ORNs-D-M exerts a protective effect against TAA-induced liver injury, which may be associated with its anti-inflammatory effects, inhibition of overexpression of mRNA cytokines, and direct effects on the metabolism of the toxin.

Keywords: oligoribonucleotides-D-mannitol complexes; thioacetamide-induced hepatotoxicity; hepatoprotective effect

1. Introduction

The liver acts as the main metabolic organ where the major biochemical processes involved in maintaining the homeostasis of an organism are integrated. Being a detoxifying organ, the liver is the first to make contact with xenobiotics, the action of which causes serious disorders, which lead to the development of the pathological process [1]. Toxins and drugs are among the main etiopathogenetic agents causing an acute hepatic failure. Acute toxic liver injury is characterized by membrane damage, oxidative stress, massive necrosis of hepatocytes, infiltration of parenchyma by neutrophils and activation of hepatic stellate cells, following an increased inflammation and damage to the liver [2]. This is a key event in inducing liver damage. It is generally accepted that the molecules involved in the initiation of hepatic inflammation include pro-inflammatory mediators TNF-α, cyclooxygenase-2 and IL-6, which trigger the cascade of cytokines mediating the inflammatory reactions [3]. One of the key events of acute hepatotoxicity is an activation of hepatic stellate cells (HSC). Activated stellate cells (of myofibroblast type) are characterized by a high level of proliferation, migration and contractility [4]. These activated cells are capable of expressing the major profibrotic factor-transforming growth factor β1. In addition, activated hepatic stellate cells overexpress the components of the extracellular matrix (ECM), including fibril-forming type I and III collagens, and laminin. This overexpression leads to the deposition of collagen contributing to the development of liver fibrosis [5].

Antisense RNAs, aptamers and modified nucleic acids have been used in the treatment of liver disease, which acts by binding to target nucleic acids or proteins [6]. Using antisense nucleotides targeted towards mRNA encoding TNF-α and TGF-β1 has been shown to prevent hepatic damage effectively against the action of toxic substances [7,8].

Natural oligoribonucleotides (ORNs) (total yeast RNA) have long attracted attention as pharmacological agents. They possess a wide spectrum of biological activity. It is known that the ORNs have anti-inflammatory effects investigated on local inflammation models and membrane-stabilizing action [9,10]. It was shown in a study that the oligoribonucleotides-D-mannitol complexes (ORNs-D-M) possess antiviral activity against the hepatitis C virus. Application of complexes in the treatment of hepatitis C reduces the concentration of the virus in the bloodstream and normalizes phagocytic index of monocytes [11–13]. Since hepatitis C leads to acute and chronic hepatitis, fibrosis, cirrhosis and hepatocellular carcinomas, the search for drugs with antiviral and hepatoprotective activities is promising. That is why the aim of this study was to investigate the hepatoprotective effect of the ORNs-D-M complexes at thioacetamide-induced acute hepatotoxicity.

In this study, it was discovered that the ORNs-^{D}-M have hepatoprotective effects, which are manifested in reducing the oxidative stress and inflammation.

2. Results

2.1. Influence of the ORNs-D-M on Indicators of Inflammation and Liver Damage at Acute Hepatotoxicity

It is well known that alanine aminotransferase (ALT) and γ-glutamyl transpeptidase (GGT) are sensitive biochemical markers in the serum for acute liver damage. Results of the liver function detection are shown in Figure 1A,B. The thioacetamide (TAA)-treated group demonstrated a notable elevation of ALT and GGT levels in serum compared to the control group ($p < 0.05$). By contrast, ALT levels reduced by 53.3% and 35.6%, respectively, in the groups of animals receiving the first dose of ORNs-D-M at 0 h (ORNs-D-M 0 h) and at 12 h after the administration of toxin (ORNs-D-M 12 h). Also, treatment with ORNs-D-M contributed to a significant reduction in serum GGT levels in both experimental groups. It was also found out that the co-administering of ORNs with TAA (ORNs 0 h) reduces ALT and GGT levels. Conversely, at treatment with ORNs 12 h after the start of the study (ORNs 12 h group) and D-mannitol (D-M 0 h and D-M 12 h groups), the levels of ALT and GGT did not significantly differ from the TAA-treated group. Thus, we assume that the protective effect of ORNs-D-M in the model of TAA-induced acute liver damage is due to their effect on the metabolism of the toxin.

To confirm the anti-inflammatory effects of the complexes, the myeloperoxidase (MPO) activity was investigated as an indicator of inflammatory infiltration of liver parenchyma by neutrophils [14]. The MPO activity results, after ORNs-D-M, ORNs and D-M administration into the mice of various treatment groups, are shown in Figure 2. The administration of TAA significantly increased MPO activity compared to the control group of animals. At the same time, ORNs-D-M 0 h, ORNs-D-M 12 h and ORNs 0 h groups showed a significant reduction in MPO activity by 58%, 39% and 35%, respectively, compared to the group of animals receiving TAA. Conversely, MPO activity in groups of ORNs 12 h, D-M 0 h and D-M 12 h decreased insignificantly in comparison with the TAA-treated group.

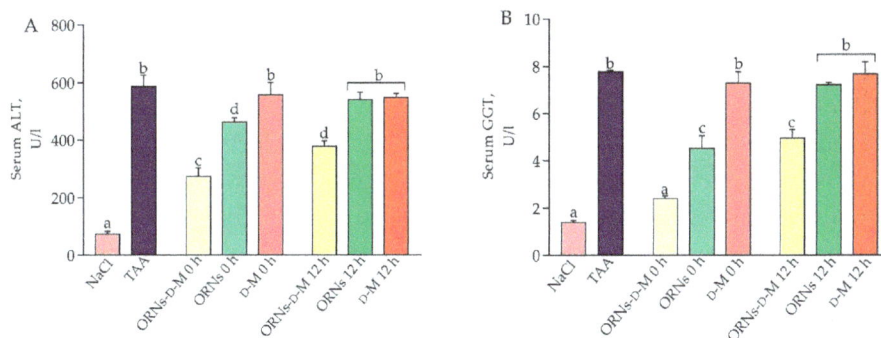

Figure 1. Effects of oligoribonucleotides-D-mannitol complexes (ORNs-D-M), natural oligoribonucleotides (ORNs) and D-mannitol (D-M) on the activities of serum ALT (**A**) and GGT (**B**) in TAA-induced liver damage mice. Data are presented as the mean $\pm$ standard deviation (SD), $n = 6$ for each group. Values marked with different letters (a, b, c, d) are statistically different, $p < 0.05$ (Student's t-test). Abbreviations: NaCl—control mice receiving a single injection of NaCl; TAA—mice receiving a single injection of TAA; ORNs-D-M 0 h—mice receiving a TAA and ORNs-D-M immediately after TAA application (i.e., 0 h) and every next 12 h for 48 h; ORNs 0 h—mice receiving a TAA and ORNs immediately after TAA application (i.e., 0 h) and every next 12 h for 48 h; D-M 0 h—mice receiving a TAA and then D-M immediately after TAA application (i.e., 0 h) and every next 12 h for 48 h; ORNs-D-M 12 h—mice receiving a TAA and ORNs-D-M after 12 h after TAA application (i.e., 12 h) and every next 12 h for 48 h; ORNs 12 h—mice receiving a TAA and ORNs after 12 h after TAA application (i.e., 12 h) and every next 12 h for 48 h; D-M 12 h—mice receiving a TAA and D-M after 12 h after TAA application (i.e., 12 h) and every next 12 h for 48 h.

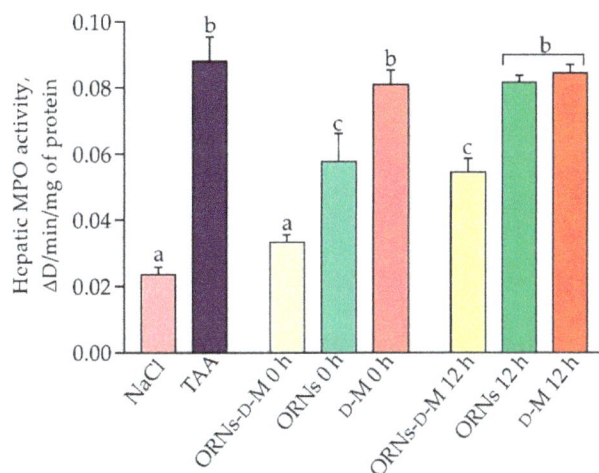

Figure 2. Effects of ORNs-D-M, ORNs and D-M on the MPO activity in TAA-induced liver damage mice. Data are presented as the mean $\pm$ SD, $n = 6$ for each group. Values marked with different letters (a, b, c, d) are statistically different, $p < 0.05$ (Student's t-test). Abbreviations: NaCl—control mice receiving a single injection of NaCl; TAA—mice receiving a single injection of TAA; ORNs-D-M 0 h—mice receiving a TAA and ORNs-D-M immediately after TAA application (i.e., 0 h) and every next 12 h for 48 h; ORNs 0 h—mice receiving a TAA and ORNs immediately after TAA application (i.e., 0 h) and every next 12 h for 48 h; D-M 0 h—mice receiving a TAA and then D-M immediately after TAA application (i.e., 0 h) and every next 12 h for 48 h; ORNs-D-M 12 h—mice receiving a TAA and ORNs-D-M after 12 h after TAA application (i.e., 12 h) and every next 12 h for 48 h; ORNs 12 h—mice receiving a TAA and ORNs after 12 h after TAA application (i.e., 12 h) and every next 12 h for 48 h; D-M 12 h—mice receiving a TAA and D-M after 12 h after TAA application (i.e., 12 h) and every next 12 h for 48 h.

2.2. Influence of the ORNs-D-M on Oxidative Stress in the Liver

Hepatotoxicity TAA requires metabolic activation with the formation of reactive metabolites S-oxide (TASO) and S,S-dioxide ($TASO_2$) [15]. Because increased levels of reactive oxygen species (ROS) induce lipid and protein oxidative damage, the levels of products of lipid peroxidation, protein carbonyl derivatives, protein thiol groups and reduced glutathione were investigated. The results of the research are shown in Figure 3. As shown in Figure 3A,B, the acute toxic liver injury was characterized by an increase in the level of TBA-reactive substances (TBARS) and protein carbonyl derivatives by 6.1 and 3.97 times, respectively, compared with the control group. At the same time, the levels of protein thiol groups and reduced glutathione (GSH) in TAA-induced mice livers were found to be 91.9% and 67.5% lower than the control group (Figure 3C,D). However, the treatment with ORNs-D-M 0 h, ORNs-D-M 12 h, ORNs 0 h and ORNs 12 h significantly ($p < 0.05$) reduced TBARS and protein carbonyl derivatives compared to the TAA group (Figure 3A,B). The levels of protein thiol groups and GSH significantly increased in ORNs-D-M 0 h and ORNs-D-M 12 h groups in comparison with the TAA-treated group (Figure 3C,D). In turn, ORNs 0 h and ORNs 12 h did not have a significant effect on the levels of protein thiol groups and reduced glutathione.

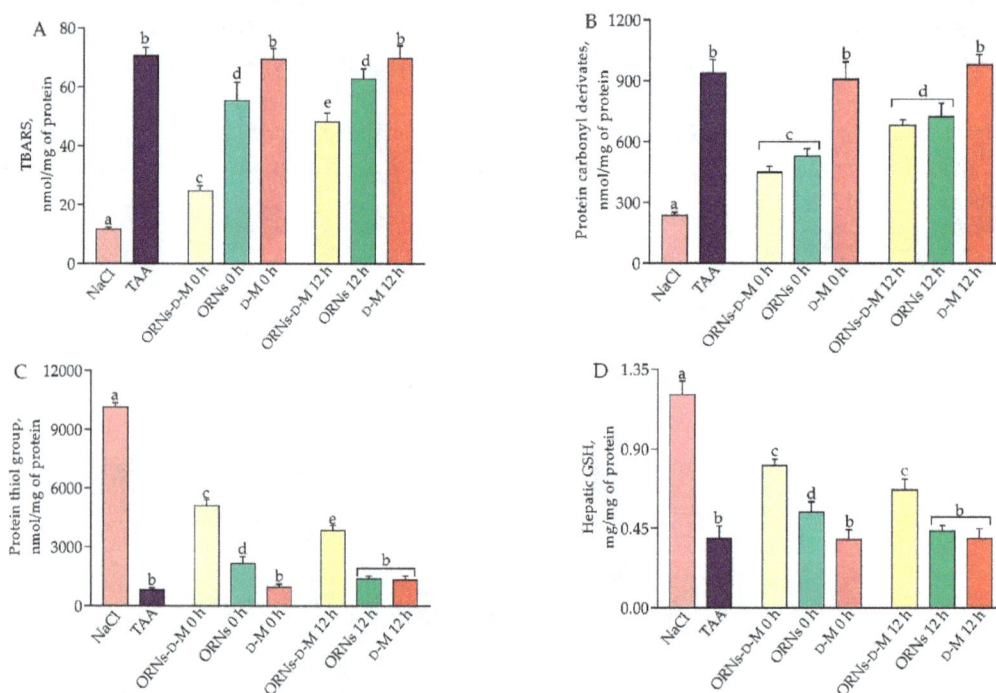

Figure 3. Effects of ORNs-D-M, ORNs and D-M on the levels of thiobarbituric acid reactive substances (TBARS) (**A**), protein carbonyl derivatives (**B**), protein thiol groups (**C**) and glutathione (GSH) (**D**) in TAA-induced liver damage mice. Data are presented as the mean ± SD, $n = 6$ for each group. Values marked with different letters (a, b, c, d, e) are statistically different, $p < 0.05$ (Student's *t*-test). Abbreviations: NaCl—control mice receiving a single injection of NaCl; TAA—mice receiving a single injection of TAA; ORNs-D-M 0 h—mice receiving a TAA and ORNs-D-M immediately after TAA application (i.e., 0 h) and every next 12 h for 48 h; ORNs 0 h—mice receiving a TAA and ORNs immediately after TAA application (i.e., 0 h) and every next 12 h for 48 h; D-M 0 h—mice receiving a TAA and then D-M immediately after TAA application (i.e., 0 h) and every next 12 h for 48 h; ORNs-D-M 12 h—mice receiving a TAA and ORNs-D-M after 12 h after TAA application (i.e., 12 h) and every next 12 h for 48 h; ORNs 12 h—mice receiving a TAA and ORNs after 12 h after TAA application (i.e., 12 h) and every next 12 h for 48 h; D-M 12 h—mice receiving a TAA and D-M after 12 h after TAA application (i.e., 12 h) and every next 12 h for 48 h.

2.3. Influence of the ORNs-D-M on GST and GPx Activities at Acute Toxic Liver Injury

After 48 h of intoxication of mice with TAA and treatment with ORNs-D-M, ORNs and D-M, the activities of glutathione S-transferase (GST) and glutathione peroxidase (GPx) were investigated. As shown in Table 1, the intoxication of mice with TAA significantly decreased the activities of oxidative stress marker enzymes in the liver, including GST and GPx, by 43.8% and 46.9%, respectively, in comparison with control group. However, the downregulated activities of GST and GPx after TAA administration were significantly elevated by ORNs-D-M 0 h, ORNs-D-M 12 h and ORNs 0 h. Conversely, the activities of GST and GPx remained unchanged in groups of the treated mice with ORNs 12 h, D-M 0 h and D-M 0 h in comparison with the control.

Table 1. Effects of ORNs-D-M, ORNs and D-M on the activities glutathione peroxidase (GPx) and glutathione S-transferase (GST) in TAA-induced liver damage mice.

Group	GPx Activity in Liver, nmol/min/mg of Protein	GST Activity in Liver, μnmol/min/mg of Protein
NaCl	276.66 ± 19.68 [a]	1.21 ± 0.13 [a]
TAA	146.62 ± 17.79 [b]	0.68 ± 0.15 [b]
TAA + ORNs-D-M 0 h	221.14 ± 21.70 [c]	1.00 ± 0.16 [c]
TAA + ORNs 0 h	201.31 ± 13.29 [c]	0.92 ± 0.08 [d]
TAA + D-M 0 h	135.19 ± 7.67 [b]	0.58 ± 0.09 [b]
TAA + ORNs-D-M 12 h	186.44 ± 4.40 [d]	0.91 ± 0.07 [d]
TAA + ORNs 12 h	158.18 ± 17.60 [b]	0.64 ± 0.14 [b]
TAA + D-M 12 h	139.69 ± 15.91 [b]	0.54 ± 0.08 [b]

Data are presented as the mean $\pm$ SD, $n = 6$ for each group. Values marked with different letters (a, b, c, d) are statistically different, $p < 0.05$ (Student's t-test). Abbreviations: NaCl—control mice receiving a single injection of NaCl; TAA—mice receiving a single injection of TAA; ORNs-D-M 0 h—mice receiving a TAA and ORNs-D-M immediately after TAA application (i.e., 0 h) and every next 12 h for 48 h; ORNs 0 h—mice receiving a TAA and ORNs immediately after TAA application (i.e., 0 h) and every next 12 h for 48 h; D-M 0 h—mice receiving a TAA and then D-M immediately after TAA application (i.e., 0 h) and every next 12 h for 48 h; ORNs-D-M 12 h—mice receiving a TAA and ORNs-D-M after 12 h after TAA application (i.e., 12 h) and every next 12 h for 48 h; ORNs 12 h—mice receiving a TAA and ORNs after 12 h after TAA application (i.e., 12 h) and every next 12 h for 48 h; D-M 12 h—mice receiving a TAA and D-M after 12 h after TAA application (i.e., 12 h) and every next 12 h for 48 h.

2.4. Influence of the ORNs-D-M on Expression of IL-6, TNF-α, TGF-B1, COL1A1 and α-SMA mRNA at Acute Hepatotoxicity

It is known that oxidative stress stimulates the pro-inflammatory reactions in liver parenchyma, and therefore, the expression of IL-6 and TNF-α genes expressed by resident macrophages of the liver and recruited cells of the immune system [16] has been investigated. Single administration of TAA was detected to increase the mRNA level of the pro-inflammatory cytokines IL-6 and TNF (Figure 4A,B). However, ORNs-D-M suppressed the increase of these cytokines induced by the acute toxic dose of TAA, depending on the time of treatment with complexes. The TNF-α and IL-6 levels were significantly different between ORNs-D-M 0 h, ORNs-D-M 12 h and TAA groups ($p < 0.05$).

The activation of stellate cells of liver is defined as the central event in the development of liver fibrosis. TGF-β1 acts as one of the major profibrotic cytokines in liver disease [17]. We detected an increase in the expression of this gene by 15.1 times in TAA-injured livers compared with the control group (Figure 5). However, in the ORNs-D-M 0 h and ORNs-D-M 12 h groups, the TGF-β1 mRNA expression level was significantly decreased by 57% and 28.4%, respectively, in comparison with the TAA-treated group.

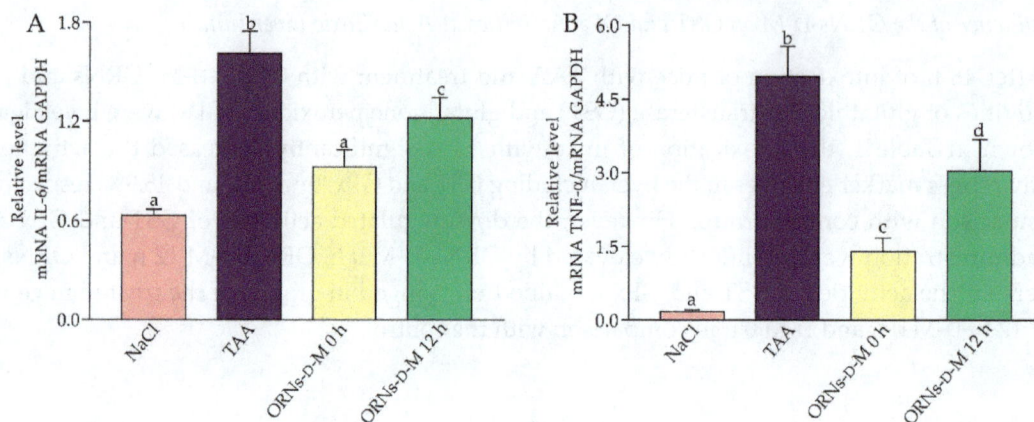

Figure 4. Effects of ORNs-D-M on the expression of IL-6 (**A**) and TNF-α (**B**) mRNA in TAA-induced liver damage mice. The investigated mRNA levels were normalized to GAPDH as a control. Data are presented as the mean ± SD, $n = 6$ for each group. Values marked with different letters (a, b, c, d) are statistically different, $p < 0.05$ (Student's t-test). Abbreviations: NaCl—control mice receiving a single injection of NaCl; TAA—mice receiving a single injection of TAA; ORNs-D-M 0 h—mice receiving a TAA and ORNs-D-M immediately after TAA application (i.e., 0 h) and every next 12 h for 48 h; ORNs-D-M 12 h—mice receiving a TAA and ORNs-D-M after 12 h after TAA application (i.e., 12 h) and every next 12 h for 48 h.

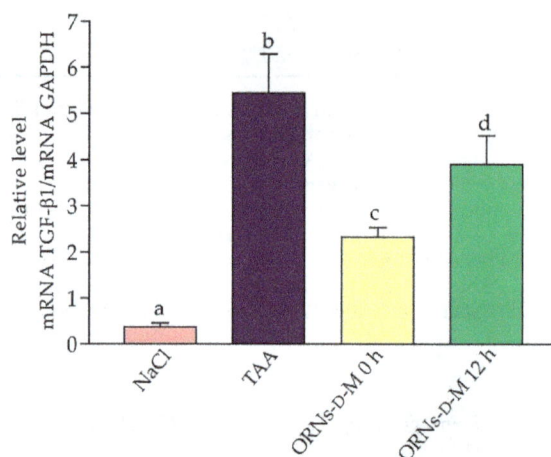

Figure 5. Effect of ORNs-D-M on the expression of TGF-β1 mRNA in TAA-induced liver damage mice. The investigated mRNA levels were normalized to GAPDH as a control. Data are presented as the mean ± SD, $n = 6$ for each group. Values marked with different letters (a, b, c, d) are statistically different, $p < 0.05$ (Student's t-test). Abbreviations: NaCl—control mice receiving a single injection of NaCl; TAA—mice receiving a single injection of TAA; ORNs-D-M 0 h—mice receiving a TAA and ORNs-D-M immediately after TAA application (i.e., 0 h) and every next 12 h for 48 h; ORNs-D-M 12 h—mice receiving a TAA and ORNs-D-M after 12 h after TAA application (i.e., 12 h) and every next 12 h for 48 h.

Analysis of hepatic collagen mRNA expression revealed a strong induction of collagen after 48 h in the animal group, which received a single TAA injection. Nevertheless, in ORNs-D-M 0 h and ORNs-D-M 12 h groups, this figure was significantly ($p < 0.05$) lower than in the TAA-treated group (Figure 6A). Additionally, the expression of the α-SMA gene, which is expressed by activated stellate cells, has been investigated. Toxin administration increased the expression mRNA level of α-SMA by 59.7 times compared with the control group (Figure 6B). In contrast, the ORNs-D-M 0 h and ORNs-D-M

12 h reduced the expression mRNA level of α-SMA after TAA application, depending on the time of treatment with complexes.

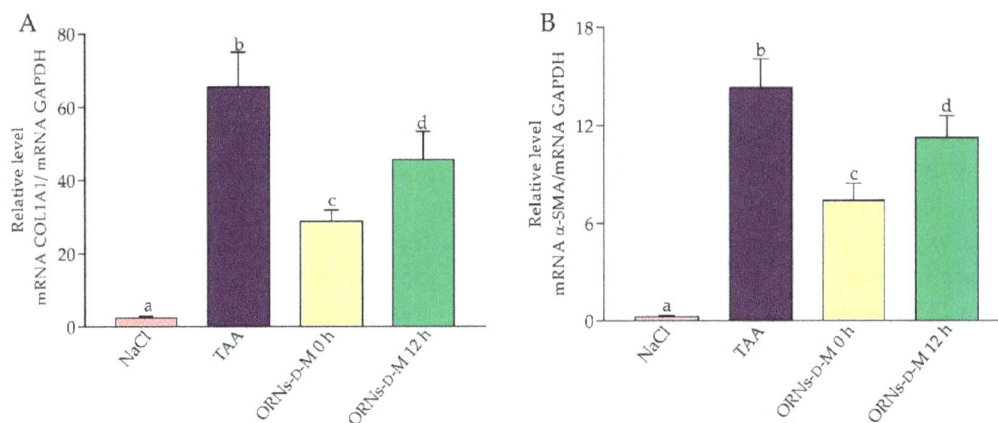

Figure 6. Effects of ORNs-D-M on the expression of COL1A1 (**A**) and α-SMA (**B**) mRNA in TAA -induced liver damage mice. The investigated mRNA levels were normalized to GAPDH as a control. Data are presented as the mean ± SD, $n = 6$ for each group. Values marked with different letters (a, b, c, d) are statistically different, $p < 0.05$ (Student's t-test). Abbreviations: NaCl—control mice receiving a single injection of NaCl; TAA—mice receiving a single injection of TAA; ORNs-D-M 0 h—mice receiving a TAA and ORNs-D-M immediately after TAA application (i.e., 0 h) and every next 12 h for 48 h; ORNs-D-M 12 h—mice receiving a TAA and ORNs-D-M after 12 h after TAA application (i.e., 12 h) and every next 12 h for 48 h.

3. Discussion

The liver is the main metabolic and detoxifying organ that first contacts and neutralizes xenobiotics [18]. Despite the presence in the hepatocytes of the cellular system of detoxification (cytochrome P450, flavin-containing monooxygenase, glutathione transferase, glucuronyltransferase), which provide biotransformation of xenobiotics, the metabolic transformations of some of them can lead to the formation of toxic intermediates, resulting in a liver toxic injury [19]. TAA is an organosulfur compound, which today is used as a fungicidal agent and organic solvent in the leather, textile and paper industries [20]. At the same time, it acts as hepatotoxin for the induction of acute hepatic failure. The mechanism by which TAA causes the liver injury involves its biotransformation using the cytochrome P450 enzyme system. These enzymes convert TAA to thioacetamide sulfoxide (TAASO), a reactive intermediate with toxic nature, and then to a more reactive thioacetamide-S,S-dioxide (TAASO$_2$), causing severe damage to the liver [21,22].

Liver injury can be assessed by monitoring sensitive biochemical markers such as ALT and GGT, which are released from the hepatocytes into the circulatory system by changing membrane permeability. In this study, TAA leads to increased GGT and ALT activities in blood serum of mice, indicating a loss of functional integrity of hepatocytes [23]. When ORNs-D-M was applied, the levels of these marker enzymes were restored, depending on the start time of the complexes' administration (at 0 h or 12 h after hepatotoxin application). ORNs-D-M treatment from the beginning of the study (ORNs-D-M 0 h) showed a profound hepatoprotective effect that was not observed in ORNs 12 h and D-mannitol groups (D-M 0 h and D-M 12 h). These data allow us to argue that ORNs-D-M, but not ORNs, have a protective effect in the model of TAA-induced liver damage. Restoring lesions may be due to hepatocyte repair and stabilization of the cell membrane by the ORNs-D-M. Previously, it had been shown that ORNs-D-M have membrane-stabilizing properties in the in-vitro system [10]. Therefore, we assume that ORNs-D-M can stabilize the structural integrity of the hepatocellular membrane at TAA-induced liver damage.

TAA treatment promotes necrosis and apoptosis of hepatocytes [22], which in turn is accompanied by the recruitment of neutrophils to liver parenchyma. One of the major molecules released after the recruitment of neutrophils is myeloperoxidase, an important enzyme involved in the generation of active forms of oxygen, and it may further damage the parenchyma [24]. It has been found that treatment with ORNs-D-M, starting at 0 and 12 h after the administration of hepatotoxin, significantly reduced MPO activity in liver parenchyma, but not ORNs and D-M. The obtained results suggest that ORNs-D-M can reduce inflammatory infiltration of parenchyma by neutrophils.

The active intermediates TAA (TAASO, TAASO$_2$) formed by the pro-oxidant free-radical mechanism lead to the formation of adducts of proteins, lipids and nucleic acids. The formation of reactive oxygen species (ROS), which is the result of the TAA activation, leads to the initiation of processes of lipid and protein peroxidation, damage to mitochondria and violation of energy generation [25,26]. We evaluated the ability of the ORNs-D-M to affect the levels of oxidative stress markers in TAA-damaged livers, and detected that ORNs-D-M treatment from 0 h after TAA administration decreases the levels of oxidative stress markers in TAA-treated mice. Interestingly, the treatment with complexes starting from 12 h after TAA administration showed a weaker protective effect compared with the group receiving complexes from the beginning of the study (ORNs-D-M 0 h). It is known that the ORNs-D-M based on total yeast RNA possesses anti-inflammatory properties, inhibits oxidative processes in cell membranes and contributes to the normalization of inducible nitric oxide synthase activity [9,10,27]. Therefore, on the one hand, we assume that the resulting effect may be related to the above-mentioned ORNs-D-M properties. On the other hand, the resulting effect in the ORNs-D-M 12 h group leads us to believe that complexes can directly affect the metabolism of TAA, thus preventing the development of hepatotoxicity.

One of the main mechanisms of TAA-induced liver injury is the formation of free radicals in TAA metabolism [20]. Consequently, antioxidant activity and inhibition of free-radical production are important for protecting cells from TAA-induced hepatotoxicity. GSH is a known antioxidant, which by binding covalently to free radicals and enhancing the activity of glutathione peroxidase and glutathione reductase plays an important role against TAA-induced acute liver damage [28,29]. Our results have shown that TAA overdose results in the depletion of a GSH pool. However, treatment with ORNs-D-M, starting at 0 and 12 h after the administration of hepatotoxin, significantly increased GSH levels compared to the TAA-treated group. Antioxidant enzymes such as GPx and GST perform important functions in protection mechanisms against the harmful effects of free radicals in the liver. This study showed that the ORNs-D-M protects the liver from free radical oxidation by enhancing the activity of the glutathione-related antioxidant defense system. The ORNs-D-M probably acted by increasing the level of reduced glutathione. Depletion of the glutathione pool by oxidative stress affects the activity of glutathione-dependent enzymes that neutralize ROS. The ORNs-D-M could restore depleted levels of GSH and thereby increase the GPx and GST activities. Thus, this study showed that ORNs-D-M effectively protects the liver by improving the enzymatic and nonenzymatic protection against acute toxic liver damage.

The series of factors that are involved in the liver injury pathogenesis include oxidative stress, inflammation and immune responses. Cytokines act as central mediators that link with specific receptors on the cell membrane of targeting cells, thereby causing a cascade of reactions leading to induction, amplification or inhibition of the activity of the genes regulated by them [30]. TNF-α and IL-6 are important hepatotoxic mediators when liver is damaged by the toxins. It has been shown that the use of TAA induces the production of the nuclear factor-kappa B (NF-κB), which leads to the production of various inflammatory factors, including TNF-α and IL-6 [31,32]. NF-κB activation would contribute to massive hepatocyte death, inflammation, and activation of hepatic stellate cells [33]. TNF-α acts as an important inflammatory mediator that is able to modulate the effects of other cytokines, such as IL-6 [34]. In this study, treatment with ORNs-D-M, starting with both 0 and 12 h after the administration of hepatotoxin, reduced the increased expression of both the TNF-α and IL-6 mRNA. Reduced expression of TNF-α mRNA by the action of complexes indicates a reduced activation of Kupffer cells and liver infiltration by immune system cells, which has been confirmed by biochemical parameters (MPO activity). Since NF-κB is a central transcription mediator, which regulates the expression of inflammatory cytokines (TNF-α, IL-6), we assume that complexes may suppress NF-kb activation, which leads to reducing TNF-α and IL-6 mRNA expression.

HSC activation is recognized as a central event in the development of hepatic fibrosis and occurs early in response to liver injury. Therefore, in the model of acute TAA-induced liver injury, the activation of stellate liver cells was also described as a critical event by us and others [35,36]. Activated hepatic stellate cells are capable of ECM overproduction, including collagen I and III, hyaluronic acid and laminin, decreasing the collagenase activity and collagen degradation [37,38]. Expression of α-SMA is a representative sign of activated stellate liver cells. An equally important role in the development of fibrosis is played by TGF-β1, which acts as the major profibrotic cytokine synthesized mainly by stellate liver cells [39]. The results of this study showed that the treatment with ORNs-D-M starting at 0 h after TAA administration is more effective in reducing the expression of α-SMA mRNA compared to the ORNs-D-M 12 h group. Also, our study showed a significant decrease in TGF-β1 and COL1A1 mRNAs that play a crucial role in the development of fibrosis. These results suggest that ORNs-D-M can have a protective effect on the formation of fibrosis after acute TAA-induced liver injury.

ORNs-D-M are complexes of total yeast RNA with a dominant fraction of 5–8 nucleotides and D-mannitol [40]. In our studies, we found that ORNs-D-M treatment has a protective effect in the model of TAA-induced acute toxic damage of the liver. We assume that the main mechanisms by which the complexes protect the liver from toxic damage are associated with their anti-inflammatory properties [10] and the ability to modulate some signaling pathways (including NF-κB signaling) [41] that are involved in the development of hepatotoxicity. We also believe that ORNs-D-M can directly affect the key molecules (including CYP2E1, CYP1A2, CYP2C6, CYP3A2) that are involved in TAA biotransformation. On the other hand, ORNs-D-M are capable of nonspecific binding to target molecules [42], so we assume that the complexes also can bind to a toxin, thereby preventing the development of hepatotoxicity. It is abundantly clear that the demonstration of the interdependence between our established effect and the possible ability of ORNs-D-M to affect both the signaling pathways involved in the development of hepatotoxicity and the TAA metabolism should be the subject of our further research.

4. Materials and Methods

4.1. Chemicals and Reagents

TAA was purchased from Sigma Aldrich, St. Louis, MO, USA.

ORNs-D-M complexes are compounds consisting of oligoribonucleotides (highly purified total yeast RNA) without protein and DNA impurities with a dominant fraction of 3–8 nucleotides and D-mannitol. The ratio of oligoribonucleotides to D-mannitol is 2.5:1 [40,43]. ORNs-D-M was purchased from the company "BioCell", Kyiv, Ukraine.

All other chemicals were received from standard commercial suppliers (Sigma Chemical Co, Acros Organics, St. Louis, MO, USA; Thermo Fisher Scientific, Macherey Nagel, Berlin, Germany).

4.2. Animals and Experimental Design

All procedures that were performed in studies were in accordance with ethical standards (Federalwide Assurance No 00019663) and carried out within the guidelines of the European Convention for the Protection of Vertebrate Animals Used for Experimental and Other Scientific Purposes (Strasbourg, France, 1986) and with regard to the NIH Guide for the Care and Use of Laboratory Animals [44]. The experimental animals were female C57BL/6J mice of 2–2.5 months of age, with body mass of 20–22 g. Acute thioacetamide-induced hepatotoxicity was used to model toxic lesions of the liver in mice [45]. 200 mg/kg body weight dose of ORNs-D-M was chosen, as it was previously proven to be protective against oxidative damage caused by TAA in mice [46]. The animals ($n = 6$) were randomly divided into 4 experimental groups:

1. NaCl control group—the animals were administered normal saline (0.9% NaCl) by a single intraperitoneal injection.
2. TAA—the animals were given 500 mg/kg body weight of TAA by a single intraperitoneal injection.
3. ORNs-D-M 0 h—the animals were administered 500 mg/kg body weight of TAA by a single intraperitoneal injection, and then 200 mg/kg doses of ORNs-D-M (per os) immediately after TAA application (i.e., 0 h) and every next 12 h for 48 h (12, 24, 36, 48 h).
4. ORNs 0 h—the animals were administered 500 mg/kg body weight of TAA by a single intraperitoneal injection, and then 143 mg/kg (the quantity of ORNs in 200 mg/kg of the ORNs-D-M) doses of ORNs (per os) immediately after TAA application (i.e., 0 h) and every next 12 h for 48 h (12, 24, 36, 48 h).
5. D-M 0 h—the animals were administered 500 mg/kg body weight of TAA by a single intraperitoneal injection, and then 57 mg/kg (the quantity of D-M in 200 mg/kg of the ORNs-D-M) doses of D-M (per os) immediately after TAA application (i.e., 0 h) and every next 12 h for 48 h (12, 24, 36, 48 h).
6. ORNs-D-M 12 h—the animals were administered 500 mg/kg body weight of TAA by a single intraperitoneal injection, and then 200 mg/kg doses of ORNs-D-M (per os) after 12 h after TAA application (i.e., 12 h) and every next 12 h for 48 h (24, 36, 48 h).
7. ORNs 12 h—the animals were administered 500 mg/kg body weight of TAA by a single intraperitoneal injection, and then 143 mg/kg doses of ORNs (per os) after 12 h after TAA application (i.e., 12 h) and every next 12 h for 48 h (24, 36, 48 h).
8. D-M 12 h—the animals were administered 500 mg/kg body weight of TAA by a single intraperitoneal injection, and then 57 mg/kg doses of D-M (per os) after 12 h after TAA application (i.e., 12 h) and every next 12 h for 48 h (24, 36, 48 h).

At the end of the experimental period, the animals were anesthetized intraperitoneally with a ketamine–xylazine solution and euthanized after 48 h of TAA administration.

4.3. Biochemical Determinations

GGT and ALT enzymatic activities were determined in mouse serum using a kit from Felicit Diagnostics (Felicit Diagnostics, Dnipro, Ukraine), according to the manufacturer's instructions and expressed as U/l. MPO activity as an indicator of infiltration of parenchyma by neutrophils was determined by the method [47].

The evaluation of oxidative destruction of biomolecules was carried out on the basis of the determination of the levels of TBARS, protein carbonyl derivatives, protein thiol groups, and the level of reduced glutathione in the liver tissue. TBARS level was determined by a method [48] that is based on reaction between product of lipid peroxidation and thiobarbituric acid with production of a pink pigment with a 532-nm absorption maximum. TBARS content was expressed as nmol/mg of protein. The level of protein carbonylation was assayed with method [49]. This method is based on the reaction of protein carbonyls with 2,4-dinitrophenylhydrazine which leads to formation of a stable dinitrophenylhydrazone product. Carbonyl group levels was expressed as nmol/mg of protein. Protein thiol groups in liver were determined by reaction with Ellman's reagent that produces yellow 2-nitro-5-thiobenzoate anion [50]. Hepatic reduced glutathione level was measured according to the method of Ellman [51].

An evaluation of the functional activity of the antioxidant system was analyzed for the enzymatic activity of glutathione peroxidase and glutathione-S-transferase. GPx activity in the liver was determined by method [52] and expressed in nmol/min/mg protein. GST activity was determined through the conjugation of GSH with 1-chloro-2,4-dinitrobenzene (CDNB) with a 340 nm absorption maximum [53].

Protein concentration was determined using the method of Lowry et al. [54].

4.4. RNA Preparation and Quantitative Real-Time PCR

The isolation of total RNA was performed using the NucleoMag RNA Kit (Macherey Nagel, Duren, Germany) and BeadRetriever system (Invitrogen, Carlsbad, CA, USA) according to the manufacturer's protocol. The amount of isolated RNA and the presence of protein and carbohydrate impurities in it were determined by the absorbence of solutions at 260 nm and by the ratio A260/A280 using a MaestroNano Pro Micro-Volume MN-913 spectrophotometer (Maestrogen, Hsinchu, Taiwan). The integrity of total RNA was determined by the ratio of the intensity of the 28S/18S rRNA bands in the electrophoregram after electrophoresis using the Microchip electrophoresis system (MCE-202/MultiNA Shimadzu, Berlin, Germany). Synthesis of cDNA was performed in a final volume of 20 µL with a total RNA concentration of 2 µg using the Maxima H Minus First Strand cDNA Synthesis Kit (Thermo Scientific, Waltham, MA, USA). The reverse-transcription reaction was performed on Thermal Cycler CFX96 Real-Time system (Bio-Rad, Singapore) with the reaction parameters: 42 °C 60 min, 25 °C 5 min, 42 °C 60 min, 70 °C 5 min. Quantitative evaluation of IL-6, TNF-α, TGF-β1, COL1A1 and α-SMA gene transcription was performed by real-time polymerase chain reaction in a Thermal Cycler CFX96 Real-Time system (Bio-Rad, Singapore) using the BioRad CFX Manager software. The amplification was performed in the mode: 95 °C 10 min, 39 cycles: 95 °C 40 s, 60 °C 30 s, 72 °C 30 s, including the plate scanning. As a reference housekeeping gene used to normalize mRNA expression, we employed GAPDH. This gene gave excellent reproducibility, never varying in its Ct value by more than 0.5 units. To calculate the relative expression, the method $2^{-\Delta\Delta Ct}$ was used [55]. The primers sequenced were designed on GenBank database and were synthesized (Invitrogen, Carlsbad, CA, USA). Primers used for quantitative analysis of mRNA expression are shown in Table 2.

Table 2. Primers used in this study.

Primer Name	Primer Sequence (5′→3′)
IL-6_for	5′-GTCACAGAAGGAGTGGC
IL-6_rev	5′-CTGACCACAGTGAGGAA
TNF-α_for	5′-CCTCCCTCTCATCAGTTCTA
TNF-α_rev	5′-CTTTGAGATCCATGCCG
TGF-β1_for	5′-GGCTACCATGCCAACTT
TGF-β1_rev	5′-ACCCACGTAGTAGACGA
COL1A1_for	5′-CCTCAGAAGAACTGGTACATCA
COLA1_rev	5′-GGCCTCGGTGGACATTA
α-SMA_for	5′-TCTGGCACCACTCTTTCTATAAC
α-SMA_rev	5′-TAGCCACATACATGGCGG
GAPDH_for	5′-TCAACAGCAACTCCCACTCTTCCA
GAPDH_rev	5′-ACCCTGTTGCTGTAGCCGTATTCA

4.5. Statistical Analysis

All data are expressed as the mean $\pm$ SD. Student's t-tests were used to compare different groups. The differences were considered significant if $p \leq 0.05$.

Author Contributions: Data curation, I.S. and Z.T.; Formal analysis, T.M. and T.Y.; Investigation, T.M. and T.Y.; Methodology, T.M. and I.S.; Project administration, Z.T.; Resources, I.S. and Z.T.; Validation, Z.T.; Visualization, T.M.; Writing–original draft, T.M.; Writing—review & editing, Z.T.

Funding: This research received no external funding.

References

1. Jaeschke, H.; Gores, G.J.; Cederbaum, A.I.; Hinson, J.A.; Pessayre, D.; Lemasters, J.J. Mechanisms of Hepatotoxicity. *Toxicol. Sci.* **2002**, *65*, 166–176. [CrossRef] [PubMed]

2. Luo, M.; Dong, L.; Li, J.; Wang, Y.; Shang, B. Protective Effects of Pentoxifylline on Acute Liver Injury Induced by Thioacetamide in Rats. *Int. J. Clin. Exp. Pathol.* **2015**, *8*, 8990–8996. [PubMed]

3. Hermenean, A.; Mariasiu, T.; Navarro-González, I.; Vegara-Meseguer, J.; Miuţescu, E.; Chakraborty, S.; Pérez-Sánchez, H. Hepatoprotective Activity of Chrysin is Mediated Through TNF-α in Chemically-Induced Acute Liver Damage: An in vivo Study and Molecular Modeling. *Exp. Ther. Med.* **2017**, *13*, 1671–1680. [CrossRef] [PubMed]

4. Friedman, S.L. Molecular Regulation of Hepatic Fibrosis, an Integrated Cellular Response to Tissue Injury. *J. Biol. Chem.* **2000**, *275*, 2247–2250. [CrossRef] [PubMed]

5. Tsuchida, T.; Friedman, S.L. Mechanisms of Hepatic Stellate Cell Activation. *Nat. Rev. Gastroenterol. Hepatol.* **2017**, *14*, 397–411. [CrossRef] [PubMed]

6. Sehgal, A.; Vaishnaw, A.; Fitzgerald, K. Liver as a Target for Oligonucleotide Therapeutics. *J. Hepatol.* **2013**, *59*, 1354–1359. [CrossRef] [PubMed]

7. Ponnappa, B.C.; Israel, Y.; Aini, M.; Zhou, F.; Russ, R.; Cao, Q.N.; Hu, Y.; Rubin, R. Inhibition of Tumor Necrosis Factor Alpha Secretion and Prevention of Liver Injury in Ethanol-Fed Rats by Antisense Oligonucleotides. *Biochem. Pharmacol.* **2005**, *69*, 569–577. [CrossRef] [PubMed]

8. Kyung-Oh, D. Effects of TGF-beta1 Ribbon Antisense on CCl(4)-Induced Liver Fibrosis. *Korean J. Physiol. Pharmacol.* **2008**, *12*, 1–6. [CrossRef] [PubMed]

9. Tkachuk, Z. Compound, Composition and Method for Treatment of Inflammatory and Inflammatory-Related Disorders. U.S. Patent 6,737,271, 18 May 2004.

10. Tkachuk, Z.Y.; Tkachuk, V.V.; Tkachuk, L.V. The Study on Membrane-Stabilizing and Anti-Inflammatory Actions of Yeast RNA in vivo and in vitro. *Biopolym. Cell* **2006**, *12*, 109–116. [CrossRef]

11. Frolov, V.M.; Sotskaya, Y.A.; Kruglova, O.V.; Tkachuk, Z.Y. Estimation of Nuclex Effectivity at the Treatment of the Patients with Chronic Viral Hepatitis C. *Ukr. Med. Alm.* **2012**, *15*, 157–164.

12. Frolov, V.M.; Sotska, Y.A.; Kruglova, O.V.; Tkachuk, Z.Y. Influence of Antiviral Drug Nuclex on the Cellular Immunity at the Patients with Chronic Viral Hepatitis C. *Ukr. Morpholog. Alm.* **2012**, *10*, 99–105.

13. Tkachuk, Z.; Dykyi, B.; Kondryn, A.; Prishliak, O.; Vaskul, N. Application of Preparation of Nuclex in Therapy of Hepatitis. *Ukr. Med. Alm.* **2011**, *14*, 200–203.

14. Rensen, S.S.; Slaats, Y.; Nijhuis, J.; Jans, A.; Bieghs, V.; Driessen, A.; Malle, E.; Greve, J.W.; Buurman, W.A. Increased Hepatic Myeloperoxidase Activity in Obese Subjects with Nonalcoholic Steatohepatitis. *Am. J. Pathol.* **2009**, *175*, 1473–1482. [CrossRef] [PubMed]

15. Chilakapati, J.; Shankar, K.; Korrapati, M.C.; Hill, R.A.; Mehendale, H.M. Saturation Toxicokinetics of Thioacetamide: Role in Initiation of Liver Injury. *Drug Metab. Dispos.* **2005**, *33*, 1877–1885. [CrossRef] [PubMed]

16. Huang, W.; Wang, Y.; Jiang, X.; Sun, Y.; Zhao, Z.; Li, S. Protective Effect of Flavonoids from Ziziphus jujuba cv. Jinsixiaozao against Acetaminophen-Induced Liver Injury by Inhibiting Oxidative Stress and Inflammation in Mice. *Molecules* **2017**, *22*, 1781. [CrossRef] [PubMed]

17. Fabregat, I.; Moreno-Càceres, J.; Sánchez, A.; Dooley, S.; Dewidar, B.; Giannelli, G.; Ten, D.P. TGF-β Signalling and Liver Disease. *FEBS J.* **2016**, *283*, 2219–2232. [CrossRef] [PubMed]

18. Pandit, A.; Barna, P.; Sachdeva, T. Drug-Induced Hepatotoxicity: A Review. *J. Appl. Pharm. Sci.* **2012**, *2*, 233–243. [CrossRef]

19. Robin, S.; Sunil, K.; Rana, A.C.; Nidhi, S. Different Models of Hepatotoxicity and Related Liver Diseases: A Review. *Int. Res. J. Pharm.* **2012**, *3*, 86–95.

20. Akhtar, T.; Sheikh, N. An Overview of Thioacetamide-Induced Hepatotoxicity. *Toxin Rev.* **2013**, *32*, 43–46. [CrossRef]

21. Rahman, T.M.; Hodgson, H.J. Animal models of acute hepatic failure. *Int. J. Exp. Pathol.* **2000**, *81*, 145–157. [CrossRef] [PubMed]

22. Hajovsky, L.; Hu, G.; Koen, Y.; Sarma, D.; Cui, W.; Moore, D.S.; Staudinger, J.L.; Hanzlik, R.P. Metabolism and Toxicity of Thioacetamide and Thioacetamide S-Oxide in Rat Hepatocytes. *Chem. Res. Toxicol.* **2012**, *25*, 1955–1963. [CrossRef] [PubMed]

23. Everhart, J.E.; Wright, E.C. Association of γ-Glutamyl Transferase (GGT) Activity with Treatment and Clinical Outcomes in Chronic Hepatitis C (HCV). *Hepatology* **2013**, *57*, 1725–1733. [CrossRef] [PubMed]

24. Amanzada, A.; Malik, I.A.; Nischwitz, M.; Sultan, S.; Naz, N.; Ramadori, G. Myeloperoxidase and Elastase are Only Expressed by Neutrophils in Normal and in Inflamed Liver. *Histochem. Cell Biol.* **2011**, *135*, 305–315. [CrossRef] [PubMed]

25. Ramaiah, S.K.; Apte, U.; Mehendale, H.M. Cytochrome P4502E1 Induction Increases Thioacetamide Liver Injury in Diet-Restricted Rats. *Drug Metab. Dispos.* **2001**, *29*, 1088–1095. [PubMed]

26. Wang, T.; Shankar, K.; Ronis, M.J.; Mehendale, H.M. Potentiation of Thioacetamide Liver Injury in Diabetic Rats is Due to Induced CYP2E1. *J. Pharm. Exp. Ther.* **2000**, *294*, 473–479.

27. Toropchin, V.I. Influence of Nuclex and Enerliv Combination at Lipoperoxidation Index at the Patients with Nonalcoholic Steatohepatitis on Background Chronic Fatigue Syndrome. *Ukr. Morpholog. Almanah.* **2011**, *9*, 124–128.

28. Birben, E.; Sahiner, U.M.; Sackesen, C.; Erzurum, S.; Kalayci, O. Oxidative Stress and Antioxidant Defense. *World Allergy Organ. J.* **2012**, *5*, 9–19. [CrossRef] [PubMed]

29. Kurutas, E.B. The Importance of Antioxidants which Play the Role in Cellular Response against Oxidative/Nitrosative Stress: Current State. *Nutr. J.* **2016**, *15*, 71. [CrossRef] [PubMed]

30. Ramadori, G.; Armbrust, T. Cytokines in the Liver. *Eur. J. Gastroenterol. Hepatol.* **2001**, *13*, 777–784. [CrossRef] [PubMed]

31. Kang, J.S.; Wanibuchi, H.; Morimura, K.; Wongpoomchai, R.; Chusiri, Y.; Gonzalez, F.J.; Fukushima, S. Role of CYP2E1 in Thioacetamide-Induced Mouse Hepatotoxicity. *Toxicol. Appl. Pharmacol.* **2008**, *228*, 295–300. [CrossRef] [PubMed]

32. Amanzada, A.; Moriconi, F.; Mansuroglu, T.; Cameron, S.; Ramadori, G.; Malik, I.A. Induction of Chemokines and Cytokines Before Neutrophils and Macrophage Recruitment in Different Regions of Rat Liver After TAA Administration. *Lab. Investig.* **2014**, *94*, 235–247. [CrossRef] [PubMed]

33. Shen, H.; Sheng, L.; Chen, Z.; Jiang, L.; Su, H.; Yin, L.; Omary, M.B.; Rui, L. Mouse Hepatocyte Overexpression of NF-κB-Inducing Kinase (NIK) Triggers Fatal Macrophage-Dependent Liver Injury and Fibrosis. *Hepatology* **2014**, *60*, 2065–2076. [CrossRef] [PubMed]

34. Simeonova, P.P.; Gallucci, R.M.; Hulderman, T.; Wilson, R.; Kommineni, C.; Rao, M.; Luster, M.I. The Role of Tumor Necrosis Factor-Alpha in Liver Toxicity, Inflammation, and Fibrosis Induced by Carbon Tetrachloride. *Toxicol. Appl. Pharmacol.* **2001**, *177*, 112–120. [CrossRef] [PubMed]

35. Palacios, R.S.; Roderfeld, M.; Hemmann, S.; Rath, T.; Atanasova, S.; Tschuschner, A.; Gressner, O.A.; Weiskirchen, R.; Graf, J.; Roeb, E. Activation of Hepatic Stellate Cells is Associated with Cytokine Expression in Thioacetamide-Induced Hepatic Fibrosis in Mice. *Lab. Investig.* **2008**, *88*, 1192–1203. [CrossRef] [PubMed]

36. Zhou, Z.; Park, S.; Kim, J.W.; Zhao, J.; Lee, M.; Choi, K.C.; Lim, C.W.; Kim, B. Detrimental Effects of Nicotine on Thioacetamide-Induced Liver Injury in Mice. *Toxicol. Mech. Methods* **2017**, *27*, 501–510. [CrossRef] [PubMed]

37. Friedman, S.L. Mechanisms of Hepatic Fibrogenesis. *Gastroenterology* **2008**, *134*, 1655–1669. [CrossRef] [PubMed]

38. Wang, T.; Wu, D.; Li, P.; Zhang, K.; Tao, S.; Li, Z.; Li, J. Effects of Taohongsiwu Decoction on the Expression of α-SMA and TGF-β1 mRNA in the Liver Tissues of a Rat Model of Hepatic Cirrhosis. *Exp. Ther. Med.* **2017**, *14*, 1074–1080. [CrossRef] [PubMed]

39. Friedman, S.L. Hepatic Stellate Cells: Protean, Multifunctional, and Enigmatic Cells of the Liver. *Physiol. Rev.* **2008**, *88*, 125–172. [CrossRef] [PubMed]

40. Melnichuk, N.; Semernikova, L.; Tkachuk, Z. Complexes of Oligoribonucleotides with D-Mannitol Inhibit Hemagglutinin–Glycan Interaction and Suppress Influenza A Virus H1N1 (A/FM/1/47) Infectivity In Vitro. *Pharmaceuticals* **2017**, *10*, 71. [CrossRef] [PubMed]

41. Melnichuk, N.; Kashuba, V.; Rybalko, S.; Tkachuk, Z. Tkachuk Complexes of Oligoribonucleotides with D-Mannitol Modulate the Innate Immune Response to Influenza A Virus H1N1 (A/FM/1/47) In Vivo. *Pharmaceuticals* **2018**, *11*, 73. [CrossRef] [PubMed]

42. Vivcharyk, M.; Iakhnenko, M.; Levchenko, S.; Chernykh, S.; Tkachuk, Z. Monitoring of Interferon-α (peg) Conformational Changes Caused by Yeast RNA. In Proceedings of the 7th International Conference Physics of Liquid Matter: Modern Problems (PLM MP), Kyiv, Ukraine, 27–30 May 2016.

43. Vivcharyk, M.M.; Ilchenko, O.O.; Levchenko, S.M.; Yu, Z. Tkachuk Complexation of RNA with D-Mannitol, Its Spectral Characteristics and Biological Activity. *Dopov. Nac. Acad. Nauk. Ukr.* **2016**, *10*, 78–83. [CrossRef]

44. National Research Council (US) Committee. *Guide for the Care and Use of Laboratory Animals*, 8th ed.; The National Academies Press: Washington, DC, USA, 2011.

45. Shmarakov, I.O.; Borschovetska, V.L.; Marchenko, M.M.; Blaner, W.S. Retinoids Modulate Thioacetamide-Induced Acute Hepatotoxicity. *Toxicol. Sci.* **2014**, *139*, 284–292. [CrossRef] [PubMed]

46. Shmarakov, I.; Marchyshak, T.; Borschovetska, V.; Marchenko, M.; Tkachuk, Z. Hepatoprotective Activity of Exogenous RNA. *Ukr. Biochem. J.* **2015**, *87*, 37–44. [CrossRef] [PubMed]

47. Schierwagen, C.; Bylund-Fellenius, A.C.; Lundberg, C. Improved Method for Quantification of Tissue PMN Accumulation Measured by Myeloperoxidase Activity. *J. Pharmacol. Methods* **1990**, *23*, 179–186. [CrossRef]

48. Ohkawa, H.; Ohishi, N.; Yagi, K. Assay for Lipid Peroxides in Animal Tissues by Thiobarbituric Acid Reaction. *Anal. Biochem.* **1979**, *95*, 351–358. [CrossRef]

49. Levine, R.L.; Garland, D.; Oliver, C.N.; Amici, A.; Climent, I.; Lenz, A.G.; Ahn, B.W.; Shaltiel, S.; Stadtman, E.R. Determination of Carbonyl Content in Oxidatively Modified Proteins. *Methods Enzymol.* **1990**, *186*, 464–478. [PubMed]

50. Murphy, M.E.; Kehrer, J.P. Oxidation State of Tissue Thiol Groups and Content of Protein Carbonyl Groups in Chickens with Inherited Muscular Dystrophy. *Biochem. J.* **1989**, *260*, 359–364. [CrossRef] [PubMed]

51. Ellman, G.L. Tissue Sulfhydryl Groups. *Arch. Biochem. Biophys.* **1959**, *82*, 70–77. [CrossRef]

52. Wendel, A. Glutathione Peroxidase. *Methods Enzymol.* **1981**, *77*, 325–333. [PubMed]

53. Habig, W.H.; Pabst, M.J.; Jakoby, W.B. Glutathione S-transferases. The first Enzymatic Step in Mercapturic Acid Formation. *J. Biol. Chem.* **1974**, *249*, 7130–7139. [PubMed]

54. Waterborg, J.H.; Matthews, H.R. The Lowry Method for Protein Quantitation. *Methods Mol. Biol.* **1984**, *1*, 1–3. [PubMed]

55. Livak, K.J.; Schmittgen, T.D. Analysis of relative gene expression data using real-time quantitative PCR and the $2^{-\Delta\Delta CT}$ Method. *Methods* **2001**, *25*, 402–408. [CrossRef] [PubMed]

3

Synthesis, Evaluation of Cytotoxicity and Molecular Docking Studies of the 7-Acetamido Substituted 2-Aryl-5-bromo-3-trifluoroacetylindoles as Potential Inhibitors of Tubulin Polymerization

Malose J. Mphahlele [1],* 🆔 and Nishal Parbhoo [2]

[1] Department of Chemistry, College of Science, Engineering and Technology, University of South Africa, Private Bag X06, Florida 1710, South Africa

[2] Department of Life & Consumer Sciences, College of Agriculture and Environmental Sciences, University of South Africa, Private Bag X06, Florida 1710, South Africa; parbhn1@unisa.ac.za

* Correspondence: mphahmj@unisa.ac.za

Abstract: The 3-trifluoroacetyl–substituted 7-acetamido-2-aryl-5-bromoindoles **5a–h** were prepared and evaluated for potential antigrowth effect in vitro against human lung cancer (A549) and cervical cancer (HeLa) cells and for the potential to inhibit tubulin polymerization. The corresponding intermediates, namely, the 3-unsubstituted 7-acetyl-2-aryl-5-bromoindole **2a–d** and 7-acetamido-2-aryl-5-bromoindole **4a–d** were included in the assays in order to correlate both structural variations and cytotoxicity. No cytotoxicity was observed for compounds **2a–d** and their 3-trifluoroacetyl–substituted derivatives **5a–d** against both cell lines. The 7-acetamido derivatives **4–d** exhibited modest cytotoxicity against both cell lines. All of the 3-trifluoroacetyl–substituted 7-acetamido-2-aryl-5-bromoindoles **5e–h** were found to be more active against both cell lines when compared to the chemotherapeutic drug, Melphalan. The most active compound, **5g**, induced programmed cell death (apoptosis) in a caspase-dependent manner for both A549 and HeLa cells. Compounds **5e–h** were found to significantly inhibit tubulin polymerization against indole-3-carbinol and colchicine as reference standards. Molecular docking of **5g** into the colchicine-binding site suggests that the compounds bind to tubulin by different type of interactions including pi-alkyl, amide-pi stacked and alkyl interactions as well as hydrogen bonding with the protein residues to elicit anticancer activity.

Keywords: 7-acetamido-2-aryl-5-bromoindoles; trifluoroacetylation; cytotoxicity; apoptosis; tubulin polymerization; molecular docking

---

1. Introduction

Microtubule targeting agents have an established history of utility in the treatment of cancer and have been instrumental as biological probes to identify the nature of tubulin and the role of tubulin dynamics in mitosis [1]. Colchicine is known to bind to tubulin and block the formation of microtubules while the other anticancer agents stabilize the tubulin structure and, therefore, prevent microtubule disassembly [2]. Nitrogen-containing heterocycles such as indoles with anticancer properties have the potential to inhibit tubulin polymerization by binding to colchicine-binding site [3–5]. The methoxy-substituted 2-aryl-3-formylindoles (**a**) shown in Figure 1, for example, have been found to completely block the microtubule assembly at micromolar concentrations, which suggests a correlation between cytotoxicity and the microtubule system [3]. Structure–activity relationship (SAR) studies of indole derivatives revealed that a hydrogen bond donor NH at position 1 is essential for their antiproliferative activity [3]. A nitrogen-containing group on the fused benzo ring of the indole derivatives, on the other hand, was found to lead to increased cytotoxicity against the HeLa and A549 cell lines as well as HIV-1 inhibition activity [6]. Likewise, the presence of a lipophilic bromine atom on the fused benzo ring of an indole framework was found to impart significant anti-tumour activity in both the synthetic [7] and the naturally [8] occurring indole derivatives. Aplicyanin A (b) shown in Figure 1, for example, is a 5-bromoindole–based compound previously isolated from ascidian *Aplidium cyaneum* and this compound has been found to exhibit increased antiproliferative activity against MDA-MB-231, A549 and HT-29 cancer cell lines [8]. A hydrogen bond acceptor such as a formyl group at position 3 of the indole framework of compound (a), for example, facilitates interaction with biological receptors and therefore enhance anticancer activity [9]. Thomas et al. have previously isolated N-[(5-{[(4-methylphenyl)sulfonyl]amino}-3-(trifluoroacetyl)-1H-indol-1-yl)acetyl]-L-leucine (NTRC-824) shown in Figure 1 as an impurity and found it to be 90-fold more active (IC_{50} = 38 nM) and selective for the neurotesin receptor type 2 (NTS2 *versus* NTS1) than the expected C-3 unsubstituted analogue (IC_{50} = 3322 nM) [10]. The enhanced activity of NTRC-824 due to the presence of a trifluoroacetyl group is presumably due to the increased electron withdrawing effect of the trifluoromethyl group. Literature precedents revealed that the presence of a trifluoromethyl group at the C-3 position of an indole framework results in increased affinity for lipids (lipophilicity) and metabolic stability of the molecule as well as its activity profile more so than the 3-unsubstituted or 3-acetyl analogues [2,11–13].

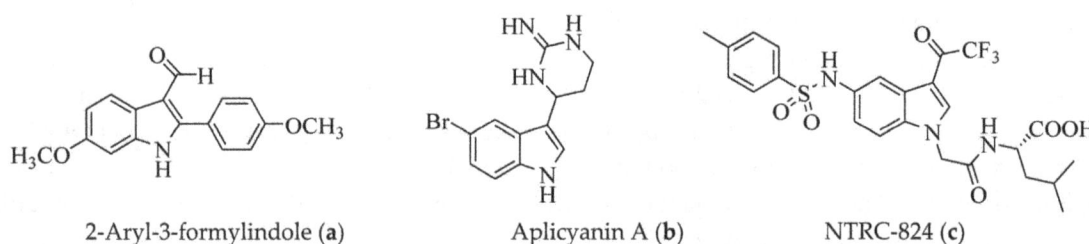

2-Aryl-3-formylindole (a)   Aplicyanin A (b)   NTRC-824 (c)

Figure 1. Structures of 3-formyl substituted 2-arylindole (a), aplicyanin A (b) and NTRC-824 (c).

We considered the antiproliferative properties of the 2-arylindoles [14] in combination with the above literature SAR analysis to introduce a trifluoroacetyl group at position-3 of the 7-acetyl-2-aryl-5-bromoindoles and the 7-acetamido-2-aryl-5-bromoindoles. The main aim was to evaluate the effect of incorporating a trifluoroacetyl group on the biological activity of the polysubstituted indole derivatives. The prepared 3-trifluoroacetyl–substituted indole derivatives and the corresponding synthetic intermediates, namely, the 7-acetyl-2-aryl-5-bromoindoles and the 7-acetamido-2-aryl-5-bromoindoles were evaluated for cytotoxicity against the human lung cancer (A549) and cervical cancer (HeLa) cell lines in order to correlate between both structural variations and cytotoxicity. The pro-apoptotic properties of the analogous indole-3-carbinol [15] encouraged us to elucidate their mechanism of cancer cell death and for their ability to inhibit tubulin polymerization.

2. Results and Discussion

2.1. Chemistry

The title compounds were prepared via a series of steps involving different intermediate products as shown in Scheme 1 and the corresponding yields are listed in Table 1. We first subjected the 3-arylalkynylated 2-amino-5-bromoacetophenone derivatives **1a–d** to palladium chloride-mediated endo-dig cyclization to afford the 7-acetyl-2-aryl-5-bromoindoles **2a–d** in high yields. The indole derivatives **2a–d** were, in turn, reacted with a hydroxylamine hydrochloride- pyridine mixture in ethanol under reflux to afford the oxime derivatives **3a–d**. The ^{1}H-NMR spectra of the indole derivatives **2a–d** revealed the presence of two singlets around δ 6.90 and 11.10 ppm, which correspond to H-3 and NH, respectively. The oxime nature of **3a–d**, on the other hand, was confirmed by the additional singlet around δ 11.6 ppm and carbon signal significantly upfield around $\delta_{C=N}$ 154 ppm in their ^{1}H-NMR and ^{13}C-NMR spectra, respectively. The oxime derivatives **3a–d** were, in turn, subjected to trifluoroacetic acid (TFA)-mediated Beckmann rearrangement in acetonitrile under reflux for 2 h to afford the corresponding 7-acetamido-2-aryl-5-bromoindoles **4a–d** (Scheme 1, Table 1). The NH proton of the amide group resonates as a singlet around δ 9.70 ppm in the proton NMR spectra of these compounds. The methyl protons of these compounds resonate significantly up-field around δ 2.18 ppm compared to those in the ^{1}H-NMR spectra of **2** (around δ 2.79 ppm) and **3** (around δ 2.30 ppm). Their carbonyl carbon resonates significantly up-field ($\delta_{C=O}$ 170 ppm) than that of the corresponding precursors **2** ($\delta_{C=O}$ 200 ppm) and more downfield than the oxime substrates **3** ($\delta_{C=N}$ 154 ppm). The observed significant up-field shift of the methyl protons and the carbonyl carbon of **4a–d** compared to **2a–d** confirm the formation of the amide derivatives to be the result of an aryl carbon migration. Trifluoroacetic anhydride (TFAA) has previously been found to affect the regioselective Friedel-Crafts trifluoroacetylation of the N-benzyl substituted 2-methyl-5-nitroindole [16], the N-unprotected 2-arylindoles [17], and their indole-chalcone derivatives [18] at the C-3 position without competitive formation of the 1-acylated and/or the 1,3-diacylated products. A series of fluoromethyl indol-3-yl ketones has also been prepared via Friedel-Craft fluoroacetylation of indoles with fluorinated acetic acids (3 equiv.) in dichloroethane at 100 °C in the absence of catalyst or additive [19]. Compounds **2a–d** and **4a–d** were subjected to TFAA (1.2 equiv.) in THF under reflux for 5 h to afford the corresponding 7-acetyl **5a–d** and 7-acetamido substituted 5-bromo-3-trifluoroacetylindoles **5e–h** in moderate to high yields.

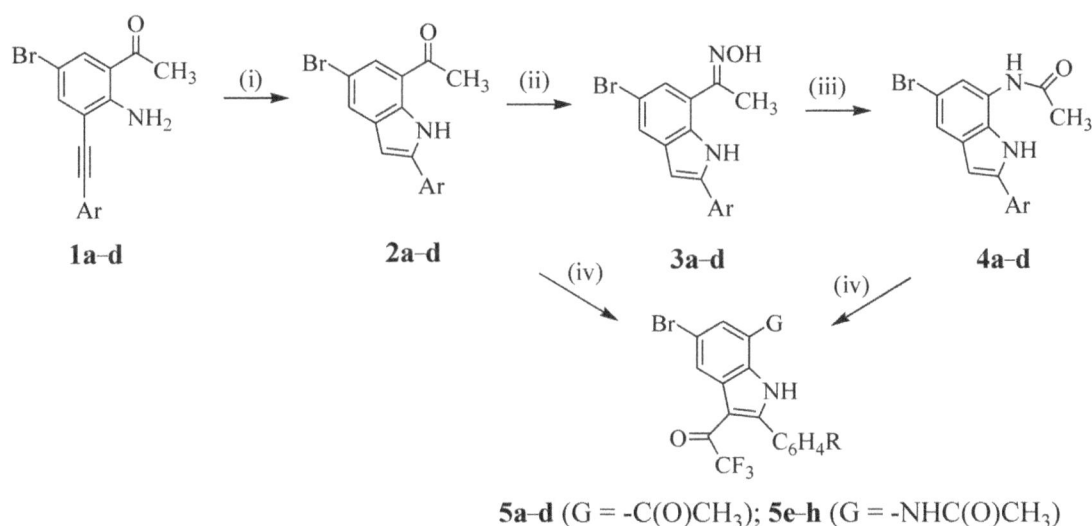

5a–d (G = -C(O)CH$_3$); **5e–h** (G = -NHC(O)CH$_3$)

Scheme 1. Reaction steps involved in the synthesis of compounds **5a–h**. Reagents and conditions: (i) PdCl$_2$, CH$_3$CN, reflux, 3 h; (ii) NH$_2$OH.HCl, pyridine, EtOH, reflux, 5 h; (iii) TFA, CH$_3$CN, reflux, 2 h; (iv) (CF$_3$CO)$_2$O, THF, reflux 5 h.

Table 1. Percentage yields of the compounds **5a–h** and the corresponding reaction intermediates **2–4**.

Ar	2	3	4	5a–d	5e–h
C$_6$H$_5$-	92 (**2a**)	90 (**3a**)	81 (**4a**)	92 (**5a**)	84 (**5e**)
4-FC$_6$H$_4$-	84 (**2b**)	87 (**3b**)	76 (**4b**)	84 (**5b**)	78 (**5f**)
3-ClC$_6$H$_4$-	85 (**2c**)	82 (**3c**)	73 (**4c**)	85 (**5c**)	80 (**5g**)
4-MeOC$_6$H$_4$-	77 (**2d**)	80 (**3d**)	76 (**4d**)	77 (**5d**)	52 (**5h**)

2.2. Biological Evaluation

As a prelude to the 3-trifluoroacetyl–substituted 2-arylindole derivatives with potential anticancer properties, we screened compounds **5a–h** for in vitro antiproliferative properties against human lung cancer (A549) and cervical cancer (HeLa) cell lines, which have been found to be the main causes of cancer death in males and females worldwide. The corresponding intermediates, namely, the 3-unsubstituted 7-acetyl-2-aryl-5-bromoindole **2a–d** and 7-acetamido-2-aryl-5-bromoindole **4a–d** precursors were also included in the assays in order to correlate between both structural variations and cytotoxicity.

2.2.1. In Vitro Cytotoxicity Studies of Indole Derivatives 2a–d, 4a–d and 5a–h

The HeLa and A549 cancer cells were initially exposed to two concentrations of each test compound (10 μM and 100 μM) for 48 h with a well-known chemotherapeutic drug, Melphalan, used as a reference standard at the same concentrations (Tables 2 and 3). Acquisition was performed using the ImageXpress Micro XLS Widefield Microscope and the acquired images were analyzed using the MetaXpress software and Multi-Wavelength Cell Scoring Application Module (see Figure S2 in the Supplementary Information for cell viability percentages for each compound). The structure activity relationship (SAR) of these compounds has been evaluated with respect to the substitution patterns on the 2-phenyl ring, C-3 and C-7 positions. The acetyl derivatives **2a–d** were found to be generally inactive against the two cancer cell lines at both concentrations (Table 2). The presence of an acetamido moiety at the 7-position, on the other hand, led to modest cytotoxicity against the two cell lines for the 2-(4-fluorophenyl)- **4b**, 2-(3-chlorophenyl)- **4c** and 2-(4-methoxyphenyl)-substituted 7-acetamido-5-bromoindole **4d** (Table 2). The presence of the amide moiety on the fused benzo ring has previously been found to enhance the biological activity of indole-based compounds [6,10,12]. Lack of cytotoxicity for the 2-phenyl substituted derivative **4a** against both cancer cell lines, on the other hand, presumably reflects the importance of a lipophilic substituent (halogen or methoxy group) on the 2-phenyl ring of compounds **4b–d** on biological activity.

Table 2. IC$_{50}$ values of compounds **2a–d**, **4a–d** and Melphalan against the A549 and HeLa cells.

2a–d (G = -C(O)CH₃); 4a–d (G = -NHC(O)CH₃)   Melphalan

Compound	G	Ar	Cancer Cells IC$_{50}$ (μM) (A549)	HeLa
2a	-C(O)CH$_3$	C$_6$H$_5$-	>200	>200
2b	-C(O)CH$_3$	4-FC$_6$H$_4$-	>200	>200
2c	-C(O)CH$_3$	3-ClC$_6$H$_4$-	>200	>200
2d	-C(O)CH$_3$	4-MeOC$_6$H$_4$-	>200	>200
4a	-NHC(O)CH$_3$	C$_6$H$_5$-	>200	>200
4b	-NHC(O)CH$_3$	4-FC$_6$H$_4$-	116.2 ± 0.78	122.4 ± 1.02
4c	-NHC(O)CH$_3$	3-ClC$_6$H$_4$-	154.6 ± 0.90	126.9 ± 1.00
4d	-NHC(O)CH$_3$	4-MeOC$_6$H$_4$-	146.8 ± 1.00	125.0 ± 0.88
Melphalan	-	-	30.66 ± 0.76	37.16 ± 0.22

Diminished activity against both cell lines was observed for all the 2-aryl-5-bromoindoles **5a–d** bearing a combination of the 7-acetyl and 3-trifluoroacetyl groups (Table 3). A combination of a 7-acetamido and 3-trifluoroacetyl groups in compounds **5e–h**, on the other hand, resulted in increased cytotoxicity against both cancer cell lines and more so than the chemotherapeutic drug, Melphalan, used as a positive control at the same concentrations (see Supplementary Information (Figure S3) for the corresponding dose response curves). Within this series, the trend in IC$_{50}$ values (Table 4) against the lung cancer (A549) cell line is as follows: **5g** (2.72 μM) > **5h** (3.26 μM) > **5f** (5.03 μM) > **5e** (9.94 μM) with the following trend in activity against the cervical cancer (HeLa) cells: **5f** (7.95 μM) > **5g** (8.74 μM) > **5h** (10.72 μM) > **5e** (12.89 μM). These preliminary cytotoxicity results suggest that a combination of the 7-acetamido and 3-trifluoroacetyl group is desirable for cytotoxicity of the 2-aryl-5-bromoindoles against both cancer cell lines. The slight antiproliferative activity observed for the corresponding C-3 unsubstituted 7-acetamido-5-bromoindoles **4a–d**, which significantly increased upon incorporation of a 3-trifluoroacetyl in derivatives **5e–h** further confirm the importance of a strong hydrogen bond acceptor at this position 3 of the indole framework to facilitate interaction with biological receptors in analogy with the literature precedents [9,10]. The presence of a strong electron-withdrawing trifluoromethyl group ($-CF_3$) has previously been found to increase the activity profile of indole derivatives [11,13]. The combined electron-withdrawing and hydrogen bonding effects of the trifluromethyl and carbonyl fragments of the 3-trifluoroacetyl group probably account for the observed increased cytotoxicity of compounds **5e–h**.

Table 3. IC_{50} values of compounds **5a–h** against A549 and HeLa cells.

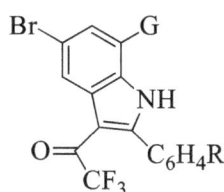

5a–d (G = -C(O)CH₃); **5e–h** (G = -NHC(O)CH₃)

Compound	G	Ar	Cancer Cells IC_{50} (μM)	
			(A549)	HeLa
5a	-C(O)CH₃	C₆H₅-	>200	>200
5b	-C(O)CH₃	4-FC₆H₄-	>200	>200
5c	-C(O)CH₃	3-ClC₆H₄-	>200	>200
5d	-C(O)CH₃	4-MeOC₆H₄-	>200	>200
5e	-NHC(O)CH₃	C₆H₅-	9.94 ± 0.99	12.89 ± 1.11
5f	-NHC(O)CH₃	4-FC₆H₄-	5.03 ± 0.71	7.95 ± 0.90
5g	-NHC(O)CH₃	3-ClC₆H₄-	2.72 ± 0.43	8.74 ± 0.94
5h	-NHC(O)CH₃	4-MeOC₆H₄-	3.26 ± 0.51	10.72 ± 1.03
Melphalan	-		30.66 ± 0.76	37.16 ± 0.22

In vitro studies indicated that indole derivatives such as indole-3-carbinol inhibit cell proliferation, caused cell cycle arrest at the G1 phase and induced apoptosis [15]. Deregulation of apoptosis plays a significant role in the development of cancer [20]. Cytotoxicity, on the other hand, does not define a specific cellular death mechanism (necrosis or apoptosis). We considered the pro-apoptotic properties of indole-3-carbinol [15] and selected compounds **4c** and **5g** as representative examples for further evaluation regarding the mechanism of action of the 3-trifluoroacetylated 2-arylindole derivatives **5e–h** in the A549 and HeLa cells.

2.2.2. Evaluation of Cell Death Pathways

Several distinctive mechanisms of cancer cell death such as apoptosis, necrosis, autophagy and cornification have been identified, and these are characterized by differences in morphology and biochemical changes [21]. A major biochemical feature of apoptosis is the activation of caspases, which plays a central role in the morphological changes associated with apoptosis [21–23]. Caspase activation was determined using immunochemical methods and the antibodies against activated caspase 8 and caspase 3. As an initiator caspase, caspase 8 is first activated through a death signal suggesting a cellular response to an external signal for cell death. Activated caspase 8 can be used as a convenient indicator of involvement of the extrinsic death receptor pathway of apoptosis [24]. Executioner caspases including caspase 3 are, in turn, activated by the initiator caspases.

This protein is either partially or totally responsible for the cleavage of many key proteins such as PARP, DNA protein kinases and retinoblastoma protein [25]. Figures 2 and 3 show the results of caspase activation analysis and it is evident that clear increases in the percentage of mean fluorescence intensity of the untreated control occurred when the HeLa and A549 cells were treated with **4c** and Melphalan. A decrease in percentage was noticed when HeLa cells were treated with **5g**, but the expected increase was evident in A549 cells. This was true for both activated caspase 8 and 3. A more distinct increase was evident with caspase 3 albeit less pronounced than that of **4c** and the increase was expected as caspase 3 is activated by initiator caspase including caspase 8, which is a later event in apoptosis. It is evident from the observed results that **5g** induces apoptosis in a caspase-dependent manner in both cancer cell lines and this effect is more pronounced for the A549 cells, which also showed increased sensitivity towards this compound in the cytotoxicity assays than the HeLa cells. Prolonged treatment of the cells with compounds **5e–h** for 48 h or more, for example, would probably result in significant effects. We also evaluated compound **5g** for potential to induce other key apoptotic biochemical features such as phosphatidylserine (PS) translocation, cell cycle arrest and mitochondrial membrane depolarization. However, the compound failed to induce PS translocation, cell cycle arrest and mitochondrial membrane depolarization in both cell lines after 24 h (data not included).

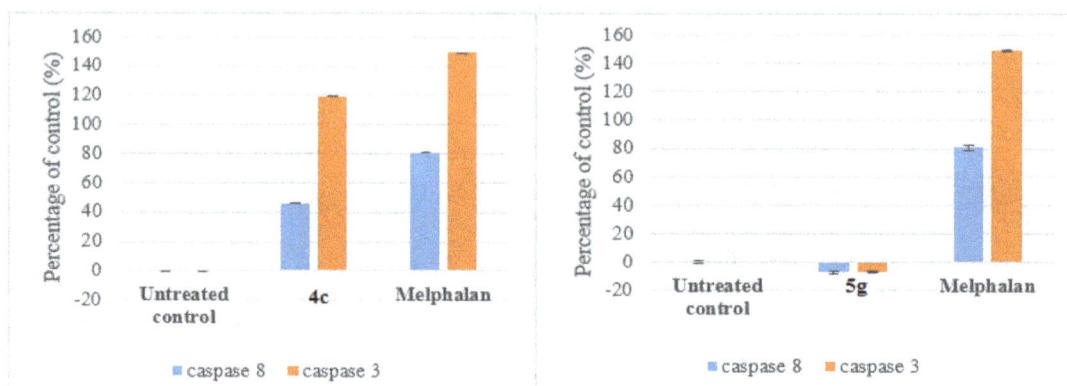

Figure 2. Caspase 8 and 3 activation as indicated by % changes in the mean integrated fluorescence intensity of the untreated control using HeLa cells after 24 h of exposure to compounds **4c** and **5g** (IC_{50} values) using Melphalan as a positive control. Bar graph represents the average of one individual experiment performed in quadruplicate. The standard deviations are represented as error bars.

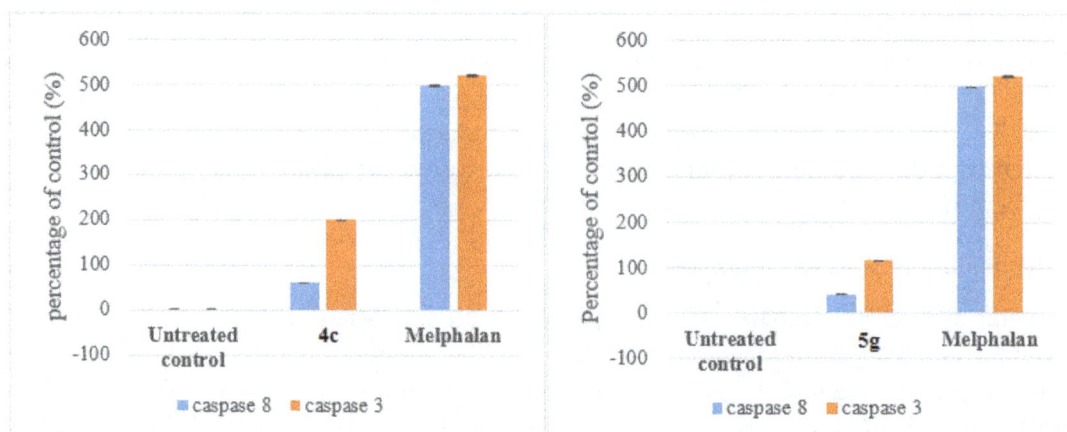

Figure 3. Caspase 8 and 3 activation as indicated by % changes in the mean integrated fluorescence inensity of the untreated control using A549 cells after 24 h of exposure to **4c** and **5g** (IC_{50} values) using Melphalan as a positive control. Bar graph represents the average of one individual experiment performed in quadruplicate. The standard deviations are represented as error bars.

Recourse to the literature revealed that a series of analogous indole-bearing combretastatin derivatives prepared by condensing indole-3-acetic acid with aldehydes prevent tubulin polymerization as confirmed by immunofluorescence confocal microscopy [26]. Molecular docking revealed that the compounds bind to the colchicine binding site which is situated at α and β interface of tubulin [26]. This literature precedent encouraged us to evaluate the 3-trifluoroacetyl substituted derivatives **5e–h** for potential to inhibit tubulin polymerization.

2.3. Effect of Compounds **5e–h** on Tubulin Polymerization

In order to determine if the antiproliferative activity of compounds **5e–h** was related to their capacity to destabilize tubulin, we evaluated them in a tubulin polymerization assay using colchicine and indole-3-carbinol as reference standards. Kinetics of inhibition of tubulin polymerization of compounds **5e–h** at 0.25 μM against colchicine and indole-3-carbinol as reference standards (Figure 4) revealed that these compounds significantly interfere with tubulin polymerization by lowering the rate of microtubule assembly. The IC$_{50}$ values for compounds **5a–e** and the corresponding reference standards (Table 3) were obtained at the following concentrations: 0.1, 1.0 and 10 μM. These results are in agreement with the antiproliferative activity in the cell culture.

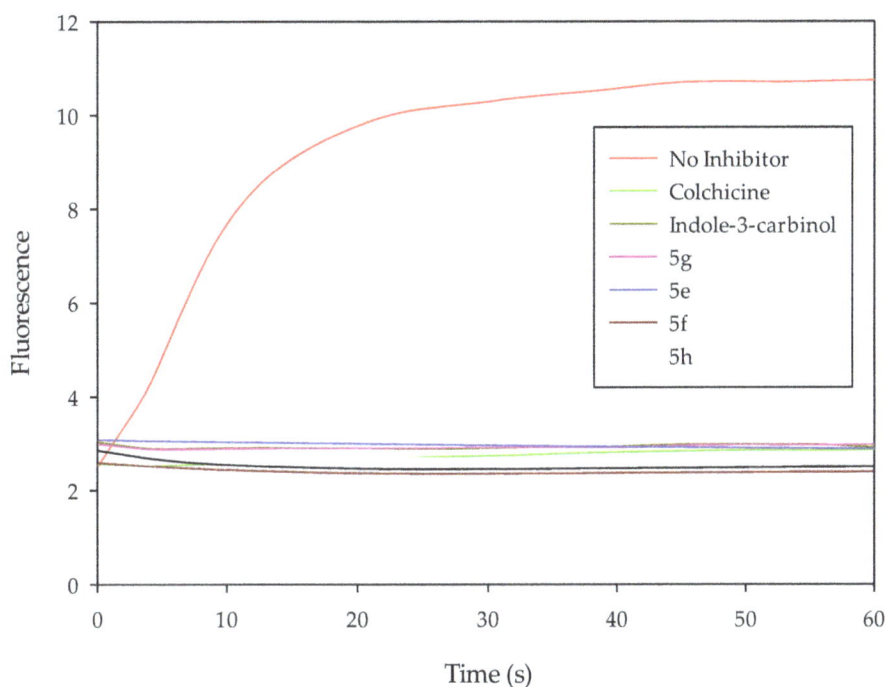

Figure 4. Kinetics of inhibition of tubulin polymerization by **5e–h** at 0.25 μM against colchicine (green) and indole-3-carbinol (yellow) and in the absence of an inhibitor (red). Fluorescence at 450 nm was measured every three seconds over a period of 1 h at 37 $°$C.

Table 4. IC$_{50}$ values of **5e–h** against tubulin using indol-3-carbinol and colchicine as positive controls.

Compound	IC$_{50}$ (μM)	S.D.
5e	3.18×10^{-5}	± 0.06
5f	3.28×10^{-7}	± 0.66
5g	2.42×10^{-5}	± 0.01
5h	4.86×10^{-6}	± 0.08
Indole-3-carbinol	9.76×10^{-5}	± 0.27
Colchicine	9.88×10^{-5}	± 0.17

The increased cytotoxicity and inhibition of tubulin polymerization of compounds **5e–h** are probably due to strong hydrogen bond interactions between the trifluoroacetyl group of the ligands with the receptor's protein residues. The propensity of the amide moiety for hydrogen bonding cannot be over ruled because it plays an important role in the interaction of bioactive compounds with the receptors [27]. In order to prove these assumptions and further ass sit us to rationalize the structure activity relationship (SAR), we subjected the most active compound **5g** to molecular docking into the colchicine-binding site of tubulin.

2.4. Molecular Docking Studies of **2a**, **4a** *and* **5g** *into Tubulin*

To help us understand the anticancer activity of the 3-trifluoroacetyl indole derivatives **5e–h** and further rationalize SAR, we docked **5g** and the corresponding parent compounds **2a** and **4a** into tubulin (Figure 5). The crystal structure of tubulin employed in this investigation was obtained from the protein data bank (PDB ID: 1TUB). Compounds **2a**, **4a** and **5g** were docked between the two subunits of the tubulin heterodimer as shown in Figure 5.

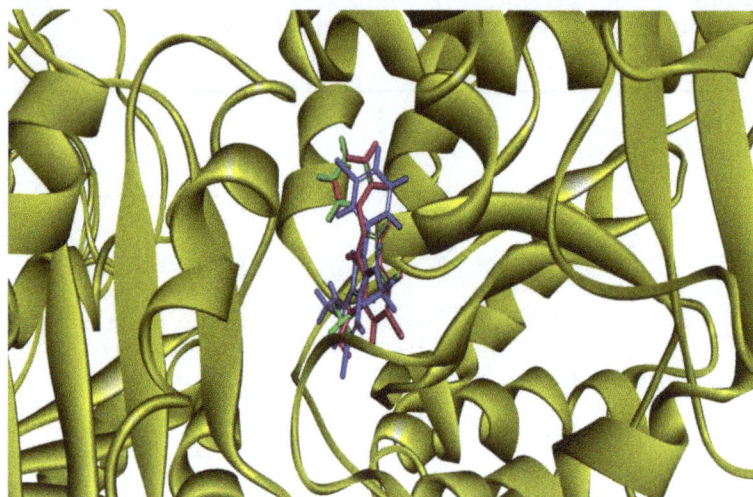

Figure 5. Compounds **2a** (green), **4a** (pink) and **5g** (blue) were docked at the interface of a tubulin heterodimer (PDB code: 1TUB), which is coloured yellow.

Figure 6 reveals the presence of pi-alkyl, amide-pi stacked and alkyl interactions between these aromatic compounds and the active site residues, for example, Ala12, Val177, Val182, Leu248, Ile171 and Tyr224. There is no hydrogen bonding between the acetyl group of **2a** and any of the protein residues. The results of molecular docking and cytotoxicity evaluation against the two cancer cell lines seem to suggest that an acetyl group at the 7-position of the fused benzo ring is less desirable for cytotoxicity. However, the presence of a carbonyl (formyl or acetyl) group was previously found to enhance the antiproliferative properties of the indoles when attached to the C-3 position [9]. Molecular docking of **4a** into the colchicine binding site, on the other hand, revealed a hydrogen bond between the amide functionality and the protein residue Ala12. The propensity of the amide moiety for hydrogen bonding plays a significant role in the interaction of bioactive compounds with the receptors [27] and this may account for the observed slight cytotoxicity of compounds **4b–d** against the two cancer cell lines when compared to **2a–d**. A combination of the hydrophobic and hydrogen bond interactions are responsible for the strong binding of compound **5g** in the colchicine-binding site of tubulin between the two heterodimers [28]. The presence of the trifluoroacetyl group in **5g** resulted in hydrogen bonding between the carbonyl group (2.6 Å) and fluorine atoms (3.5 Å) with amide group of the amino acid residue, Asn20. Additional hydrogen bond interaction is observed between the acetamido group of compound **5g** and the amide group of Asn101 (2.5 Å) with π-π stacking interaction between the protein residue Tyr224 and the 3-chlorophenyl group. These interactions probably help to stabilize the binding of compounds **5a–h** in the colchicine-binding domain of α,β-tubulin interface. A 3-trifluoroacetyl moiety in the 7-acetamido-2-aryl-5-bromoindoles **5e–h** in our view enhances the binding of these compounds to tubulin in the colchicine-binding domain of α,β-tubulin interface Such binding would probably lead to cancer cell death (apoptosis).

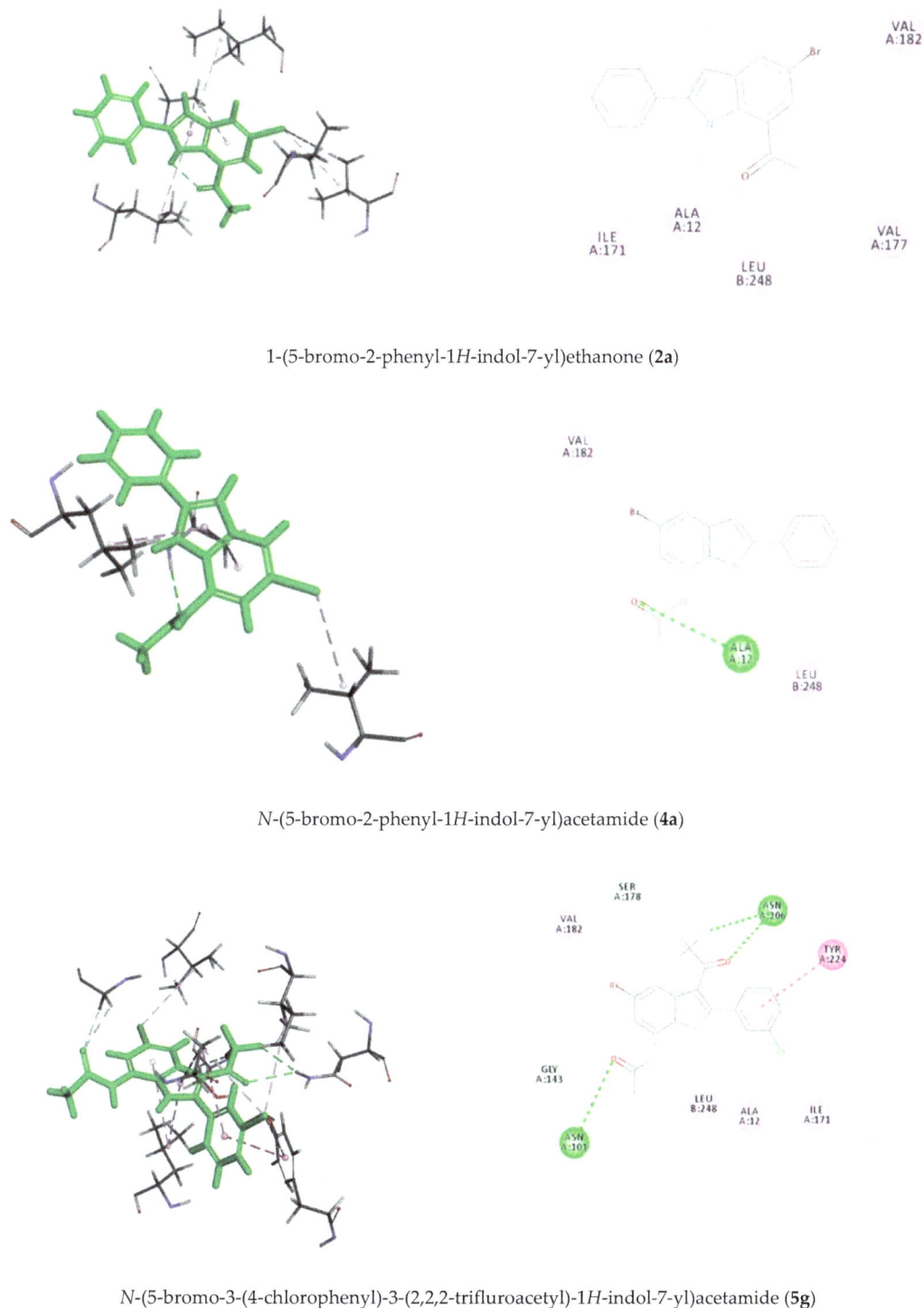

1-(5-bromo-2-phenyl-1*H*-indol-7-yl)ethanone (**2a**)

N-(5-bromo-2-phenyl-1*H*-indol-7-yl)acetamide (**4a**)

N-(5-bromo-3-(4-chlorophenyl)-3-(2,2,2-trifluroacetyl)-1*H*-indol-7-yl)acetamide (**5g**)

Figure 6. 2D interaction diagrams for the binding of tubulin (PDB code 1TUB) with **2a**, **4a** and **5g**. Residues are annotated with their 3-letter amino acid code The various interactions are annotated by color; alkyl/pi-alkyl (pink), carbon hydrogen bond (light green) and conventional hydrogen bond.

3. Materials and Methods

3.1. General

The melting point values of the prepared compounds were recorded on a Thermocouple digital melting point apparatus and are uncorrected. Their IR spectra were recorded as powders on a Bruker VERTEX 70 FT-IR Spectrometer (Bruker Optics, Billerica, MA, USA) with a diamond ATR (attenuated total reflectance) accessory by using the thin-film method. Merck kieselgel 60 (0.063–0.200 mm) (Merck KGaA, Frankfurt, Germany) was used as stationary phase for column chromatography. The ^{1}H-NMR and ^{13}C-NMR spectra were obtained as DMSO-d_6 solutions using Agilent 300 MHz NMR (Agilent Technologies, Oxford, UK) spectrometer and the chemical shifts are quoted relative to the TMS peak. The high-resolution mass spectra were recorded at an ionization potential of 70 eV using Waters Synapt G2 Quadrupole Time-of-flight mass spectrometer (Waters Corp., Milford, MA, USA) at the University of Stellenbosch Central Analytical Facility (CAF). The synthesis and analytical data of compounds **1a–d** have been described before [14].

3.2. Typical Procedure for the PdCl$_2$-Mediated Heteroannulation of **1a–d**

A stirred mixture of **1** (1 equiv.) and PdCl$_2$ (0.2 equiv.) in acetonitrile (15 mL/mmol of **1**) was heated at 80 °C under an argon atmosphere for 3 h. The mixture was evaporated to dryness on a rotary evaporator and the residue was dissolved in chloroform. The organic solvent was washed with brine and then dried over anhydrous MgSO$_4$. The salt was filtered off and the solvent was evaporated under reduced pressure on a rotary evaporator. The residue was purified by column chromatography on a silica gel using 10% EtOAc-hexane as eluent to afford **2** as a solid. Compounds **2a–d** were prepared in this fashion.

1-(5-Bromo-2-phenyl-1H-indol-7-yl)ethanone (**2a**). A mixture of **1a** (1.00 g, 3.18 mmol) and PdCl$_2$ (0.11 g, 0.64 mmol) in acetonitrile (50 mL) afforded **2a** as a solid (0.92 g, 92%), R_f 0.36, mp. 139–142 °C; ν_{max} (ATR) 550, 596, 671, 750, 849, 961, 1043, 1163, 1230, 1251, 1322, 1360, 1448, 1490, 1516, 1595, 1650, 3436 cm^{-1}; ^{1}H-NMR: 2.71 (3H, s, CH$_3$), 6.98 (1H, s, 3-H), 7.38 (1H, t, J = 7.5 Hz, 4′-H), 7.47 (2H, t, J = 7.5 Hz, 3′,5′-H), 7.89 (2H, d, J = 7.5 Hz, 2′,6′-H), 7.94 (1H, d, J = 1.2 Hz, 4-H), 8.05 (1H, d, J = 1.2 Hz, 6-H), 11.14 (1H, s, NH); ^{13}C-NMR: 27.6, 99.5, 111.7, 122.1, 126.4, 127.4, 128.6, 128.9, 129.4, 131.3, 132.6, 134.0, 141.3, 199.2; HRMS (ES): found 314.0191. C$_{16}$H$_{13}$NO^{79}Br$^+$ requires 314.0181. *Anal* calcd for C$_{16}$H$_{12}$NOBr: C, 61.17; H, 3.85; N, 4.46. Found: C, 61.02; H, 3.79; N, 4.52.

1-[5-Bromo-2-(4-fluorophenyl)-1H-indol-7-yl]ethanone (**2b**). A mixture of **1b** (1.00 g, 3.01 mmol) and PdCl$_2$ (0.11 g, 0.60 mmol) in acetonitrile (50 mL) afforded **2b** as a solid (0.84 g, 84%), R_f 0.35, mp. 171–173 °C; ν_{max} (ATR) 549, 749, 786, 835, 925, 1006, 1043, 1162, 1231, 1251, 1321, 1360, 1449, 1491, 1578, 1595, 1650, 3436 cm^{-1}; ^{1}H-NMR: 2.69 (3H, s, CH$_3$), 6.91 (1H, s, 3-H), 7.29 (2H, t, J = 8.7 Hz, 3′,5′-H), 7.91–7.95 (3H, m, 4-H and 2′,6′-H), 8.01 (1H, d, J = 1.2 Hz, 6-H), 11.19 (1H, s, NH); ^{13}C-NMR: 27.6, 99.4, 111.7, 116.2 (d, $^2J_{CF}$ = 21.8 Hz), 122.2, 127.3, 128.0 (d, $^4J_{CF}$ = 3.5 Hz), 128.5, 128.8 (d, $^3J_{CF}$ = 8.0 Hz), 132.5, 134.0, 140.5, 162.2 (d, $^1J_{CF}$ = 243.9 Hz), 199.1; HRMS (ES) found 332.0090. C$_{16}$H$_{12}$NO^{79}FBr$^+$ requires 332.0086. *Anal* calcd for C$_{16}$H$_{11}$NOFBr: C, 57.85; H, 3.34; N, 4.22. Found: C, 57.79; H, 3.30; N, 4.12.

1-[5-Bromo-2-(3-chlorophenyl)-1H-indol-7-yl]ethanone (**2c**). A mixture of **1c** (1.00 g, 2.87 mmol) and PdCl$_2$ (0.10 g, 0.57 mmol) in acetonitrile (50 mL) afforded **2c** as a solid (0.77 g, 77%), R_f 0.34, mp. 140–143 °C; ν_{max} (ATR) 452, 542, 572, 673, 751, 785, 852, 878, 969, 1052, 1082, 1164, 1252, 1323, 1357, 1452, 1590, 1653, 3424 cm^{-1}; ^{1}H-NMR: 2.69 (3H, s, CH$_3$), 7.04 (1H, s, 3-H), 7.38–7.49 (2H, m, 4′,5′-H), 7.82–7.86 (1H, d, J = 8.7 Hz, 6′-H), 7.93 (1H, d, J = 1.2 Hz, 4-H), 8.03–8.04 (2H, m, 2′-H and 6-H), 11.33 (1H, s, NH); ^{13}C-NMR: 27.6, 100.7, 111.8, 122.4, 125.2, 126.2, 127.8, 128.4, 128.7, 131.0, 132.3, 133.4, 134.0, 134.1, 139.8, 198.9; HRMS (ES): found 347.9779. C$_{16}$H$_{12}$NO^{35}Cl^{79}Br$^+$ requires 347.9791. *Anal* calcd for C$_{16}$H$_{11}$NOClBr: C, 55.12; H, 3.18; N, 4.02. Found: C, 55.10; H, 3.33; N, 3.89.

1-[5-Bromo-2-(4-methoxyphenyl)-1H-indol-7-yl]ethanone (**2d**). A mixture of **1d** (1.00 g, 2.91 mmol) and PdCl$_2$ (0.10 g, 0.58 mmol) in acetonitrile (50 mL) afforded **2d** as a solid (0.85 g, 85%), R_f = 0.27, mp. 140–142 °C; ν_{max} (ATR) 550, 589, 749, 825, 925, 1028, 1162, 1181, 1253, 1290, 1321, 1361, 1451, 1497, 1578, 1654, 3433 cm^{-1}; ^{1}H-NMR: 2.69 (3H, s, CH$_3$), 3.80 (3H, s, OCH$_3$), 6.86 (1H, s, 3-H), 7.03 (2H, d, J = 8.7 Hz, 3′,5′-H), 7.84 (2H, d, J 8.7 Hz, 2′,6′-H), 7.90 (1H, d, J = 1.2 Hz, 4-H), 8.01 (1H, d, J = 1.2 Hz, 6-H), 11.06 (1H, s, NH); ^{13}C-NMR: 27.6, 55.7, 98.2, 111.6, 114.8, 121.9, 123.8, 126.8, 127.9, 128.2, 132.8, 133.9, 141.5, 160.0, 199.3; HRMS (ES) found 344.0289. C$_{17}$H$_{15}$NO$_2$^{79}Br$^+$ requires 344.0286. *Anal* calcd for C$_{17}$H$_{14}$NO$_2$Br: C, 59.32; H, 4.10; N, 4.07. Found: C, 59.32; H, 3.87; N, 4.10.

3.3. Typical Procedure for the Synthesis of Oxime Derivatives **3a–d** from **2a–d**

A stirred mixture of **2** (1 equivalent), hydroxylamine hydrochloride (1.5 equivalent) and pyridine (1.5 equivalent) in ethanol (20 mL/mmol of **2**) was heated at 80 °C for 5 h. The mixture was cooled to room temperature, quenched with an ice-cold water and then extracted with chloroform. The combined organic phases were washed with water and dried over anhydrous MgSO$_4$. The salt was filtered off and the solvent was evaporated under reduced pressure on a rotary evaporator. The residue was purified by column chromatography on silica gel using 20% EtOAc-hexane as an eluent to afford the oxime derivative **3** as a solid. Products **3a–d** were prepared in this fashion:

1-(5-Bromo-2-phenyl-1H-indol-7-yl)ethanone oxime (**3a**). A mixture of **2a** (0.30 g, 0.95 mmol), hydroxylamine hydrochloride (0.10 g, 1.43 mmol) and pyridine (0.11 g, 1.43 mmol) in ethanol (20 mL) afforded **3a** as a solid (0.28 g, 90%), R_f = 0.69, mp. 198–200 °C; ν_{max} (ATR) 524, 542, 634, 679, 734, 763, 839, 989, 1093, 1172, 1261, 1298, 1331, 1368, 1448, 3269, 3438 cm^{-1}; ^{1}H-NMR: 2.30 (3H, s, CH$_3$), 6.96 (1H, s, 3-H), 7.37 (1H, t, J = 7.5 Hz, 4′-H), 746–7.52 (3H, m, 6-H and 3′,5′-H), 7.78–7.81 (3H, m, 4-H and 2′,6′-H), 10.94 (1H, s, NH), 11.56 (1H, s, OH); ^{13}C-NMR: 11.2, 99.3, 112.4, 121.7, 123.4, 123.8, 125.5, 128.7, 129.6, 131.3, 131.5, 132.5, 139.2, 154.1; HRMS (ES): found 329.0276. C$_{16}$H$_{14}$N$_2$O^{79}Br$^+$ requires 329.0290.

1-(5-Bromo-2-(4-fluorophenyl)-1H-indol-7-yl)ethanone oxime (**3b**). A mixture of **2b** (0.30 g, 0.90 mmol), hydroxylamine hydrochloride (0.09 g, 1.35 mmol) and pyridine (0.11 g, 1.35 mmol) in ethanol (20 mL) afforded **3b** as a solid (0.27 g, 87%), R_f = 0.64, mp. 213–216 °C; ν_{max} (ATR) 530, 595, 651, 680, 744, 764, 828, 846, 912, 984, 1091, 1159, 1230, 1332, 1366, 1428, 1464, 1501, 3258, 3432 cm^{-1}; ^{1}H-NMR: 2.30 (3H, s, CH$_3$), 6.93 (1H, s, 3-H), 7.34 (2H, t, J = 8.7 Hz, 3′,5′-H), 7.45 (1H, d, J = 1.2 Hz, 6-H), 7.77 (1H, d, J = 1.2 Hz, 4-H), 7.84–7.87 (2H, dd, J = 5.4 and 8.7 Hz, 2′,6′-H), 10.92 (1H, s, NH), 11.56 (1H, s, OH); ^{13}C-NMR: 11.3, 99.3, 112.5, 116.5 (d, $^2J_{CF}$ = 21.8 Hz), 121.8, 123.4, 123.7, 127.7 (d, $^3J_{CF}$ = 9.1 Hz), 128.3 (d, $^4J_{CF}$ = 3.5 Hz), 131.3, 132.5, 138.4, 154.0, 162.4 (d, $^1J_{CF}$ = 243.9 Hz); HRMS (ES): found 347.0179. C$_{16}$H$_{13}$N$_2$OF^{79}Br$^+$ requires 347.0195.

1-(5-Bromo-2-(3-chlorophenyl)-1H-indol-7-yl)ethanone oxime (**3c**). A mixture of **2c** (0.30 g, 0.86 mmol), hydroxylamine hydrochloride (0.09 g, 1.29 mmol) and pyridine (0.10 g, 1.29 mmol) in ethanol (20 mL) afforded **3c** as a solid (0.26 g, 82%), R_f = 0.63, mp. 204–206 °C; ν_{max} (ATR) 454, 532, 631, 673, 742, 784, 847, 876, 947, 985, 1094. 1167, 1268, 1268, 1296, 1334, 1368, 1421, 1463, 3203, 3392 cm^{-1}; ^{1}H-NMR: 2.32 (3H, s, CH$_3$), 7.09 (1H, s, 3-H), 7.44–7.55 (3H, m, 6-H and 4′,5′-H), 7.78–7.81 (2H, m, 4-H and 6′-H), 7.92 (1H, s Hz, 2′-H), 11.02 (1H, s, NH), 11.60 (1H, s, OH); ^{13}C-NMR: 11.5, 100.5, 112.6, 122.1, 123.8, 123.9, 124.2, 125.1, 128.3, 131.1, 131.4, 132.7, 133.4, 134.4, 137.7, 153.8; HRMS (ES): found 362.9893. C$_{16}$H$_{13}$N$_2$O^{35}Cl^{79}Br$^+$ requires 362.9900.

1-(5-Bromo-2-(4-methoxyphenyl)-1H-indol-7-yl)ethanone oxime (**3d**). A mixture of **2d** (0.30 g, 0.87 mmol), hydroxylamine hydrochloride (0.09 g, 1.31 mmol) and pyridine (0.10 g, 1.31 mmol) in ethanol (20 mL) afforded **3d** as a solid (0.25 g, 80%), R_f = 0.45, mp. 202–204 °C; ν_{max} (ATR) 521, 585, 612, 653, 671, 755, 796, 826, 984, 1017, 1172, 1185, 1246, 1323, 1372, 1439, 1460, 1497, 3372, 3518 cm^{-1}; ^{1}H-NMR: 2.30 (3H, s, CH$_3$), 3.80 (3H, s, OCH$_3$), 6.80 (1H, s, 3-H), 7.04 (2H, d, J = 8.7 Hz, 3′,5′-H), 7.42 (1H, d, J = 1.2 Hz, 6-H), 7.70 (3H, m, 4-H and 2′,6′-H), 10.84 (1H, s, NH), 11.57 (1H, s, OH); ^{13}C-NMR: 11.3, 55.7, 98.0,

112.3, 115.0, 121.4, 122.9, 123.4, 124.2, 126.9, 131.6, 132.2, 139.4, 154.2, 159.8; HRMS (ES): found 359.0293. $C_{17}H_{16}N_2O_2{}^{79}Br^+$ requires 359.0395.

3.4. Typical Procedure for the Beckmann Rearrangement of 3a–d

A stirred mixture of **3** (1 equiv.) and TFA (1.2 equiv.) in acetonitrile (10 mL/mmol of **3**) was heated at 80 °C for 2 h. The mixture was cooled to room temperature, quenched with ice-cold water and the product was extracted with chloroform (3 × 20 mL). The combined organic layers were dried over anhydrous MgSO$_4$ and the salt was filtered off. The solvent was evaporated under reduced pressure on a rotary evaporator and the residue was purified by column chromatography on a silica gel using 60% EtOAc-hexane as an eluent to afford **4**. The following compounds were prepared in this fashion:

N-(5-Bromo-2-phenyl-1H-indol-7-yl)acetamide (**4a**). A mixture of **3a** (0.20 g, 0.61 mmol) and TFA (0.08 g, 0.73 mmol) in acetonitrile (15 mL) afforded **4a** as solid (0.16 g, 81%), R_f = 0.56, mp. 243–244 °C; ν_{max} (ATR) 518, 562, 600, 688, 740, 760, 842, 998, 1184, 1273, 1315, 1404, 1425, 1455, 1530, 1623, 1651, 3267, 3319 cm^{-1}; ^{1}H-NMR: 2.19 (3H, s, CH$_3$), 6.88 (1H, s, 3-H), 7.38 (1H, t, J = 7.5 Hz, 4′-H), 7.46–7.52 (3H, m, 4-H and 3′,5′-H), 7.82 (2H, d, J = 7.5 Hz, 2′,6′-H), 7.88 (1H, d, J = 1.2 Hz, 6-H), 9.76 (1H, s, NH), 11.28 (1H, s, NH); ^{13}C-NMR: 24.5, 99.5, 112.1, 115.5, 118.2, 125.5, 125.7, 127.3, 128.5, 129.5, 131.6, 131.9, 139.0, 169.1; HRMS (ES): found 329.0265. $C_{16}H_{14}N_2O^{79}Br^+$ requires 329.0289. *Anal* calcd for $C_{16}H_{13}N_2OBr$: C, 58.38; H, 3.98; N, 8.51. Found: C, 58.24; H, 3.93; N, 8.47.

N-[5-Bromo-2-(4-fluorophenyl)-1H-indol-7-yl]acetamide (**4b**). A mixture of **3b** (0.20 g, 0.58 mmol) and TFA (0.08 g, 0.69 mmol) in acetonitrile (15 mL) afforded **4b** as solid (0.14 g, 76%); R_f = 0.53, mp. 263–265 °C; ν_{max} (ATR) 519, 576, 695, 744, 780, 837, 1000, 1163, 1231, 1274, 1318, 1438, 1474, 1502, 1542, 1624, 1654, 3267, 3355 cm^{-1}; ^{1}H-NMR: 2.17 (3H, s, CH$_3$), 6.84 (1H, s, 3-H), 7.34 (2H, t, J = 8.7 Hz, 3′,5′-H), 7.44 (1H, d, J = 1.2 Hz, 4-H), 7.82–7.86 (3H, m, 6-H and 2′,6′-H), 9.71 (1H, s, NH), 11.23 (1H, s, NH); ^{13}C-NMR: 24.5, 99.4, 112.2, 115.7, 116.5 (d, $^2J_{CF}$ = 21.8 Hz), 118.3, 125.4, 127.5, 127.8 (d, $^3J_{CF}$ = 8.0 Hz), 128.6 (d, $^4J_{CF}$ = 3.4 Hz), 131.5, 138.1, 162.3 (d, $^1J_{CF}$ = 243.9 Hz), 169.1; HRMS (ES): found 347.0168. $C_{16}H_{13}N_2OF^{79}Br^+$ requires 347.0195. *Anal* calcd for $C_{16}H_{12}N_2OFBr$: C, 55.35; H, 3.48; N, 8.07. Found: C, 55.22; H, 3.39; N, 7.89.

N-(5-Bromo-2-(3-chlorophenyl)-1H-indol-7-yl)acetamide (**4c**). A mixture of **3c** (0.30 g, 0.55 mmol) and TFA (0.08 g, 0.66 mmol) in acetonitrile (15 mL) afforded **4c** as solid (0.15 g, 73%), R_f = 0.54, mp. 261–263 °C; ν_{max} (ATR) 562, 598, 668, 680, 751, 775, 846, 1010, 1095, 1277, 1317, 1445, 1462, 1538, 1573, 1622, 1650, 3268, 3397 cm^{-1}; ^{1}H-NMR: 2.18 (3H, s, CH$_3$), 6.97 (1H, s, 3-H), 7.38–7.53 (3H, m, 4-H and 4′,5′-H), 7.77 (1H, d. J = 8.7 Hz, 6′-H), 7.87–7.90 (2H, m, 6-H and 2′-H), 9.70 (1H, s, NH), 11.28 (1H, s, NH); ^{13}C-NMR: 24.6, 100.6, 112.3, 116.2, 118.5, 124.4, 125.0, 125.5, 127.8, 128.1, 131.3, 131.4, 134.0, 134.4, 137.3, 169.1; HRMS (ES): found 362.9890. $C_{16}H_{13}N_2O^{35}Cl^{79}Br^+$ requires 362.9900. *Anal* calcd for $C_{16}H_{12}N_2OClBr$: C, 52.85; H, 3.33; N, 7.70. Found: C, 52.78; H, 3.41; N, 7.59.

N-[5-Bromo-2-(4-methoxyphenyl)-1H-indol-7-yl]acetamide (**4d**). A mixture of **3d** (0.30 g, 0.56 mmol) and TFA (0.08 g, 0.67 mmol) in acetonitrile (15 mL) afforded **4d** as solid (0.16 g, 76%), R_f = 0.36, mp. 226–228 °C; ν_{max} (ATR) 559, 584, 694 786, 834, 1021, 1179, 1244, 1320, 1398, 1439, 1500, 1612, 1658, 3300, 3403 cm^{-1}; ^{1}H-NMR: 2.18 (3H, s, CH$_3$), 3.80 (3H, s, OCH$_3$), 6.74 (1H, s, 3-H), 7.06 (2H, d, J = 8.7 Hz, 3′,5′-H), 7.41 (1H, d, J = 1.2 Hz, 4-H), 7.74 (2H, d, J = 8.7 Hz, 2′,6′-H), 7.83 (1H, d, J = 1.2 Hz, 6-H), 9.71 (1H, s, NH), 11.14 (1H, s, NH); ^{13}C-NMR: 24.6, 55.7, 98.2, 112.0, 114.9 (2C), 115.1, 117.9, 124.5, 125.2, 127.1, 131.8, 139.1, 159.7, 169.1; HRMS (ES): found 359.0393. $C_{17}H_{16}N_2O_2{}^{79}Br^+$ requires 359.0395. *Anal* calcd for $C_{17}H_{15}N_2O_2Br$: C, 56.84; H, 4.21; N, 7.80. Found: C, 56.79; H, 4.13; N, 7.56.

3.5. Typical Procedure for the Trifluoroacetylation of 2a–d and 4a–d

A mixture of **2/4** (1 equivalent) and TFAA (1.5 equivalent) in THF (15 mL/mmol of **1/4**) was heated at 60 °C for 5 h. The mixture was cooled to room temperature and quenched with saturated sodium hydrogen carbonate solution. The mixture was extracted with chloroform (3 × 20 mL) and the combined organic layers were dried with anhydrous $MgSO_4$. The salt was filtered off and the solvent was evaporated under reduced pressure on a rotary evaporator. The residue was purified by column chromatography on a silica gel using 20% or 60% EtOAc-hexane as eluent to afford **5a**–**d** or **5e**–**h** as solids, respectively. Compounds **5a**–**h** were prepared in this fashion.

1-(7-Acetyl-5-bromo-2-phenyl-1H-indol-3-yl)-2,2,2-trifluoroethanone (**4a**). A mixture of **2a** (0.30 g, 0.95 mmol) and TFAA (0.30 g, 1.43 mmol) in THF (15 mL) afforded **5a** as solid (0.30 g, 78%); R_f 0.86, mp. 175–176 °C; ν_{max} (ATR) 515, 647, 671, 697, 746, 767, 861, 911, 994, 1083, 1143, 1203, 1275, 1358, 1433, 1450, 1660, 3401 cm^{-1}; ^{1}H-NMR: 2.70 (3H, s, CH$_3$), 7.47–7.55 (5H, m, Ph), 8.14 (1H, d, J = 1.2 Hz, 4-H), 8.42 (1H, d, J = 1.2 Hz, 6-H), 12.52 (1H, s, NH); ^{13}C-NMR: 27.8, 107.3, 115.6, 116.2 (q, $^1J_{CF}$ 288.5 Hz), 123.7, 128.1, 128.3, 129.3, 130.4, 130.5 (2C), 130.7, 132.3, 151.6, 176.6 (q, $^2J_{CF}$ 35.6 Hz), 198.3; HRMS (ES): found 410.0015. C$_{18}$H$_{12}$NO$_2$F$_3$^{79}Br$^+$ requires 410.0003. *Anal* calcd for C$_{18}$H$_{11}$NO$_2$F$_3$Br: C, 52.71; H, 2.70; N, 3.41. Found: C, 52.62; H, 2.35; N, 3.39.

1-[7-Acetyl-5-bromo-2-(4-fluorophenyl)-1H-indol-3-yl]-2,2,2-trifluoroethanone (**5b**). A mixture of **2b** (0.30 g, 0.90 mmol) and TFAA (0.28 g, 1.35 mmol) in THF (15 mL) afforded **5b** as solid (0.26 g, 69%); R_f 0.86, mp. 168–171 °C; ν_{max} (ATR) 518, 587, 645, 667, 706, 746, 842, 911, 999, 1082, 1142, 1205, 1244, 1274, 1435, 1489, 1606, 1662, 3401 cm^{-1}; ^{1}H-NMR: 2.70 (3H, s, CH$_3$), 7.33 (2H, t, J 8.5 Hz, 3',5'-H), 7.62 (2H, t, J = 6.9 Hz, 2',6'-H), 8.14 (1H, d, J = 1.2 Hz, 4-H), 8.42 (1H, d, J = 1.2 Hz, 6-H), 12.61 (1H, s, NH); ^{13}C-NMR: 27.8, 107.4, 115.1 (d, $^2J_{CF}$ = 21.8 Hz), 115.7, 116.3 (q, $^1J_{CF}$ = 288.6 Hz), 123.6, 127.1 (d, $^4J_{CF}$ = 3.5 Hz), 128.4, 129.4, 130.3, 132.2, 133.2 (d, $^3J_{CF}$ = 8.0 Hz), 150.7, 163.6 (d, $^1J_{CF}$ = 246.2 Hz), 176.3 (q, $^2J_{CF}$ = 35.5 Hz), 198.3; HRMS (ES): found 427.9721. C$_{18}$H$_{11}$NO$_2$F$_4$^{79}Br$^+$ requires 427.9909. *Anal* calcd for C$_{18}$H$_{10}$NO$_2$F$_4$Br: C, 50.49; H, 2.35; N, 3.27. Found: C, 50.44; H, 2.31; N, 3.30.

1-[7-Acetyl-5-bromo-2-(3-chlorophenyl)-1H-indol-3-yl]-2,2,2-trifluoroethanone (**5c**). A mixture of **2c** (0.30 g, 0.86 mmol) and TFAA (0.27 g, 1.29 mmol) in THF (15 mL) afforded **5c** as solid (0.21 g, 56%); R_f 0.86, mp. 138–141 °C; ν_{max} (ATR) 581, 661, 702, 728, 769, 795, 870, 903, 913, 946, 997, 1074, 1147, 1209, 1281, 1316, 1433, 1462, 1651, 3257 cm^{-1}; ^{1}H-NMR: 2.70 (3H, s, CH$_3$), 7.51–7.52 (2H, m, 4',5'-H), 7.60–7.62 (1H, m, 6'-H), 7.67 (1H, s, 2'-H), 8.15 (1H, d, J = 1.2 Hz, 4-H), 8.42 (1H, d, J = 1.2 Hz, 6-H), 12.72 (1H, s, NH); ^{13}C-NMR: 27.9, 107.5, 115.7, 116.3 (q, $^1J_{CF}$ 288.6 Hz), 123.7, 128.4, 129.6, 129.7, 129.9, 130.1, 130.2, 130.5, 132.2, 132.6, 132.7, 149.9, 176.2 (q, $^2J_{CF}$ 35.5 Hz), 198.3; HRMS (ES): found 443.9623. C$_{18}$H$_{11}$NO$_2$F$_3$^{35}Cl^{79}Br$^+$ requires 443.9614. *Anal* calcd for C$_{18}$H$_{10}$NO$_2$F$_3$ClBr: C, 48.62; H, 2.27; N, 3.15. Found: C, 48.47; H, 2.26; N, 2.98.

1-[7-Acetyl-5-bromo-2-(4-methoxyphenyl)-1H-indol-3-yl]-2,2,2-trifluoroethanone (**5d**). A mixture of **2d** (0.30 g, 0.87 mmol) and TFAA (0.27 g, 1.31 mmol) in THF (15 mL) afforded **5d** as solid (0.29 g, 75%); R_f 0.70, mp. 170–173 °C; ν_{max} (ATR) 615, 642, 660, 746, 836, 910, 1028, 1082, 1140, 1173, 1202, 1262, 1437, 1489, 1607, 1657, 3392 cm^{-1}; ^{1}H-NMR: 2.70 (3H, s, CH$_3$), 3.83 (3H, s, OCH$_3$), 7.05 (2H, d, J = 8.7 Hz, 3',5'-H), 7.52 (2H, d, J = 8.7 Hz, 2',6'-H), 8.11 (1H, d, J = 1.2 Hz, 4-H), 8.38 (1H, d, J = 1.2 Hz, 6-H), 12.32 (1H, s, NH); ^{13}C-NMR: 27.9, 107.0, 113.7, 115.5, 116.3 (q, $^1J_{CF}$ = 289.7 Hz), 122.8, 123.0, 123.5, 128.2, 129.2, 130.5, 132.2, 132.4, 151.8, 161.2, 176.7 (q, $^2J_{CF}$ = 35.6 Hz), 198.5; HRMS (ES): found 440.0110. C$_{19}$H$_{14}$NO$_3$F$_3$^{79}Br$^+$ requires 440.0109. *Anal* calcd for C$_{19}$H$_{13}$NO$_3$F$_3$Br: C, 51.84; H, 2.98; N, 3.18. Found: C, 51.78; H, 2.93; N, 3.14.

N-[5-Bromo-2-phenyl-3-trifluoroacetyl-1H-indol-7-yl]acetamide (**5e**). A mixture of **4a** (0.30 g, 0.91 mmol) and TFAA (0.29 g, 1.37 mmol) in THF (15 mL) afforded **5e** as solid (0.32 g, 84%); R_f 0.49, mp. 141–144 °C; ν_{max} (ATR) 502, 582, 659, 699, 738, 773, 863, 882, 922, 1010, 1143, 1199, 1269, 1334, 1389, 1434, 1449, 1546, 1627, 1655, 3210, 3329 cm^{-1}; ^{1}H-NMR: 2.11 (3H, s, CH$_3$), 7.53–7.63 (5H, m, Ar), 7.94 (1H, d, J = 1.2 Hz, 4-H), 7.96 (1H, d, J = 1.2 Hz, 6-H), 9.74 (1H, s, NH), 12.53 (1H, s, NH); ^{13}C-NMR: 24.3, 107.2, 116.2, 116.6 (q, $^1J_{CF}$ = 295.5 Hz), 118.8, 126.2, 126.3, 126.8, 128.6, 129.5, 130.3, 130.6, 131.3, 149.2, 169.3, 175.9 (q, $^2J_{CF}$ = 35.6 Hz); HRMS (ES): found 425.0107. C$_{18}$H$_{13}$N$_2$O$_2$F$_3$^{79}Br$^+$ requires 425.0112. *Anal* calcd for C$_{18}$H$_{12}$N$_2$O$_2$F$_3$Br: C, 50.85; H, 2.84; N, 6.99. Found: C, 50.52; H, 2.87; N, 6.94.

N-[5-Bromo-2-(4-fluorophenyl)-3-trifluoroacetyl-1H-indol-7-yl]acetamide (**5f**). A mixture of **4b** (0.30 g, 0.86 mmol) and TFAA (0.27 g, 1.30 mmol) in THF (15 mL) afforded **5f** as solid (0.29 g, 78%); R_f 0.50, mp. 195–197 °C; ν_{max} (ATR) 515, 611, 732, 844, 884, 924, 1011, 1044, 1146, 1198, 1224, 1271, 1330, 1447, 1497, 1631, 1659, 3196, 3286 cm^{-1}; ^{1}H-NMR: 2.12 (3H, s, CH$_3$), 7.41 (2H, t, J = 9.0 Hz, 3',5'-H), 7.69 (2H, d, J = 8.7 Hz, 2',6'-H), 7.93 (1H, d, J = 1.2 Hz, 4-H), 7.94 (1H, d, J = 1.2 Hz, 6-H), 9.77 (1H, s, NH), 12.54 (1H, s, NH); ^{13}C-NMR: 24.2, 107.4, 115.7 (d, $^2J_{CF}$ 21.8 Hz), 116.1, 116.5 (q, $^1J_{CF}$ 288.6 Hz), 118.7, 118.8, 126.2, 126.9, 127.6 (d, $^4J_{CF}$ = 3.5 Hz), 129.4, 133.8 (d, $^3J_{CF}$ = 9.1 Hz), 148.2, 163.6 (d, $^1J_{CF}$ = 246.2 Hz), 169.3, 176.6 (q, $^2J_{CF}$ = 35.5 Hz); HRMS (ES): found 443.0020. C$_{18}$H$_{13}$N$_2$O$_2$F$_4$^{79}Br$^+$ requires 443.0020. *Anal* calcd for C$_{18}$H$_{12}$N$_2$O$_2$F$_4$Br: C, 48.78; H, 2.50; N, 6.32. Found: C, 48.59; H, 2.39; N, 6.30.

N-[5-Bromo-2-(3-chlorophenyl)-3-trifluoroacetyl-1H-indol-7-yl]acetamide (**5g**). A mixture of **4c** (0.30 g, 0.83 mmol) and TFAA (0.26 g, 1.23 mmol) in THF (15 mL) afforded **5g** as solid (0.19 g, 52%); R_f 0.50, mp. 172–174 °C; ν_{max} (ATR) 541, 570, 685, 746, 794, 851, 913, 1010, 1039, 1083, 1143, 1198, 1260, 1369, 1441, 1542, 1630, 1660, 3217, 3356 cm^{-1}; ^{1}H-NMR: 2.12 (3H, s, CH$_3$), 7.60–7.66 (3H, m, Ar), 7.75 (1H, s, 2'-H), 8.28 (1H, d, J = 1.2 Hz, 4-H), 8.29 (1H, d, J = 1.2 Hz, 6-H), 9.77 (1H, s, NH), 12.61 (1H, s, NH); ^{13}C-NMR: 24.3, 107.4, 116.2, 116.5 (q, $^1J_{CF}$ = 289.7 Hz), 118.9, 126.3, 127.2, 129.3, 129.9, 130.5, 133.2, 133.4, 147.3, 169.3, 175.6 (q, $^2J_{CF}$ = 34.4 Hz); HRMS (ES): found 458.9731. C$_{18}$H$_{12}$F$_3$N$_2$O$_2$^{35}Cl^{79}Br$^+$ requires 458.9723. *Anal* calcd for C$_{18}$H$_{11}$F$_3$N$_2$O$_2$ClBr: C, 47.03; H, 2.41; N, 6.09. Found: C, 47.10; H, 2.36; N, 6.05.

N-[5-Bromo-2-(4-methoxyphenyl)-3-trifluoroacetyl-1H-indol-7-yl]acetamide (**5h**). A mixture of **4d** (0.30 g, 0.83 mmol) and TFAA (0.26 g, 1.25 mmol) in THF (15 mL) afforded **5h** as solid (0.30 g, 80%); R_f 0.23, mp. 179–182 °C; ν_{max} (ATR) 520, 573, 643, 751, 838, 884, 922, 1009, 1031, 1154, 1191, 1250, 1415, 1448, 1499, 1538, 1629, 1645, 3211, 3369 cm^{-1}; ^{1}H-NMR: 2.08 (3H, s, CH$_3$), 3.80 (3H, s, OCH$_3$), 7.07 (2H, d, J = 8.7 Hz, 3',5'-H), 7.52 (2H, d, J = 8.7 Hz, 2',6'-H), 7.86 (1H, d, J = 1.2 Hz, 4-H), 9.91 (1H, d, J = 1.2 Hz, 6-H), 9.74 (1H, s, NH), 12.39 (1H, s, NH); ^{13}C-NMR: 24.2, 55.8, 107.0, 114.1, 116.0, 116.6 (q, $^1J_{CF}$ = 289.7 Hz), 118.4, 118.6, 123.2, 126.3, 126.8, 129.6, 131.9, 149.5, 161.2, 169.2, 176.9 (q, $^2J_{CF}$ = 35.5 Hz); HRMS (ES): found 455.0195. C$_{19}$H$_{15}$N$_2$O$_3$F$_3$^{79}Br$^+$ requires 455.0219. *Anal* calcd for C$_{19}$H$_{14}$N$_2$O$_3$F$_3$Br: C, 50.13; H, 3.10; N, 6.15. Found: C, 49.95; H, 3.20; N, 6.00.

3.6. Evaluation for Cytotoxicity

3.6.1. Screening Protocol

The human cervical cancer cell line, HeLa, and lung cancer cell line, A549 were used for the screening assay. HeLa cells were grown and maintained in RPMI 1640 medium supplemented with 10% fetal bovine serum (FBS) and A549 cells were grown and maintained in EMEM supplemented with 10% FBS and 10% non-essential amino acids. In the case of screening experiments, the cells were seeded into 96 well microtiter plates at a density of 6000 cells/well to a total volume of 200 μL per well. The microtiter plates were incubated at 37 °C, 5% CO$_2$, and 100% relative humidity for 24 h to allow for cell attachment. Each of the test compounds was first reconstituted in DMSO at a concentration of 40 mM and then stored at 4 °C prior to use and final dilution to working concentrations with culture complete medium on the day of treatment. Two hundred microliters aliquots of the diluted compound in fresh medium was used to treat cells after aspiration of seeding medium. Each of the cell lines was incubated for 48 h at 37 °C in a humidified incubator under 5% CO$_2$ atmosphere. Treatment medium was aspirated from all wells and replaced with 100 μL of Hoechst 33342 nuclear dye (5 μg/mL) and incubated for 10 min at room temperature. Thereafter, cells were stained with propidium iodide (PI) at 100 μg/mL in order to enumerate the proportion of dead cells within the population. Cells were imaged immediately after addition of PI using the ImageXpress Micro XLS Widefield Microscope (Separations, Randburg, South Africa).

3.6.2. Dose Response Analysis and Determination of IC_{50} Values

Cells were seeded as described in above. The compounds were tested at a concentration range of 0–100 μM to determine their respective IC_{50} values on lung cancer (A549) cells and cervical cancer (HeLa) cells. The medium was aspirated and replaced with 200 μL fresh medium containing the dilution of the respective test compound. The test sample were added to each well and the plates were incubated for a further 48 h at 37 °C under 5% CO_2 atmosphere in a humidified incubator. After this incubation period, the medium was removed and then replaced with 100 μL fresh culture medium containing MTT at a final concentration of 0.5 mg/mL. The 96-well plates were returned to the incubator and incubated for an additional 3 h. The medium was removed and the MTT crystals were solubilized in 100 μL DMSO and the absorbance was measured at 560 nm using a Labsystems Multiwell Scanning spectrophotometer (Thermo Fischer Scientific, Edenvale, South Africa).

3.6.3. Data Analysis

Quantification of live and dead cells for the screening assay was performed using the ImageXpress Micro XLS Widefield Microscope and acquired images analysed using the MetaXpress software and Multi-Wavelength Cell Scoring Application Module. Acquired data was transferred to an EXCEL spreadsheet and relative cell viability was determined using quadruplicate wells for each concentration. Untreated cells were considered to have 100% cell viability (i.e., the mean OD of the untreated wells = 100% viability). Cell viabilities in other test wells were calculated relative to the untreated control and expressed as a percentage. Dose response analysis was performed using the statistical software GraphPad Prism and IC_{50} values calculated from the concentration-response data using a mathematical Hill function. If the concentration range selected did not produce 100% inhibition, a lower concentration equal to zero was included to allow IC_{50} determination.

3.7. Evaluation of Mode of Cell Death

3.7.1. Caspace Activation

Compounds **4c** and **5g** were selected for mechanism studies and these test compounds were reconstituted in dimethyl sulphoxide (DMSO) to give a final concentration of 40 mM. Samples were stored at 4 °C until required. Cells were seeded and treated as described in 3.6.1 Cells were first fixed and permeabilized using the IntraPrep kit as per manufacturer's instructions (Beckman Coulter). This kit allows for the immunological detection of intracellular antigens by creating apertures in the cell membrane without affecting the morphology of the cell. Cleaved caspase-8 (Asp 391) and cleaved caspase-3 (Asp 175) monoclonal antibodies (Cell Signaling Technology, Danvers, MA, USA) were used to determine the presence of activated caspase-8 and caspase-3, respectively. Cells were first blocked using PBS containing 0.5% BSA and thereafter incubated with the antibodies separately (1:200 for caspase-8 and 1:100 for caspase-3) for 1 h at 37 °C. The cells were washed and incubated with the Alexa 647 conjugated secondary antibody (1:1000) for 30 min at 37 °C in the dark. Both cell lines were incubated at 37 °C in a humidified 5% CO_2 and then treated with the IC_{50} values of each compound for 24 h. 200 μL Aliquots of the diluted compound in fresh medium was used to treat cells after aspiration of seeding medium. Treatment medium was aspirated from all wells and replaced with 100 μL of Hoechst 33342 nuclear dye (5 μg/mL) and incubated for 10 min at RT.

3.7.2. Data Quantification

Quantification of live and dead cells for the assay was performed using the ImageXpress Micro XLS Widefield Microscope and acquired images analysed using the MetaXpress software and Multi-Wavelength Cell Scoring Application Module and the Cell Cycle Module. Acquired data was transferred to an EXCEL spreadsheet and data was analysed and processed.

3.8. Tubulin Polymerization Assay

Tubulin polymerization assays were conducted using the tubulin polymerization assay kit following the manufacturer's instructions (Cytoskeleton, Inc., Denver, CA, USA). Briefly, 50 μL of 1.3 mg/mL tubulin (>99% pure) proteins in G-PEM buffer (consisting of 80 mmol/L PIPES 2 mmol/L MgCl$_2$, 0.5 mmol/L EGTA, 1 mmol/L GTP, and 15% glycerol at pH 6.9,) was placed in a quartz cuvette in the presence of the test agent (concentration: 0.25 μM). Polymerization was measured at every 3 s for 1 h using an Applied Photophysics Chirascan spectroflourimeter (excitation at 360 nm and emission at 420 nm) at 37 °C.

3.9. Methodology for Docking Studies

Docking of the compounds **2a**, **4a** and **5e–h** was performed to the crystal structure of a tubulin heterodimer (PDB code:1TUB) [29]. using the CDOCKER protocol [30] in Discovery Studio 2017. Prior to performing the docking, compounds were drawn using Discovery Studio and prepared using the 'Prepare Ligand' protocol. The protein structure was obtained from the Protein Data Bank, prepared using the 'Prepare Protein' protocol in Discovery Studio which included: removing any existing ligands bound to the model and binding sites defined from receptor cavities as well as all water molecules, protonate the protein at pH 7.5, The receptor cavity in this tubulin structure is present between the two monomers of the tubulin dimer structure. Docking was performed using CHARMm force field and the best conformation of the ligand selected and evaluated.

4. Conclusions

The observed increased cytotoxicity of compounds **5e–h** against the A549 and HeLa cell lines and their strong inhibitory effect against tubulin polymerization suggest that a combination of the strong hydrogen bonding 7-acetamido and the 3-trifluoroacetyl groups on the 2-aryl-5-bromoindole framework is desirable for biological activity. An acetamido group elicited some cytotoxicity in derivatives **4b–d** against both cell lines, which increased significantly upon incorporation of a trifluoroacetyl group in **5e–h**. This observation suggests the importance of a nitrogen-based substituent on the fused benzo ring of indole derivatives in analogy with the literature precedence on the increased cytotoxicity of analogues indoles against the HeLa and A549 cell lines as well as HIV-1 inhibition activity [6]. The lack of cytotoxicity for the C-3 unsubstituted 2-arylindoles **2a-d** or their 3-trifluoroacetyl derivatives **5a–d** in our view suggest that an acetyl group attached to the fused benzo ring of a 2-arylindole framework is not desirable for the cytotoxicity of polysubstituted indole derivatives. The immunochemical experiments, on the other hand, revealed that the 3-trifluoroacetyl derivatives **5e–h** may induce apoptosis in a caspase-dependent manner for both cell lines. Experimental and molecular docking of **5e–h** into the colchicine-binding site of tubulin suggest that these compounds have potential to inhibit tubulin polymerization to elicit anticancer activity. These results pave the way for the development of the 3-trifluoroacetyl substituted indole derivatives as anticancer agents.

Author Contributions: M.J.M. coordinated the study, reviewed the literature, interpreted the data and results, and written the manuscript. N.P. assayed the compounds for inhibitory effects against tubulin polymerization and performed molecular docking studies.

Acknowledgments: We are grateful to the following institutions: University of South Africa and the National Research Foundation for financial assistance and the University of Stellenbosch Central Analytical Facility (CAF) for mass spectrometric and elemental analyses. We acknowledge M.M. Mmonwa and M.M. Maluleka for technical assistance. The cytotoxicity assays were performed by M. Van De Venter and L. Venables of the Nelson Mandela Metropolitan University (Summerstrand Campus South).

References

1. Lu, Y.; Chen, J.; Xiao, M.; Li, W.; Miller, D.D. An overview of tubulin inhibitors that interact with the colchicine binding site. *Pharm. Res.* **2012**, *29*, 2943–2971. [CrossRef] [PubMed]

2. Jordan, M.A. Anti-cancer agents. *Curr. Med. Chem.* **2002**, *2*, 1–17.

3. Gastpar, R.; Goldbrunner, M.; Marko, D.; Von Angerer, E. Methoxy-substituted 3-formyl-2-phenylindoles inhibit tubulin polymerization. *J. Med. Chem.* **1998**, *41*, 4965–4972. [CrossRef] [PubMed]

4. Dong, M.; Liu, F.; Zhou, H.; Zhai, S.; Yan, B. Novel natural product- and privileged scaffold-based tubulin inhibitors targeting the colchicine binding site. *Molecules* **2016**, *21*, 1375. [CrossRef] [PubMed]

5. Kaur, R.; Kaur, G.; Gill, R.K.; Soni, R.; Bariwal, J. Recent developments in tubulin polymerization inhibitors: An overview. *Eur. J. Med. Chem.* **2014**, *87*, 89–124. [CrossRef] [PubMed]

6. Hu, H.; Wu, J.; Ao, M.; Wang, H.; Zhou, T.; Xue, Y.; Qiu, Y.; Fang, M.; Wu, Z. Synthesis, structure–activity relationship studies and biological evaluation of novel 2,5-disubstituted indole derivatives as anticancer agents. *Chem. Biol. Drugs Des.* **2016**, *88*, 766–778. [CrossRef] [PubMed]

7. Cooper, L.C.; Chicchi, G.G.; Dinnell, K.; Elliott, J.M.; Hollingworth, G.J.; Kurtz, M.M.; Locker, K.L.; Morrison, D.; Shaw, D.E.; Tsao, K.-L.; et al. 2-Aryl indole NK1 receptor antagonists: Optimisation of indole substitution. *Bioorg. Med. Chem. Lett.* **2001**, *11*, 1233–1236. [CrossRef]

8. Sisa, M.; Pla, D.; Altuna, M.; Francesch, A.; Cuevas, C.; Albericio, F.; Alvarez, M. Total synthesis and antiproliferative activity screening of (±)-Aplicyanins A, B and E and related analogues. *J. Med. Chem.* **2009**, *52*, 6217–6223. [CrossRef] [PubMed]

9. Watterson, S.H.; Dhar, T.G.M.; Ballentine, S.K.; Shen, Z.; Barrish, J.C.; Cheney, D.; Fleener, C.A.; Roleau, K.A.; Townsend, R.; Hollenbaugh, D.L.; et al. Novel indole-based inhibitors of IMPDH: Introduction of hydrogen bond acceptors at indole C-3. *Bioorg. Med. Chem. Lett.* **2003**, *13*, 1273–1276. [CrossRef]

10. Thomas, J.B.; Giddings, A.M.; Wiethe, R.W.; Olepu, S.; Warner, K.R.; Sarret, P.; Gendron, L.; Longpre, J.-M.; Zhang, Y.; Runyon, S.P.; et al. Identification of *N*-[(5-{[(4-methylphenyl)sulfonyl]amino}-3-(trifluoroacetyl)-1*H*-indol-1-yl)acetyl]-L-leucine (NTRC-824), a neurotensin-like nonpeptide compound selective for the neurotensin receptor type 2. *J. Med. Chem.* **2014**, *57*, 7472–7477. [CrossRef] [PubMed]

11. Usachev, B.I. 1-/2-/3-Fluoroalkyl-substituted indoles, promising medicinally and biologically beneficial compounds: Synthetic routes, significance and potential applications. *J. Fluor. Chem.* **2016**, *185*, 118–167. [CrossRef]

12. Cade, H.C.; Blocker, M.; Shaik, A. Synthesis of indole-derived fluorine-containing amino acids. *J. Nat. Sci.* **2015**, *1*, e169.

13. Lo'pez, S.E.; Salazar, J. Trifluoroacetic acid: Uses and recent applications in organic synthesis. *J. Fluor. Chem.* **2013**, *156*, 73–100. [CrossRef]

14. Mphahlele, M.J.; Mmonwa, M.M.; Makhafola, T.J. In vitro cytotoxicity of novel 2,5,7-tricarbo-substituted indoles derived from 2-amino-5-bromo-3-iodoacetophenone. *Bioorg. Med. Chem.* **2016**, *24*, 4576–4586. [CrossRef] [PubMed]

15. Choi, H.-S.; Cho, M.-C.; Lere, H.G.; Yoon, D.-Y. Indole-3-carbinol induces apoptosis through p53 and activation of caspase-8 pathway in lung cancer A549 cells. *Food Chem. Toxicol.* **2010**, *48*, 883–890. [CrossRef] [PubMed]

16. Mphahlele, M.J.; Maluleka, M.M. Trifluoroacetylation of indole-chalcones derived from the 2-amino-3-(arylethynyl)-5-bromo-iodochalcones. *J. Fluor. Chem.* **2016**, *189*, 88–95. [CrossRef]

17. Mphahlele, M.J.; Mmonwa, M.M.; Choong, Y.S. Synthesis and evaluation of *N*-(3-trifluoroacetyl-indol-7-yl)acetamides for potential in vitro antiplasmodial properties. *Molecules* **2017**, *22*, 1099. [CrossRef] [PubMed]

18. Yao, S.-J.; Ren, Z.-H.; Wang, Y.-Y.; Guan, Z.-H. Friedel–Crafts fluoroacetylation of indoles with fluorinated acetic acids for the synthesis of fluoromethyl indol-3-yl ketones under catalyst- and additive-free conditions. *J. Org. Chem.* **2016**, *81*, 4226–4234. [CrossRef] [PubMed]

19. Owa, T.; Yokoi, A.; Yamazaki, K.; Yoshimatsu, K.; Yamori, T.; Nagasu, T. Array-based structure and gene expression relationship study of antitumor sulfonamides including *N*-[2-[(4-hydroxyphenyl)amino]-3-pyridinyl]-4-methoxybenzenesulfonamide and *N*-(3-chloro-7-indolyl)-1,4-benzenedisulfonamide. *J. Med. Chem.* **2002**, *45*, 4913–4922. [CrossRef] [PubMed]

20. Kroemer, G.; Galluzzi, L.; Vandenabeele, P.; Abrams, J.; Alnemri, E.S.; Baehrecke, E.H.; Blagosklonny, M.V.; El-Deiry, W.S.; Golstein, P.; Green, D.R.; et al. Classification of cell death: Recommendations of the Nomenclature Committee on Cell Death 2009. *Cell Death Differ.* **2009**, *16*, 3–11. [CrossRef] [PubMed]

21. Fischer, U.; Janicke, R.U.; Schulze-Osthoff, K. Many cuts to ruin: A comprehensive update of caspase substrates. *Cell Death Differ.* **2003**, *10*, 76–100. [CrossRef] [PubMed]

22. Fulda, S.; Debatin, K.-A. Extrinsic versus intrinsic apoptosis pathways in anticancer chemotherapy. *Oncogene* **2006**, *25*, 4798–4811. [CrossRef] [PubMed]

23. Taylor, R.C.; Cullen, S.P.; Martin, S.J. Apoptosis: Controlled demolition at the cellular level. *Nat. Rev. Mol. Cell Biol.* **2008**, *9*, 231–241. [CrossRef] [PubMed]

24. Cohen, G.M. Caspases; the executioners of apoptosis. *Biochem. J.* **1997**, *326*, 1–16. [CrossRef] [PubMed]

25. Kool, E.T. Hydrogen bonding, base stacking, and steric effects in DNA replication. *Annu. Rev. Biophys. Biomol. Struct.* **2001**, *30*, 1–22. [CrossRef] [PubMed]

26. Kumar, S.; Mehndiratta, S.; Nepali, K.; Gupta, M.K.; Koul, S.; Sharma, P.R.; Saxena, A.K.; Dhar, K.L. Novel indole-bearing combretastatin analogues as tubulin polymerization inhibitors. *Org. Med. Chem. Lett.* **2013**, *3*, 3. [CrossRef] [PubMed]

27. Hadzi, D.; Kidric, J.; Koller, J.; Mavri, J. The role of hydrogen bonding in drug-receptor interactions. *J. Mol. Struct.* **1990**, *237*, 139–150. [CrossRef]

28. Farce, A.; Loge, C.; Gallet, S.; Lebegue, N.; Carato, P.; Chavatte, P.; Berthelot, P.; Lesieur, D. Docking study of ligands into colchicine binding site of tubulin. *J. Enzym. Inhib. Med. Chem.* **2004**, *19*, 541–547. [CrossRef] [PubMed]

29. Nogales, E.; Wolf, S.G.; Downing, K.H. Structure of the β-tubulin dimer by electron crystallography. *Nature* **1998**, *391*, 199–203. [CrossRef] [PubMed]

30. Wu, G.; Robertson, D.H.; Brooks, C.L., III; Vieth, M. Detailed analysis of grid-based molecular docking: A case study of CDOCKER-A CHARMm-based MD docking algorithm. *J. Comput. Chem.* **2003**, *24*, 1549–1562. [CrossRef] [PubMed]

4

Targeted Molecular Imaging using Aptamers in Cancer

Sorah Yoon [1],[*] (iD) and John J. Rossi [1],[2],[*]

[1] Department of Molecular and Cellular Biology, Beckman Research Institute of City of Hope, Duarte, CA 91010, USA

[2] Irell and Manella Graduate School of Biological Sciences, Beckman Research Institute of City of Hope, Duarte, CA 91010, USA

[*] Correspondence: syoon@coh.org (S.Y.); jrossi@coh.org (J.J.R.)

Abstract: Imaging is not only seeing, but also believing. For targeted imaging modalities, nucleic acid aptamers have features such as superior recognition of structural epitopes and quick uptake in target cells. This explains the emergence of an evolved new class of aptamers into a wide spectrum of imaging applications over the last decade. Genetically encoded biosensors tagged with fluorescent RNA aptamers have been developed as intracellular imaging tools to understand cellular signaling and physiology in live cells. Cancer-specific aptamers labeled with fluorescence have been used for assessment of clinical tissue specimens. Aptamers conjugated with gold nanoparticles have been employed to develop innovative mass spectrometry tissue imaging. Also, use of chemically conjugated cancer-specific aptamers as probes for non-invasive and high-resolution imaging has been transformative for in vivo imaging in multiple cancers.

Keywords: aptamer; targeted imaging; live cells; tissue; in vivo; cancer

1. Introduction

Recent decades have seen remarkable progress in molecular imaging, which is an indispensable tool for bench to bedside applications [1,2]. The array of imaging techniques currently available include optical imaging (fluorescence and bioluminescence), magnetic resonance imaging (MRI), positron-emission tomography (PET), single-photon emission computed tomography (SPECT), computed tomography (CT), and ultrasound (US), which are used in detection and characterization of cancers and assessment of responses for therapeutic intervention. To achieve satisfactory imaging, many factors have to be considered; suitable probes that have low target-to-background-noise signals, low toxicity, and suitable stability are indispensable [3]. To achieve this, antibodies or their derivatives targeted to specific antigens are typically employed [4]. However, in terms of target specificity and stability for imaging probes, aptamers are better tools, with greater advantages over antibodies, including target-specific recognition, high target-binding affinity, low immunogenicity, structural stability, and comparably smaller size (~3 nm vs. 10–15 nm for antibodies) [5]. Their excellent functions as imaging probes are demonstrated by super-resolution microscopy, showing superior and brighter targeted imaging of membrane receptors and intracellular organelles than antibodies [6]. In a comparison study of ^{111}Indium (In)-labeled aptamers with ^{111}In-antibodies using SPECT/CT images, ^{111}In-labeled aptamers showed better tumor-specific uptake than ^{111}In-antibodies after intravenous injection at 4 h [7], because of their smaller size relative to antibodies. As these two studies clearly show, aptamers have improved function over antibodies, and they have quickly emerged as molecular imaging probes for both subcellular and in vivo applications. Thus, in this review, we focus on several types of aptamer-guided imaging techniques based on recently released research, covering subcellular imaging to in vivo imaging in cancer.

2. Cell Imaging

Cell imaging is considered essential for understanding cellular physiology. Historically, green fluorescent protein (GFP) has been central to cellular imaging applications by way of being tagged onto endogenously coding genes to investigate the expression, interaction, localization, and role of target proteins in cells [8,9]. However, the vast amount of research in the RNA field has started to expand the role of RNAs, leading to development of innovative tools for intracellular imaging. This includes fluorogenic aptamers that activate fluorescence upon binding of their target fluorophores; e.g., Spinach [10], Broccoli [11], Mango [12], and Corn [13]. For in vitro applications, these fluorogenic aptamers can be engineered as biosensors to detect intracellular metabolites or imaging tags to investigate the dynamics of intracellular RNAs in living cells by microscopy. To date, no in vivo imaging has been conducted with these fluorogenic aptamers. However, these fluorogenic aptamers have great potential for in vivo imaging. Thus, in this section, we will discuss fluorogenic aptamers and their in vitro applications.

2.1. Green Fluorogenic Aptamers: Spinach and Broccoli

The "Spinach" fluorogenic RNA aptamer activates green fluorescence upon the binding of the small-molecule fluorophore 3,5-difluoro-4-hydroxybenzylidene imidazolinone (DFHBI) and its variants (e.g., DFHBI 1T and DFHBI 2T) [10]. To investigate the precise working mechanism of fluorescence activation, the Spinach-DFHBI complex was determined by analysis of the crystal structures. The co-crystal structures of the Spinach-DFHBI complex revealed an unexpected quadruplex core connected with two G-tetrads and a mixed-base tetrad [14]. DFHBI was inserted by a base triple and confined around an unpaired guanine residue (G31) [14]. In comparison with fluorophore-free condition, the collapsed fluorophore binding site was rearranged with the base tier of the quadruplex, extruding the G31 from the helical stack [14]. The fluorogenic Spinach was a novel proof-of-concept study, but weaknesses of Spinach such as thermal instability, requirement of high magnesium concentration, misfolding, and reduced brightness [15] have limited its application for imaging. In the following studies, Spinach was mutated to multiple variants such as Spinach2 [15] and Baby Spinach [16] to increase thermal stability and folding structure.

As Spinach had some drawbacks, the microfluidic-assisted In Vitro Compartmentalization (μIVC) method was employed to screen for aptamers able to work in low bivalent concentration and the selected aptamers were minimized for in vitro application, which was named iSpinach [17]. In a comparison of iSpinach with Spinach2, iSpinach showed 1.4 times more fluorescence in the presence of potassium, better thermostability, and binding affinity than Spinach2. However, live-cell imaging was not evaluated.

For live-cell imaging, Spinach and Spinach2 were engineered as biosensors to detect cellular metabolites (S-adenosylmethionine (SAM), adenosine 5-diphosphate (ADP), and second messenger Cyclic di-AMP (cdiA)) in *Escherichia coli* (*E. coli*) and *Listeria monocytogenes* (*L. monocytogenes*) [18,19]. Spinach engineered with SAM-binding RNA aptamers via a stem sequence that acted like a transducer for a biosensor showed 6-fold increased fluorescence over 3 h, when the SAM precursor methionine was provided in DFHBI-treated *E. coli* [18]. The Spinach-ADP sensor showed a 20-fold increase of fluorescence in DFHBI-treated *E. coli* [18]. For imaging of intracellular cdiA levels in *L. monocytogenes*, the ligand-sensing domain of cdiA riboswitch (yuaA riboswitch) was combined with Spinach2, termed YuaA-Spinach2, to act as fluorescent biosensors [19]. When a plasmid encoding the biosensor was transformed into live *L. monocytogenes*, robust intracellular fluorescence was observed under fluorescence microscopy in the presence of DFHBI [19]. This clearly demonstrates that the yuaA-Spinach2 biosensor works in living cells.

To overcome the limitations of Spinach, the green fluorogenic RNA aptamer "Broccoli", which binds to the fluorophore DFHBI, was isolated using a different approach by the same group that developed Spinach [11]. The method of Broccoli isolation was designed to improve the specificity and functionality of the fluorogenic aptamer. In experimental approaches, fluorescence RNA aptamers when treated with fluorophores after first round of conventional aptamer selection method were inserted into plasmid. After transformation of cloned plasmids into *E. coli.*, fluorescence cells were isolated by fluorescence-activated cell sorting (FACS) method in the treatment of DFHBI. This approach successfully isolated the fluorogenic aptamer Broccoli, which showed robust folding in low salt concentrations, increased thermostability, and stronger fluorescence relative to Spinach2 [11]. For further in vitro imaging, Broccoli was truncated to tBroccoli and was dimerized to tdBroccoli. The dimerized tdBroccoli showed twice the fluorescence intensity compared to Broccoli in living *E. coli.* [11]. To make a biosensor, Broccoli, tBroccoli or tdBroccoli was fused to the 3′ end of 5S plasmid with or without the pAV5S tRNA scaffold. Fluorescence activation was compared in transfected HEK293T cells using microscopy. The Broccoli or dBroccoli without a tRNA scaffold showed higher fluorescence intensity than that with the tRNA scaffold [11]. What the Broccoli study suggests is that the strong thermostability and folding structure of aptamers do not require a tRNA scaffold system to support the appropriate folding of aptamers intracellularly, which is a valuable advantage for in vivo imaging in the future.

2.2. Orange Fluorogenic Aptamer: Mango

The "Mango" RNA aptamer binds to derivatives of the fluorophore thiazole orange (TO1) and shows high levels of orange fluorescence, which increase by up to 1100-fold upon the binding of TO1 [12]. The structure of Mango was predicted to be folded with two-tiered all-parallel G-quadruplexes in an A-form duplex [12]. Crystal structure analysis of the Mango-TO1 complex showed three antiparallel quinines forming G-quadruples [20]. The binding of TO1 on one of the flat faces of the G-quadruplex stabilized the Mango structure and activated orange fluorescence. For imaging applications, TO1 was directly injected into *Caenorhabditis elegans* (*C. elegans*) syncytial gonads with equimolar amounts of RNA Mango. The strong fluorescence composition was observed in the nuclei of gonad [12].

New orange fluorogenic RNA Mango aptamers were isolated by the group that isolated iSpinach using microfluidics-based selection methods [21]. This "New Mango" was brighter than enhanced green fluorescent protein (EGFP) when bound to TO1, which is a major advantage for imaging applications. For imaging sensors, New Mango was tagged by incorporating the human 5S ribosomal RNA or U6 small nuclear RNA (snRNA) into F30 folding scaffold plasmids. The RNAs of 5S-F30-New Mango or U6-F30-New Mango generated by in vitro transcription were transfected into mammalian HEK293T [21]. Subcellular co-localization and fluorescence were investigated using fluorescence microscopy. The 5S-F30-New Mango RNAs showed up to 10 bright RNA foci per cell in the cytoplasm, mainly co-localized with mitochondria [21]. The U6-F30-New Mango RNA showed a different localization; it was mainly co-localized with small nuclear protein (snRNP) Lsm3 [21]. To develop a genetically encoded imaging tag expressed in mammalian cells, New Mango was inserted into the pSLQ plasmid to express 5S rRNA under the RNA pol III promoter (pSLQ-5S-F30-New Mango) [21]. The engineered pSLQ-5S-F30-New Mango plasmid was transfected into cells. The expression of fluorescence was observed to be both nucleolar and cytoplasmic using fluorescence microscopy. pSLQ-5S-F30-New Mango was also observed to co-localize with ribosomal protein L7 [21]. These results clearly demonstrate that New Mango has the capability to be used as an imaging tag to visualize the subcellular location of target genes.

2.3. Yellow Fluorogenic Aptamer: Corn

The RNA aptamer that binds to 3,5-difluoro-4-hydroxynenzylidene imidazolinone-2-oxime (DFHO), named "Corn", activates yellow fluorescence [13]. Compared with Broccoli, Corn showed strong photostability; its fluorescence was detected at 320-ms imaging times vs. 160 ms with Broccoli [13]. In irradiation experiments, the Corn–DFHO complex exhibited minimal loss of fluorescence after as long as 10 s vs. >50% of fluorescence was lost after 200 ms with the Broccoli–DFHBI complex. Therefore, Corn was considered an emerging new fluorogenic aptamer for biosensors. To test the feasibility of Corn as a genetically encoded fluorescent RNA tag, three main subclasses of Pol III promoters (5S RNA, tRNA, and U6) with a tRNALys scaffold plasmid were constructed with the Corn aptamer. When these reporter plasmids were transfected into HEK293T cells, yellow fluorescence was observed by fluorescence microscopy after treatment with DFHO [13].

2.4. Rainbow Fluorogenic Aptamer: SRB-2

The SRB-2 aptamer, originally isolated against the fluorophore sulforhodamine B, binds to various dyes with xanthene-like cores, such as pyrosin B, pyrosin Y, acridine orange, SR-DN, and TMR-DN, and yields a "rainbow" of differently colored bright fluorescence [22]. To confirm different fluorescence by the SRB-2 aptamer upon binding of different fluorophores, a single copy of the SRB-2 aptamer sequence was inserted into tRNA scaffold plasmid. After transformation of SRB-2 inserted plasmid into *E. coli*, the activation of fluorescence was investigated using microscopy in the presence of a variety of fluorophores. The SRB2-expressing bacteria showed various colors after incubation with each fluorophore: pyrosin B (yellow color), pyrosin Y (yellow color), acridine orange (green color), SR-DN (red color), and TMR-DN (yellowish-orange color) [22]. As the SRB-2 aptamer showed various colors of fluorescence, selection of an appropriate fluorophore was investigated for subsequent no-wash and live cell imaging methods. Even though pyrosin B, pyrosin Y, and acridine orange showed differently colored fluorescence, the three fluorophores showed high signal-to-background ratio, compared with SR-DN and TMR-DN. SR-DN was previously developed as a live-cell imaging fluorophore for the SRB-2 aptamer, but it had low binding affinity ($K_d = 1.3$ μM). In contrast, TMR-DN showed higher binding affinity ($K_d = 35$ nM) for the SRB-2 aptamer. In a comparison of SR-DN and TMR-DN, SRB-2 expressing bacteria displayed 11-fold higher fluorescence intensity after incubation with TMR-DN than with SR-DN [22]. Therefore, TMR-DN was used for subsequent live cell imaging. For live-cell imaging of rRNA and mRNA in mammalian cells, 5S rRNA embedded with a single repeat of SRB-2 in a tRNA scaffold was applied in mammalian cell imaging [22]. The nuclear and cytoplasmic distribution of fluorescent 5S rRNA were clearly visualized using a 5S-SRB-2 construct in HeLa cells by microscopy [22]. For mRNA imaging in live prokaryotic cells, 6 and 15 tandem repeats of SRB-2 without a tRNA scaffold were fused to the 3'-UTR GFP mRNA. Bacteria expressing GFP-6xSRB-2 and GFP-15xSRB-2 showed significantly higher fluorescence than bacteria expressing only GFP after incubation with TMR-DN. For mRNA imaging in live eukaryotic cells, 15 repeats of SRB-2 without a tRNA scaffold were fused to 3'-UTR CFP-TM (cyan fluorescent protein). Microscopy revealed that HeLa cells transfected with CFP-TM-15xSBR-2 plasmid showed significantly higher fluorescence in TMR-DN than control cells, with mostly cytoplasmic distribution of the CFP-TM mRNAs [22].

Taken together, fluorogenic RNA aptamers such as Spinach, Broccoli, Mango, Corn, and Rainbow aptamers can be successfully applied for intracellular imaging in live cells. Thus, these fluorogenic RNA aptamers are great tools to investigate the dynamics of intracellular RNAs, as depicted in Figure 1. Theoretically, RNA aptamers can be developed to any fluorophores, and because fluorogenic RNA aptamer tags have diverse applications, we expect a variety of fluorogenic aptamers suitable for mammalian in vivo imaging will be developed in the near future.

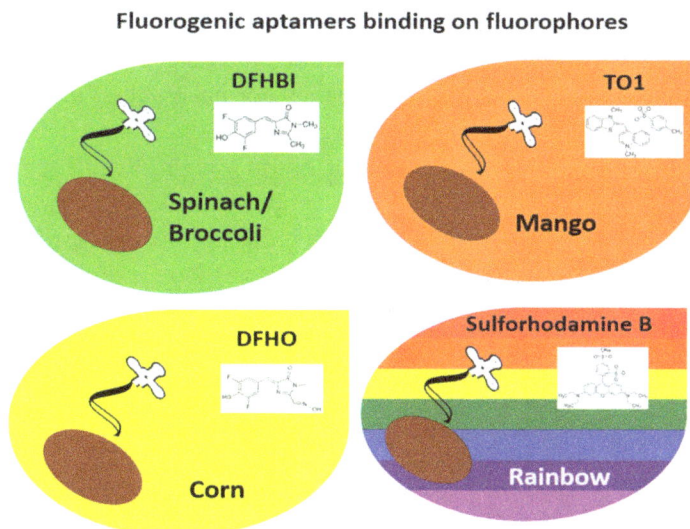

Figure 1. Live cell imaging with bioengineered aptamer tags. Fluorogenic RNA aptamers such as Mango, Corn, Broccoli, and SRB-2 Rainbow are inserted after a gene of interest, bind to their target fluorophores, and turn on fluorescence in the presence of their target fluorophores. The fluorogenic RNA aptamer tags can be used for tracking and for investigating the dynamics of a gene of interest in live cells.

3. Tissue Imaging

Tissue imaging using aptamers remains an underdeveloped research area. Because aptamers have high target specificity and cancer-specific aptamers are being continuously discovered [23], the assessment of clinical tissue specimens with labeled aptamers allows us to characterize tumors. However, to date, there are few studies investigating the use of fluorescently labeled or gold metal-conjugated aptamers to assess cancer characteristics.

The pancreatic cancer specificity of RNA aptamers isolated via cell-SELEX was assessed using Cy3-labeled RNA aptamers on human pancreatic cancer patient specimens and human normal tissues [24]. The pancreatic-cancer-specific RNA aptamers showed strong fluorescence intensity that correlated with the low survival rate of pancreatic cancer patients [24]. This implies that the target ligand of the pancreatic cancer-specific aptamer could be used a prognostic marker, when the aptamer-binding target is identified.

The DNA aptamer DML-7, which shows specific binding to metastatic prostate cancer DU145 cells, was evaluated on normal, non-metastatic, and metastatic prostate cancer (PC) tissue specimens with Cy5-labeled aptamers [25]. No fluorescence was observed on normal prostate tissues and weak fluorescence was observed on non-metastatic prostate tissues. However, moderate to strong fluorescence was observed on metastatic PC tissues [25]. This suggests that DML-7 aptamers bind to a cancer metastatic biomarker.

Mass spectrometry tissue imaging (MSI) is a very attractive imaging technique for analysis of multiple biomolecules simultaneously and biomarker discovery from tissue samples [26]. Recently, laser desorption/ionization MS (LDI-MS) techniques has been developed to analyze the distribution of nanomaterials on tissue specimens [27]. As a proof-of-concept study for tissue MSI, the anti-nucleolin aptamer AS1411 was conjugated with gold nanoparticles (GNPs) [28]. Under laser desorption/ionization, gold cluster ions (Aus) were disassociated from AS1411-gold nanoparticles and acted as signal amplifiers to detect nucleolin-positive tumor tissue images. The aptamer-guided MSI imaging was tested on human breast tumor and normal breast tissues. The tissue samples were labeled with AS1411-gold nanoparticles and LDI-MS imaging was acquired in positive-ion mode using an Autoflex III LDI TOF mass spectrometer. A SmartBeam laser (355 nm Nd: YAG) was operated at 100 Hz to irradiate the tissue slides, using conditions of laser spot diameter at 30 μm and pixel step size at 150 μm [28]. The MS images generated through monitoring of Au signal intensity clearly indicated that the tumor tissues had much stronger signal intensities than normal tissues. Furthermore, the expression and distribution of nucleolin in breast tissue by immunohistochemistry (IHC) showed consistent results with those obtained through LDI-MS. This successful imaging acquisition using aptamers has major implications for aptamers as suitable imaging probes in an MSI platform for the diagnosis of malignancies. The schematic work flow is depicted in Figure 2. However, a disadvantage of LDI-MS imaging is that it can only detect highly abundant targets on tissue samples. Therefore, it provides more valuable diagnostic information when combined with in vivo imaging.

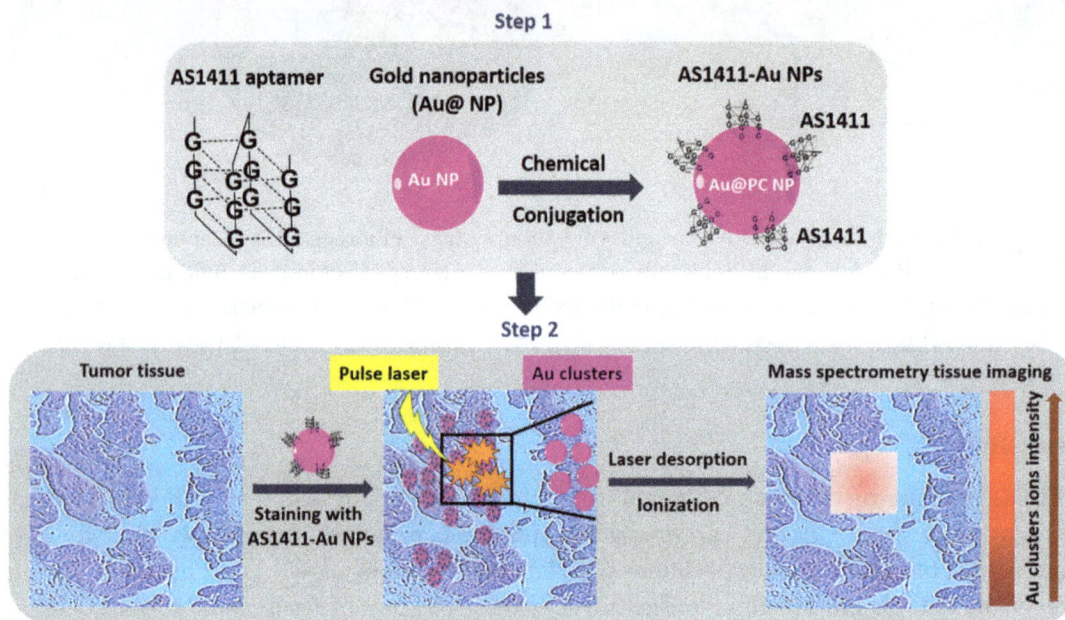

Figure 2. Mass spectrometry tissue imaging (MSI). Anti-nucleolin aptamers conjugated with gold nanoparticles are used to stain cancer tissues. Under laser desorption/ionization, gold cluster ion-amplified signal reporters are collected for laser MSI.

4. In Vivo Imaging

Identifying target-specific probes is critical to conferring specificity for in vivo imaging. In this respect, the majority of aptamers that have already been developed target cancer-specific surface antigens [23]. Therefore, these cancer-specific aptamers are great imaging probes for a variety of imaging techniques in cancer diagnostics, including fluorescence optical imaging, MRI, PET, SPECT, CT, US, and photoacoustic imaging. In this section, we will discuss cancer-specific aptamers labeled with multiple imaging dyes for targeted in vivo imaging.

4.1. Fluorescence Imaging

Fluorescence is the most adapted tool in aptamer-guided imaging because of its low cost and high sensitivity. The most commonly used fluorescent dyes are cyanine 5 (Cy 5), quantum dots (QDs), and near-infrared (NIR) dye.

Cancer cell-type-specific DNA aptamers against Ramos cells (B-cell lymphoma) were labeled with a Cy5 probe (Cy5-TD05) and the efficacy of in vivo imaging was determined in subcutaneously xenografted nude mice via tail vein injection [29]. This demonstrated that Cy5-TD05 was specifically accumulated into engrafted tumor regions by 3.5 h or later, compared with control aptamers, Cy5 dye only, or in non-targeted cells. Cy5-TD05 also showed a high signal-to background ratio at 115.50. In biodistribution assays, high fluorescence was observed in the small intestine [29]. In another cancer cell-type-specific aptamer study, DNA aptamers specific to A549 cells (lung carcinoma cells) were labeled with a Cy5 probe (Cy5-S6) for in vivo imaging [30]. In subcutaneously xenografted nude mice, Cy5-S6 showed tumor-specific accumulation between 3 to 5 h after intravenous injection. In contrast, no fluorescence was observed with a Cy5-labeled library or in non-targeted cells. Using the same approach, two other cancer cell-type-specific DNA aptamers against Bel-7404 and SMMC-7721 (human hepatocellular carcinomas) were tested in vivo. Both aptamers showed tumor-specific fluorescence accumulation by 3 h post-injection.

QDs have been studied as another fluorescence imaging dye in various cancer models. QDs are fluorescent nanoparticles that have great advantages for imaging, such as low photobleaching, high fluorescence yield, and chemical stability [31]. Fluorescence imaging using QDs has been investigated by chemical conjugation with anti-mucin 1 (MUC1) aptamers and anti-variant of epidermal growth factor receptor (EGFRvIII) aptamers in vivo. As MUC1 is highly expressed on the cancer plasma membrane, the cancer specificity of an anti-MUC1 DNA aptamer conjugated with QDs was evaluated in A549 cells [32]. Anti-MUC1 DNA aptamers labeled with QDs were injected into subcutaneously xenografted nude mice via the tail vein. Strong fluorescence was observed in the tumor specifically, but not with control QDs. EGFRvIII is selectively expressed on cancer cells, and is involved in enhancement of cancer cell proliferation, invasion, and resistance to chemotherapy and radiotherapy [33]. Therefore, it has been popularized as a target for therapeutics and imaging. The anti-EGFRvIII DNA aptamer (A32) was conjugated with streptavidin-PEG-CdSe/ZnS QDs (QD-A32 Apt). For in vivo imaging, U87 (glioma) cells and U87-EGFRvIII overexpressing cells were orthotopically xenografted into nude mice [34]. After tail-vein injection of QD-A32 Apt, fluorescence imaging was performed 6 h post-injection. Mice harboring U87-EGFRvIII overexpressing cells, but not U87 tumors, showed strong fluorescence signals in tumor areas. No significant fluorescence was observed in mice injected with unconjugated QDs. In a biodistribution assay, QD-A32 Apt showed high accumulation in the tumor region, liver, and kidneys, and low accumulation in the tumor pararegion, normal brain, spleen, heart, and lungs. In another study, anti-EGFR aptamers targeting wild-type EGFR were conjugated with lipid QDs (Apt-QLs) [35]. The feasibility of using Apt-QLs for in vivo imaging was tested in an MDA-MB-231 breast in vivo tumor model. By 4 h post-intravenous injection, it showed breast cancer-specific accumulation in engrafted mice [35].

As NIR dyes enhance sensitivity due to low background autofluorescence and higher signal-to-noise ratios, it is another suitable fluorescent dye for in vivo imaging. In PC, anti-prostate-specific membrane antigen (PSMA) RNA aptamer (A9g) was conjugated with NIR dye (IRDye 800CW) [36]. The NIR-labeled aptamer (NIR-A9g) was injected into the tail veins of mice bearing PC-3 (PSMA-positive) tumor cells. It showed intense cancer-specific fluorescence, beginning at 24 h and up to 72 h after administration [36]. In another study, a new NIR dye, which is a derivative of indocyanine green (MPA; absorbance peak at 780nm and emission peak at 810 nm), was tested in breast cancer and liver cancer animal models. Anti-MUC1 DNA aptamers were conjugated with the MPA dye (APT-MPA) or with polyethylene glycol-NIR (APT-PEG-MPA) [37]. MCF-7 breast cancer cells or HepG2 liver cancer cells were subcutaneously xenografted into nude mice. MPA, APT-MPA, or APT-PEG-MPA were injected into mice via tail-vein injection. Strong tumor-specific fluorescence by targeting of APT-MPA or APT-PEG-MPA was observed starting at 2 h up to 72 h on both breast and liver cancers in vivo. In contrast, control MPA did not show accumulation of fluorescence in the tumor-engrafted region [37]. In a biodistribution assay, the PEG-modified probe (APT-PEG-MPA) showed much quicker clearance than that of APT-MPA [37].

4.2. Magnetic Resonance Imaging (MRI)

MRI is a very powerful imaging technique used for non-invasive visualization of internal organ structures and soft tissue morphology by using a powerful magnet and radiofrequency energy [38].

Introducing MR imaging contrast agents by way of specific targeting moieties like aptamers has significantly improved the quality of imaging. The $\alpha_v \beta_3$ integrin subunit is involved in cell migration and invasion during neovascularization and/or angiogenesis in cancer. Therefore, it was targeted for molecular imaging [39]. An anti-$\alpha_v\beta_3$ aptamer (Apt $\alpha_v\beta_3$) was conjugated with magnetic nanoparticles (MNPs) for cancer-specific detection via MRI imaging [40]. The aptamer $\alpha_v\beta_3$-conjugated magnetic nanoparticles (Apt $\alpha_v\beta_3$-MNPs) were injected into epidermoid carcinoma A431 xenografted nude mice intravenously. The evaluated MR signals showed the maximum intensity at 24 h post-injection. The accumulated amount of Apt $\alpha_v\beta_3$-MNPs was 129 $\pm$ 34.3% in the tumor compared to short peptide conjugated MNPs as control.

Vascular growth factor receptor 2 (VEGFR2) is commonly overexpressed in the tumor vasculature, and could be another target-of-interest for cancer imaging. For the recognition of glioblastoma vasculature, anti-VEGFR2 aptamers were immobilized on the surface of carboxylated magnetic nanocrystals (MNCs) [41]. The molecular imaging potential of the VEGFR2 aptamer-MNCs (VEGFR2 Apt-MNCs) were assessed in an orthotopic glioblastoma nude mouse model. MRI was performed on the animal after intravenous tail veil injection of VEGFR2 Apt-MNC or unconjugated MNC with a 3.0-T MR imaging. At 4 h post-injection, MR imaging was darker in tumor sites treated with VEGFR2 Apt-MNC than in those treated with unconjugated MNC, confirming that VEGFR2 Apt-MNC enabled precise in vivo detection [41].

A common feature of solid cancer is hypoxia, which induces the activation of hypoxia-inducible factor-1α (HIF-1α) [42]. HIF-1α is also involved in the maintenance of cancer stem cells. For non-invasive imaging to identify hypoxia-induced cancer stem cells, HIF-1α aptamer-PEG-modified manganese magnetic nanoparticles, D-Fe_3O_4@Mn, were generated [43]. For in vivo imaging, PANC-1 pancreatic cancer cells were subcutaneously xenografted in nude mice. D-Fe_3O_4@Mn was injected into the mice intravenously and MRI was performed before and after injection at 2 h. Compared with images of mice without NP, the D-Fe_3O_4@Mn-injected mice showed significantly bright enhanced effects and 3.5-fold higher signal intensity in T1-weighted MRI imaging (T1W1). Upon histopathological examination, no signs of toxicity were observed in the major organs at day 10 after injection of D-Fe_3O_4@ Mn [43].

4.3. Single-Photon Emission Computed Tomography (SPECT)

Nuclear imaging techniques like SPECT and PET can monitor biological events deep within the body and provide longitudinal assessment of a patient with high detection sensitivity [44]. Therefore, development of imaging modalities for SPECT and PET with high specificity is critical. In this respect, cancer-specific aptamers are excellent detecting probes. SPECT imaging detects γ-ray emission from radioisotopes using a gamma camera. The most commonly used isotopes for SPECT imaging are ^{99m}Tc (Technetium, $t_{1/2}$: 6 h), ^{111}In (Indium, $t_{1/2}$: 2.8 d), ^{123}I (Iodine, $t_{1/2}$: 13.2 h), and ^{131}I (Iodine, $t_{1/2}$: 8.0 d) [45]. For SPECT imaging, an anti-tenascin-C aptamer (TTA1) was conjugated to the succinimidyl ester of MAG2 and radiolabeled with ^{99m}Tc (MAG2-TTA1-^{99m}Tc) [46]. To assess in vivo tumor targeting, the MAG2-TTA1-^{99m}Tc was intravenously injected into mice bearing U215 glioblastoma or MDA-MB-435 breast cancer tumors. After aptamer-based γ-camera imaging of the tumors, the U251 glioblastoma was prominently visible at 3 h, but not after application of control aptamers. The MDA-MB-435 breast tumor showed cancer-specific imaging at 20 h. Biodistribution assays showed that bladder and liver (10 min) and bladder and intestines (3 h) were predominant clearance pathways [44]. When the radiometal chelator was switched to DTPA (DTPA (^{111}In)-TTA1), the DTPA (^{111}In)-TTA1 showed persistent accumulation in the liver and kidney at 3 h.

EGFR is overexpressed in 90% of head and neck cancers [47]. For comparison studies of aptamers with antibodies, an anti-EGFR aptamer (apt) and antibody (C225) were conjugated with Hollow gold nanospheres (HAuNS), followed by radiolabeling with ^{111}In-DTPA. For in vivo imaging, the apt-HAuNS-^{111}In-DTPA, C225-HAuNS-^{111}In-DTPA, and control-HAuNS-^{111}In-DTPA were injected intravenously into OSC-19 (tongue squamous cell carcinoma cell) orthotopic xenografted nude mice. SPECT imaging was performed at 4 h and 24 h post-injection [47]. The imaging revealed that at 24 h post-injection, more apt-HAuNS-^{111}In-DTPA accumulated in the tumor than C225-HAuNS-^{111}In-DTPA. These results demonstrate that aptamers are easily uptaken into tumors, likely due to their relatively smaller size compared to antibodies, suggesting that aptamers might be better tumor-homing ligands.

In a biodistribution assay, apt-HAuNS-^{111}In-DTPA showed greater retention in blood, kidneys, and lymph nodes. In contrast, C225-HAuNS-^{111}In-DTPA showed greater retention in the liver and spleen.

Human matrix metalloprotease-9 (hMMP-9) is overexpressed in cancers, particularly in cutaneous melanomas [48]. An RNA aptamer against hMMP9 (F3B) was conjugated with ^{111}In-DOTA (^{111}In-DOTA-F3B). After intravenous injection of the ^{111}In-DOTA-F3B into mice bearing human melanoma tumors, SPECT images were acquired at 1 h. The micro-imager analysis showed that ^{111}In-DOTA-F3B induced a stronger accumulated signal than ^{111}In-DOTA-control. Signal activity was increased in a tumor grade-dependent manner in ex vivo images [49]. The biodistribution of ^{111}In-DOTA-F3B was determined at 30 min, 1 h, and 2 h post-injection. The average half-life was 11 min, which represents a rapid clearance from the blood. It also showed high uptake in kidneys and liver, but not other normal organs. The uptake of ^{111}In-DOTA-F3B in the tumor region was significantly higher at 1 h post-injection, compared with ^{111}In-DOTA-control-aptamer.

A variant of the anti-EGFRvIII DNA aptamer (U2) was labeled with rhenium radioisotope ([188]Re) [50]. The SPECT molecular imaging of [188]Re-U2 was tested in glioblastoma U87MG xenografted mice at 1 h post-injection. The [188]Re-U2 aptamer, but not control aptamer, was retained in tumors specifically. Its main route of excretion was through the urinary tract [50].

4.4. Positron-Emission Tomography (PET)

PET has at least ten-fold more sensitivity than SPECT [51]. Therefore, it has quickly emerged as a robust molecular imaging technique. For PET imaging probes, four chelators (DOTA, CB-TE2A, S-2-(4-Isothiocyanatobenzyl)-1,4,7,10-tetraazacyclododecane-tetraacetic acid [DOTA-Bn], and S-2-(4-Isothiocyanatobenzyl)-1,4,7-triazacyclononane-1,4,7-triacetic acid [NOTA-Bn]) were selected and used to label the anti-nucleolin AS1411 aptamer, along with [64]Cu [52]. In comparison studies of these chelators, ^{64}Cu-DOTA-AS1411 and ^{64}Cu-CB-TE2A-AS1411 were internalized into cells at significantly greater levels than ^{64}Cu-DOTA-Bn-AS1411 and ^{64}Cu-NOTA-Bn-AS1411. Thus, ^{64}Cu-DOTA-AS1411 and ^{64}Cu-CB-TE2A-AS1411 were chosen for further in vivo imaging. ^{64}Cu-DOTA-AS1411 or ^{64}Cu-CB-TE2A-AS1411 was injected into H460 lung cancer-bearing mice via tail-vein injection and mice were imaged at multiple time-points up to 24 h post-injection. In mice injected with ^{64}Cu-CB-TE2A-AS1411, tumors were visible from 1–24 h. However, the tumor was not detectable in mice injected with ^{64}Cu-DOTA-AS1411. This suggests that CB-TE2A is a more desirable chelator for in vivo kinetics. In biodistribution assay, ^{64}Cu-CB-TE2A-AS1411 also had faster clearance and less accumulation in the liver and kidney at 1 h post-injection than ^{64}Cu-DOTA-AS1411 [52].

Tenascin C shows a pattern of high expression in tumor stroma and plays a pivotal role in brain and breast cancer initiation and progression [53,54]. Anti-tenascin C DNA aptamers were conjugated with ^{64}Cu-NOTA to construct ^{64}Cu-NOTA-tenascin C [55]. For targeted molecular imaging of cancer, U86 MG glioma cells and H460 lung cancer cells were subcutaneously xenografted into mice and MDA-MB-435 breast cancer cells were orthotopic xenografted into the mammary glands of mice. The U86 MG and MDA-MB-435 tumors were positive for tenascin C, whereas the H460 was negative. After injection of ^{64}Cu-NOTA-tenascin C, PET images were taken at 1, 2, 6 and 24 h in the three cancer cell-engrafted mouse models. Tumor accumulation was clearly evident up to 24 h post-injection in U86 MG and MDA-MB-435 engrafted mice, but not in H460 engrafted mice [55].

Conventionally, aptamers were directly conjugated with a radioactive tracer isotope for PET imaging. As a more versatile platform for PET imaging probes, a hybridization strategy between two complementary oligonucleotides (ODN) has recently been used to label aptamers. The advantage of this platform is that the radioactive tracer isotope can be easily switched. As a proof of concept, AS1411 aptamers were hybridized with fluorine radioisotope (^{18}F)-labeled complementary ODN9 (cODN) [56]. The feasibility of hybridization-based aptamer labeling for PET imaging was tested in vivo. C6 glioma-bearing mice were injected with ^{18}F-hyAS1411 and ^{18}F-hy control C-rich aptamer (^{18}F-hyCRO) via tail-vein injection and PET imaging was performed 60 min post-injection. ^{18}F-hyAS1411 clearly showed that tumor-specific accumulation, comparing with the ^{18}F-hyCRO.

The sgc8 is a 41-nt DNA aptamer that binds to protein tyrosine kinase 7 (PTK-7) [57], which is overexpressed in several human malignancies, was conjugated with ^{18}F using click chemistry [58]. The ^{18}F-tagged DNA aptamer sgc8 was injected into nude mice bearing HCT116 colon cancer tumors, which are positive for PTK-7. ^{18}F-sgc8 clearly visualized the engrafted tumor region at 2 h post-injection. The main clearance route was reported as urinary and hepatic.

4.5. Computed Tomography (CT)

CT imaging is a commonly used technique to examine anatomical structures. However, contrast agents/probes for this modality are very limited. Recently GNPs have emerged as new nanoplatforms for CT imaging. As a proof of concept for CT imaging, anti-PSMA RNA aptamers were conjugated to gold nanoparticles and used as a CT contrast agent in PC [59]. The PSMA aptamer-conjugated gold nanoparticles showed more than 4-fold greater CT intensity for targeted LNCaP cells than that of nontargeted PC3 cells, but no in vivo imaging was carried out.

As another CT imaging approach, fluorescent gold nanoparticles were conjugated with diatrizoic acid and the anti-nucleolin AS1411 aptamer (AS1411-DA-AuNPs) [60]. The fluorescence spectrum of AS1411-DA-AuNPs showed a clear orange-red emission, with a maximum at 620 nm. In vivo molecular imaging was investigated in CLI-5 lung adenocarcinoma-bearing NOD-SCID mice via tail-vein injection of AS1411-DA-AuNPs. CT imaging was performed 30 min post-injection and showed a 106% more contrast enhancement in CLI-5 tumor-bearing mice than before-injection. In parallel, the orange-red fluorescence emitting from AS1411-DA-AuNPs in the CLI-5 tumor could also be visualized by the naked eye [60].

4.6. Ultrasound (US)

The use of gas-filled nanobubbles (NBs) constructed from poly (lactide-co-glycolic acid; PLGA), which is a biodegradable copolymer, improves US signals [61]. Therefore, it has been popularized as contrast agent for CT imaging. For targeted molecular imaging, the anti-PSMA A10-3.2 aptamer was conjugated with PLGA NBs (A10-3.2-PLGA NBs) [62]. For in vivo imaging, the A10-3.2-PLGA NBs were injected into LNCaP PC engrafted nude mice intravenously. Compared with saline control group, the distribution of contrast agent echo signals was rich and enhancement of contrast were observed in mice treated with A10-3.2-PLGA NBs [62]. The A10-3.2-PLGA NBs showed strong signal intensity, peaking at approximately 25 dB.

4.7. Photoacoustic (PA) Imaging

PA imaging has recently emerged as an alternative to MRI and X-ray tomography in the biomedical field, due to the ability to capture high resolution images at depth. However, the lack of selective probes makes its application in limit. For an experimental PA imaging by aptamers, a thrombin binding aptamer (TBA) was hybridized with IRDye 800CW-labeled (FDNA) and IRDye QC-1 quencher-labeled (QDNA) single-stranded DNA to form a DNA duplex structure for imaging probes [63]. When binding of target, it triggered the release of quencher strand and induced the relief the quenching strand. Thus, it induced the change of the PA signal at 780/725 nm. In other words, the binding of thrombin (TBA) loosed the hybridization of TBA-QDNA complexes and resulted in a release of FDNA, increase of both fluorescence and PA signals. Without thrombin, IRDye was placed next to quencher, induction of low fluorescence and PA signals.

In experimental mice imaging work, the DNA probes were injected into each flank of BALB/c mice. After then, thrombin and PBS were injected to each flank of mice. The PA images recorded at 45 min post-injection in thrombin injected mice showed a higher PA signal ratio at 780/725 than PBA or untreated mice.

4.8. Multimodal Imaging

Every molecular imaging modality has unique advantages and disadvantages. Therefore, current trend of imaging is to develop multimodal imaging to increase the diagnostic accuracy. As a proof of concept for a multimodal imaging system, multimodal nanoparticles have been developed for optical, MR, and PET imaging. For single multimodal nanoparticle imaging agent, cobalt ferrite magnetic nanoparticles surrounded by fluorescent rhodamine (termed MF) within a silica shell matrix were conjugated with anti-underglycosylated mucin-1 (uMUC-1) aptamer (MF-uMUC-1). Following step, MF-uMUC-1 was labeled by Gallium siotype ^{68}Ga (termed MFR-uMUC-1) with a p-SCN-bn-NOTA chelating agent [64]. For in vivo imaging of aptamer based multimodal imaging, MFR-uMUC-1 nanoparticles or MFR-uMUC-1 mutant (uMUC-1 mt, control) nanoparticle were injected into BT-20 breast cancer cell implanted nude mice throughout tail vein.

Three imaging modalities; fluorescence, PET, and MRI were used to take images at multi-time points such as 2, 12, 24 h after IV injection. The PET images showed significant accumulation of ^{68}Ga radioactivity in the tumor region of the MFR-uMUC-1-injected group, but not in the MFR-uMUC-1 mt-injected group. In the MFR-uMUC-1 injected group, significantly high tumor-specific fluorescence was also observed. By MR images, it showed significantly enhanced dark signals in MFR-uMUC-1-injected mice [64]. These results demonstrate a high specificity for targeting cancers using the uMUC-1 aptamer and suggest it is feasible as a single multimodal probe in vivo by aptamer guided.

Taken together, targeted molecular in vivo imaging by aptamers as depicted in Figure 3 shows cancer-specific recognition in multiple imaging modalities. Each modality has various advantages and disadvantages. Fluorescence imaging is very cost effective and shows high sensitivity, but high autofluorescence and poor tissue penetration prevent the translation of fluorescence imaging into clinics. Nuclear imaging such as SPECT and PET provide improved resolution of imaging and longitudinal assessment of deep tissues in the same patient with high sensitivity, but the expensive cost and handling of isotypes are disadvantages. MRI and CT are excellent techniques to examine anatomical body structures, so enhancement of contrast with imaging agents is a key factor. Currently, aptamer-guided molecular imaging remains in the preclinical stage, but we expect that aptamer-guided molecular imaging can be used in clinics in the near future.

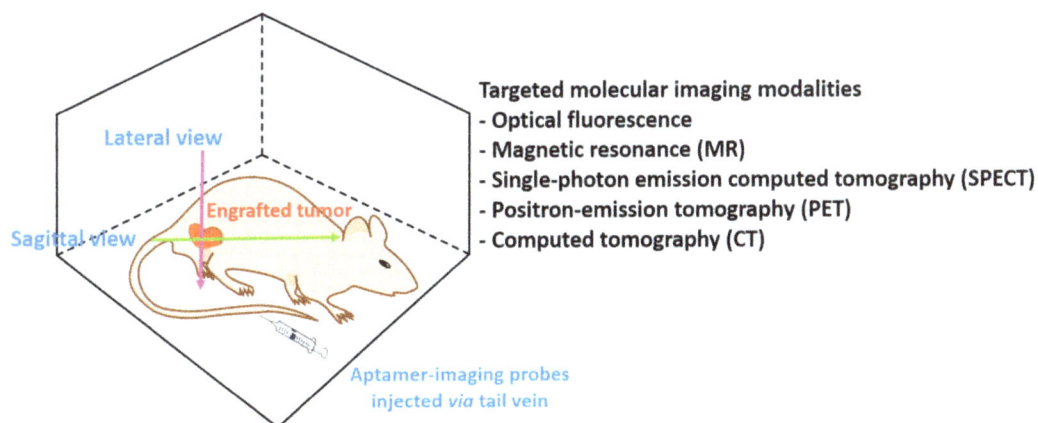

Figure 3. Targeted in vivo imaging using aptamers. Mice possessing xenografted cancer cells are injected with aptamers labeled with imaging dyes. Non-invasive imaging modalities such as fluorescence, magnetic resonance (MR), single-photon emission computed tomography (SPECT), position-emission tomography (PET), or computed tomography (CT) are used for imaging on lateral or sagittal view.

5. Clinical Trials

Clinical trials using aptamers for imaging or diagnostics are actively under investigation. For instance, the anti-PTK-7 DNA aptamer (^{68}Ga-sgc8) is under interventional clinical trial,

ClinicalTrials Identifier: NCT03385148. The aim of this study is to assess its safety and biodistribution, and to evaluate its application for PET/CT scan in colorectal patients. 10–20 mBq of ^{68}Ga-Sgc8 will be injected into colorectal cancer patients. Diagnosis efficacy of ^{68}Ga-Sgc8 PET/CT scans will be compared with those of ^{18}F-FDG PET. Patients are currently being recruited for this study.

An aptamer-based biosensor to detect a biomarker in bladder cancer is under perspective observational clinical trial, *ClinicalTrials Identifier: NCT02957370*. The aim of this trial is to discover urinary biomarkers in bladder cancer patients using a Förster resonance energy transfer (FRET) system. Patients are currently being recruiting for this study.

6. Chemical Modifications

To facilitate the translation of aptamer-guided molecular imaging, chemical modifications should be considered to increase resistance to cellular nucleases and to improve structural stability and binding affinity [65]. The most common strategies employed are depicted in Figure 4. This includes: phosphodiester backbone modifications such as phosphorothioate, methylphosphonate, and triazole linkages; base modifications such as 5-(*N*-benzycarboxyamide)-2′-deoxyuridine (5-BzdU), naphtyl, triptamino, and isobutyl in Slow Off-rate Modified aptamers (SOMAmers); sugar ring modification such as 2′-fluoro (2′-F), 2′-amino (2′-NH2), 2′-O-methyl (2′-OMe), locked nucleic acid (LNA), unlocked nucleic acid (UNA), 2′-deoxy-2′-fluoro-D-arabinonucleic acid (2′-FANA); the mirror image of L-deoxynucleotides in Spiegelmer® [65]. Such chemical modifications are mainly developed for therapeutic purposes to avoid immune responses and to increase serum resistance and potency. To date, DNA aptamers and 2′-F RNA aptamers have been proven as targeted imaging probes in tissue and in vivo imaging. We believe that introducing these chemical modifications improves the function of aptamers as targeted imaging probes, because improvement of nuclease resistance and structural stability will increase the retention time of aptamers in the body and target specificity. Indeed, the efficacy of anti-EpCAM and nucleolin LNA modified aptamer conjugated with Fe_3O_4 nanoparticles (NPs) was tested for multimodal imaging for NIR, MRI, and CT imaging in vivo [66]. After feeding the formula for 48 h, imaging was taken by three imaging modalities. Comparing with untreated control, comparatively higher fluorescence was shown by NIR imaging. Also, comparatively high contrast in tumor region was observed by NIR and CT. It suggests that chemical modifications of aptamer are well tolerated as imaging probes. On the other hand, manufacturing costs will be increased.

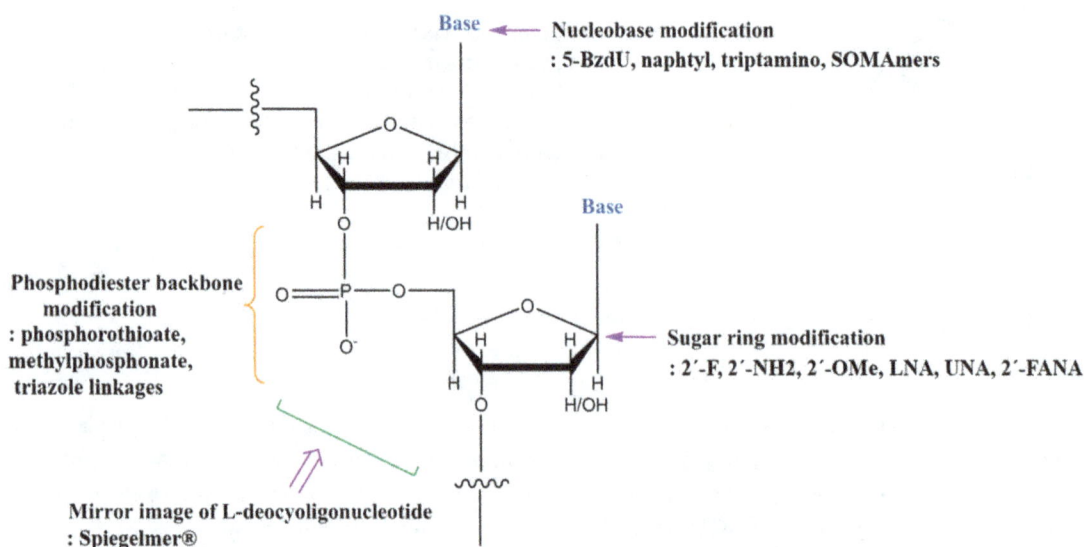

Figure 4. Strategies for chemical modification of nucleic acid aptamers to increase structural stability and nuclease resistance. The most commonly used strategies in DNA/RNA aptamers are modifications of the phosphodiester linkage, the sugar ring, and the bases.

7. Conclusions and Implications for Clinical Use

Currently, targeted molecular imaging using aptamers is an actively developing research field. For targeted imaging modalities, aptamers have shown cancer-specific recognition in tissue imaging and in vivo imaging in multiple cancer models.

For in vivo use, DNA aptamers (anti-nucleolin, anti-MUC1, anti-EGFRvIII, anti-cancer cell-type-specific aptamers) and RNA aptamers (anti-PSMA aptamer) show perform well for cancer-specific detection using various imaging techniques (e.g., fluorescence, PET, SPECT, MRI, CT, and US) at the preclinical stage. This suggests that aptamers have great potential for targeted imaging agents to differentiate disease-specific targets, which will be applicable in the clinic. As described in Section 4, every imaging technique has its own detecting mechanism, and unique pros and cons. Thus, a multimodal imaging platform might be a preferred option to fill the gap. Indeed, SPECT-CT and PET-CT are currently standard in most clinics. As for aptamer-guided multimodal imaging, optical-MR-PET imaging techniques were investigated with anti-MUC-1 aptamers [64], which showed high cancer-specific detection. Thus, construction of new multimodal imaging modalities that incorporate aptamers, such as PET-MRI, SPECT-MRI, fluorescence-PET, and US-PET, will play a leading role in developing novel, clinically relevant approaches. Regardless of what type of imaging techniques will be used, targeted molecular imaging by aptamers shows quick accumulation into target sites that gives suitable target-to-background signals. Thus, we believe that aptamer-guided imaging will improve diagnostic accuracy.

The next promising aptamer-guided imaging application to be developed is tissue MSI imaging. Aptamers conjugated with gold metal already demonstrated discrimination between cancer and normal tissues [27], suggesting that aptamers are suitable molecular probes in MSI. For the analysis of multiple biomolecules on single specimens, conjugation of multiple cancer-specific aptamers with different metals will be developed in future strategies, which can be utilized to characterize clinical human cancer specimens.

Author Contributions: S.Y. and J.J.R. conceived of and wrote the manuscript.

Funding: This work was supported by NIH grant R01 AI029329 to J.J.R.

Acknowledgments: We thank Sarah T. Wilkinson, scientific writer, at City of Hope for language editing.

References

1. Weissleder, R.; Pittet, M.J. Imaging in the era of molecular oncology. *Nature* **2008**, *452*, 580–589. [CrossRef] [PubMed]
2. James, M.L.; Gambhir, S.S. A molecular imaging primer: Modalities, imaging agents, and applications. *Physiol. Rev.* **2012**, *92*, 897–965. [CrossRef] [PubMed]
3. Chakravarty, R.; Goel, S.; Cai, W. Nanobody: The "magic bullet" for molecular imaging? *Theranostics* **2014**, *4*, 386–398. [CrossRef] [PubMed]
4. Warram, J.M.; de Boer, E.; Sorace, A.G.; Chung, T.K.; Kim, H.; Pleijhuis, R.G.; van Dam, G.M.; Rosenthal, E.L. Antibody-based imaging strategies for cancer. *Cancer Metastasis Rev.* **2014**, *33*, 809–822. [CrossRef] [PubMed]
5. Que-Gewirth, N.S.; Sullenger, B.A. Gene therapy progress and prospects: RNA aptamers. *Gene Ther.* **2007**, *14*, 283–291. [CrossRef] [PubMed]
6. Gomes de Castro, M.A.; Hobartner, C.; Opazo, F. Aptamers provide superior stainings of cellular receptors studied under super-resolution microscopy. *PLoS ONE* **2017**, *12*, e0173050. [CrossRef] [PubMed]
7. Melancon, M.P.; Zhou, M.; Zhang, R.; Xiong, C.; Allen, P.; Wen, X.; Huang, Q.; Wallace, M.; Myers, J.N.; Stafford, R.J.; et al. Selective uptake and imaging of aptamer- and antibody-conjugated hollow nanospheres targeted to epidermal growth factor receptors overexpressed in head and neck cancer. *ACS Nano* **2014**, *8*, 4530–4538. [CrossRef] [PubMed]
8. Enterina, J.R.; Wu, L.; Campbell, R.E. Emerging fluorescent protein technologies. *Curr. Opin. Chem. Biol.* **2015**, *27*, 10–17. [CrossRef] [PubMed]

9.   Mishin, A.S.; Belousov, V.V.; Solntsev, K.M.; Lukyanov, K.A. Novel uses of fluorescent proteins. *Curr. Opin. Chem. Biol.* **2015**, *27*, 1–9. [CrossRef] [PubMed]

10. Paige, J.S.; Wu, K.Y.; Jaffrey, S.R. RNA mimics of green fluorescent protein. *Science* **2011**, *333*, 642–646. [CrossRef] [PubMed]

11. Filonov, G.S.; Moon, J.D.; Svensen, N.; Jaffrey, S.R. Broccoli: Rapid selection of an RNA mimic of green fluorescent protein by fluorescence-based selection and directed evolution. *J. Am. Chem. Soc.* **2014**, *136*, 16299–16308. [CrossRef] [PubMed]

12. Dolgosheina, E.V.; Jeng, S.C.; Panchapakesan, S.S.S.; Cojocaru, R.; Chen, P.S.; Wilson, P.D.; Hawkins, N.; Wiggins, P.A.; Unrau, P.J. RNA mango aptamer-fluorophore: A bright, high-affinity complex for RNA labeling and tracking. *ACS Chem. Biol.* **2014**, *9*, 2412–2420. [CrossRef] [PubMed]

13. Song, W.; Filonov, G.S.; Kim, H.; Hirsch, M.; Li, X.; Moon, J.D.; Jaffrey, S.R. Imaging RNA polymerase III transcription using a photostable RNA-fluorophore complex. *Nat. Chem. Biol.* **2017**, *13*, 1187–1194. [CrossRef] [PubMed]

14. Huang, H.; Suslov, N.B.; Li, N.S.; Shelke, S.A.; Evans, M.E.; Koldobskaya, Y.; Rice, P.A.; Piccirilli, J.A. A G-quadruplex-containing RNA activates fluorescence in a GFP-like fluorophore. *Nat. Chem. Biol.* **2014**, *10*, 686–691. [CrossRef] [PubMed]

15. Strack, R.L.; Disney, M.D.; Jaffrey, S.R. A superfolding Spinach2 reveals the dynamic nature of trinucleotide repeat-containing RNA. *Nat. Methods* **2013**, *10*, 1219–1224. [CrossRef] [PubMed]

16. Warner, K.D.; Chen, M.C.; Song, W.; Strack, R.L.; Thorn, A.; Jaffrey, S.R.; Ferré-D'Amaré, A.R. Structural basis for activity of highly efficient RNA mimics of green fluorescent protein. *Nat. Struct. Mol. Biol.* **2014**, *21*, 658–663. [CrossRef] [PubMed]

17. Autour, A.; Westhof, E.; Ryckelynck, M. iSpinach: A fluorogenic RNA aptamer optimized for in vitro applications. *Nucleic Acids Res.* **2016**, *44*, 2491–2500. [CrossRef] [PubMed]

18. Paige, J.S.; Nguyen-Duc, T.; Song, W.; Jaffrey, S.R. Fluorescence imaging of cellular metabolites with RNA. *Science* **2012**, *335*, 1194. [CrossRef] [PubMed]

19. Kellenberger, C.A.; Wilson, S.C.; Sales-Lee, J.; Hammond, M.C. RNA-based fluorescent biosensors for live cell imaging of second messengers cyclic di-GMP and cyclic AMP-GMP. *J. Am. Chem. Soc.* **2013**, *135*, 4906–4909. [CrossRef] [PubMed]

20. Trachman, R.J., 3rd; Demeshkina, N.A.; Lau, M.W.; Panchapakesan, S.S.S.; Jeng, S.C.; Unrau, P.J.; Ferré-D'Amaré, A.R. Structural basis for high-affinity fluorophore binding and activation by RNA Mango. *Nat. Chem. Biol.* **2017**, *13*, 807–813. [CrossRef] [PubMed]

21. Autour, A.; Jeng, S.; Cawte, A.; Abdolahzadeh, A.; Galli, A.; Panchapakesan, S.S.; Rueda, D.; Ryckelynck, M.; Unrau, P.J. Fluorogenic RNA Mango aptamers for imaging small non-coding RNAs in mammalian cells. *Nat. Commun.* **2018**, *9*, 656. [CrossRef] [PubMed]

22. Sunbul, M.; Jaschke, A. SRB-2: A promiscuous rainbow aptamer for live-cell RNA imaging. *Nucleic Acids Res.* **2018**. [CrossRef] [PubMed]

23. Yoon, S.; Rossi, J.J. Emerging cancer-specific therapeutic aptamers. *Curr. Opin. Oncol.* **2017**, *29*, 366–374. [CrossRef] [PubMed]

24. Yoon, S.; Huang, K.W.; Reebye, V.; Mintz, P.; Tien, Y.W.; Lai, H.S.; Sætrom, P.; Reccia, I.; Swiderski, P.; Armstrong, B.; et al. Targeted Delivery of C/EBPα-saRNA by Pancreatic Ductal Adenocarcinoma-specific RNA Aptamers Inhibits Tumor Growth In Vivo. *Mol. Ther.* **2016**, *24*, 1106–1116. [CrossRef] [PubMed]

25. Duan, M.; Long, Y.; Yang, C.; Wu, X.; Sun, Y.; Li, J.; Hu, X.; Lin, W.; Han, D.; Zhao, Y.; et al. Selection and characterization of DNA aptamer for metastatic prostate cancer recognition and tissue imaging. *Oncotarget* **2016**, *7*, 36436–36446. [CrossRef] [PubMed]

26. Chughtai, K.; Heeren, R.M. Mass spectrometric imaging for biomedical tissue analysis. *Chem. Rev.* **2010**, *110*, 3237–3277. [CrossRef] [PubMed]

27. Chen, S.; Xiong, C.; Liu, H.; Wan, Q.; Hou, J.; He, Q.; Badu-Tawiah, A.; Nie, Z. Mass spectrometry imaging reveals the sub-organ distribution of carbon nanomaterials. *Nat. Nanotechnol.* **2015**, *10*, 176–182. [CrossRef] [PubMed]

28. Tseng, Y.T.; Harroun, S.G.; Wu, C.W.; Mao, J.Y.; Chang, H.T.; Huang, C.C. Satellite-like Gold Nanocomposites for Targeted Mass Spectrometry Imaging of Tumor Tissues. *Nanotheranostics* **2017**, *1*, 141–153. [CrossRef] [PubMed]

29. Shi, H.; Tang, Z.; Kim, Y.; Nie, H.; Huang, Y.F.; He, X.; Deng, K.; Wang, K.; Tan, W. In vivo fluorescence imaging of tumors using molecular aptamers generated by cell-SELEX. *Chem. Asian J.* **2010**, *5*, 2209–2213. [CrossRef] [PubMed]

30. Shi, H.; Cui, W.; He, X.; Guo, Q.; Wang, K.; Ye, X.; Tang, J. Whole cell-SELEX aptamers for highly specific fluorescence molecular imaging of carcinomas in vivo. *PLoS ONE* **2013**, *8*, e70476. [CrossRef] [PubMed]

31. Wu, P.; Yan, X.P. Doped quantum dots for chemo/biosensing and bioimaging. *Chem. Soc. Rev.* **2013**, *42*, 5489–5521. [CrossRef] [PubMed]

32. Zhang, C.; Ji, X.; Zhang, Y.; Zhou, G.; Ke, X.; Wang, H.; Tinnefeld, P.; He, Z. One-pot synthesized aptamer-functionalized CdTe:Zn^{2+} quantum dots for tumor-targeted fluorescence imaging in vitro and in vivo. *Anal. Chem.* **2013**, *85*, 5843–5849. [CrossRef] [PubMed]

33. Greenall, S.A.; Donoghue, J.F.; Van Sinderen, M.; Dubljevic, V.; Budiman, S.; Devlin, M.; Street, I.; Adams, T.E.; Johns, T.G. EGFRvIII-mediated transactivation of receptor tyrosine kinases in glioma: Mechanism and therapeutic implications. *Oncogene* **2015**, *34*, 5277–5287. [CrossRef] [PubMed]

34. Tang, J.; Huang, N.; Zhang, X.; Zhou, T.; Tan, Y.; Pi, J.; Pi, L.; Cheng, S.; Zheng, H.; Cheng, Y. Aptamer-conjugated PEGylated quantum dots targeting epidermal growth factor receptor variant III for fluorescence imaging of glioma. *Int. J. Nanomed.* **2017**, *12*, 3899–3911. [CrossRef] [PubMed]

35. Kim, M.W.; Jeong, H.Y.; Kang, S.J.; Choi, M.J.; You, Y.M.; Im, C.S.; Lee, T.S.; Song, I.H.; Lee, C.G.; Rhee, K.J.; et al. Cancer-targeted Nucleic Acid Delivery and Quantum Dot Imaging Using EGF Receptor Aptamer-conjugated Lipid Nanoparticles. *Sci. Rep.* **2017**, *7*, 9474. [CrossRef] [PubMed]

36. Dassie, J.P.; Hernandez, L.I.; Thomas, G.S.; Long, M.E.; Rockey, W.M.; Howell, C.A.; Chen, Y.; Hernandez, F.J.; Liu, X.Y.; Wilson, M.E.; et al. Targeted inhibition of prostate cancer metastases with an RNA aptamer to prostate-specific membrane antigen. *Mol. Ther.* **2014**, *22*, 1910–1922. [CrossRef] [PubMed]

37. Chen, H.; Zhao, J.; Zhang, M.; Yang, H.; Ma, Y.; Gu, Y. MUC1 aptamer-based near-infrared fluorescence probes for tumor imaging. *Mol. Imaging Biol.* **2015**, *17*, 38–48. [CrossRef] [PubMed]

38. Jacobs, R.E.; Papan, C.; Ruffins, S.; Tyszka, J.M.; Fraser, S.E. MRI: Volumetric imaging for vital imaging and atlas construction. *Nat. Rev. Mol. Cell Biol.* **2003**, *4*, SS10–SS16. [CrossRef]

39. Sipkins, D.A.; Cheresh, D.A.; Kazemi, M.R.; Nevin, L.M.; Bednarski, M.D.; Li, K.C. Detection of tumor angiogenesis in vivo by alphaVbeta3-targeted magnetic resonance imaging. *Nat. Med.* **1998**, *4*, 623–626. [CrossRef] [PubMed]

40. Lim, E.K.; Kim, B.; Choi, Y.; Ro, Y.; Cho, E.J.; Lee, J.H.; Ryu, S.H.; Suh, J.S.; Haam, S.; Huh, Y.M. Aptamer-conjugated magnetic nanoparticles enable efficient targeted detection of integrin alphavbeta3 via magnetic resonance imaging. *J. Biomed. Mater. Res. A* **2014**, *102*, 49–59. [CrossRef] [PubMed]

41. Kim, B.; Yang, J.; Hwang, M.; Choi, J.; Kim, H.O.; Jang, E.; Lee, J.H.; Ryu, S.H.; Suh, J.S.; Huh, Y.M.; et al. Aptamer-modified magnetic nanoprobe for molecular MR imaging of VEGFR2 on angiogenic vasculature. *Nanoscale Res. Lett.* **2013**, *8*, 399. [CrossRef] [PubMed]

42. Paolicchi, E.; Gemignani, F.; Krstic-Demonacos, M.; Dedhar, S.; Mutti, L.; Landi, S. Targeting hypoxic response for cancer therapy. *Oncotarget* **2016**, *7*, 13464–13478. [CrossRef] [PubMed]

43. Zhu, H.; Zhang, L.; Liu, Y.; Zhou, Y.; Wang, K.; Xie, X.; Song, L.; Wang, D.; Han, C.; Chen, Q. Aptamer-PEG-modified Fe$_3$O$_4$@Mn as a novel T1- and T2-dual-model MRI contrast agent targeting hypoxia-induced cancer stem cells. *Sci. Rep.* **2016**, *6*, 39245. [CrossRef] [PubMed]

44. Lu, F.M.; Yuan, Z. PET/SPECT molecular imaging in clinical neuroscience: Recent advances in the investigation of CNS diseases. *Quant. Imaging Med. Surg.* **2015**, *5*, 433–447. [PubMed]

45. Ray, P.; Viles, K.D.; Soule, E.E.; Woodruff, R.S. Application of aptamers for targeted therapeutics. *Arch. Immunol. Ther. Exp.* **2013**, *61*, 255–271. [CrossRef] [PubMed]

46. Hicke, B.J.; Stephens, A.W.; Gould, T.; Chang, Y.; Lynott, C.K.; Heil, J.; Borkowski, S.; Hilger, C.; Cook, G.; Warren, S.; et al. Tumor targeting by an aptamer. *J. Nucl. Med.* **2006**, *47*, 668–678. [PubMed]

47. Bonner, J.A.; De Los Santos, J.; Waksal, H.W.; Needle, M.N.; Trummel, H.Q.; Raisch, K.P. Epidermal growth factor receptor as a therapeutic target in head and neck cancer. *Semin. Radiat. Oncol.* **2002**, *12*, 1–20. [CrossRef]

48. Hofmann, U.B.; Westphal, J.R.; van Muijen, G.N.; Ruiter, D.J. Matrix metalloproteinases in human melanoma. *J. Investig. Dermatol.* **2000**, *115*, 337–344. [CrossRef] [PubMed]

49. Kryza, D.; Debordeaux, F.; Azéma, L.; Hassan, A.; Paurelle, O.; Schulz, J.; Savona-Baron, C.; Charignon, E.; Bonazza, P.; Taleb, J.; et al. Ex Vivo and In Vivo Imaging and Biodistribution of Aptamers Targeting the Human Matrix MetalloProtease-9 in Melanomas. *PLoS ONE* **2016**, *11*, e0149387. [CrossRef] [PubMed]

50. Wu, X.; Liang, H.; Tan, Y.; Yuan, C.; Li, S.; Li, X.; Li, G.; Shi, Y.; Zhang, X. Cell-SELEX aptamer for highly specific radionuclide molecular imaging of glioblastoma in vivo. *PLoS ONE* **2014**, *9*, e90752. [CrossRef] [PubMed]

51. Gambhir, S.S. Molecular imaging of cancer with positron emission tomography. *Nat. Rev. Cancer* **2002**, *2*, 683–693. [CrossRef] [PubMed]

52. Li, J.; Zheng, H.; Bates, P.J.; Malik, T.; Li, X.F.; Trent, J.O.; Ng, C.K. Aptamer imaging with Cu-64 labeled AS1411: Preliminary assessment in lung cancer. *Nucl. Med. Biol.* **2014**, *41*, 179–185. [CrossRef] [PubMed]

53. Oskarsson, T.; Acharyya, S.; Zhang, X.H.; Vanharanta, S.; Tavazoie, S.F.; Morris, P.G.; Downey, R.J.; Manova-Todorova, K.; Brogi, E.; Massagué, J. Breast cancer cells produce tenascin C as a metastatic niche component to colonize the lungs. *Nat. Med.* **2011**, *17*, 867–874. [CrossRef] [PubMed]

54. Leins, A.; Riva, P.; Lindstedt, R.; Davidoff, M.S.; Mehraein, P.; Weis, S. Expression of tenascin-C in various human brain tumors and its relevance for survival in patients with astrocytoma. *Cancer* **2003**, *98*, 2430–2439. [CrossRef] [PubMed]

55. Jacobson, O.; Yan, X.; Niu, G.; Weiss, I.D.; Ma, Y.; Szajek, L.P.; Shen, B.; Kiesewetter, D.O.; Chen, X. PET imaging of tenascin-C with a radiolabeled single-stranded DNA aptamer. *J. Nucl. Med.* **2015**, *56*, 616–621. [CrossRef] [PubMed]

56. Park, J.Y.; Lee, T.S.; Song, I.H.; Cho, Y.L.; Chae, J.R.; Yun, M.; Kang, H.; Lee, J.H.; Lim, J.H.; Cho, W.G.; et al. Hybridization-based aptamer labeling using complementary oligonucleotide platform for PET and optical imaging. *Biomaterials* **2016**, *100*, 143–151. [CrossRef] [PubMed]

57. Shangguan, D.; Li, Y.; Tang, Z.; Cao, Z.C.; Chen, H.W.; Mallikaratchy, P.; Sefah, K.; Yang, C.J.; Tan, W. Aptamers evolved from live cells as effective molecular probes for cancer study. *Proc. Natl. Acad. Sci. USA* **2006**, *103*, 11838–11843. [CrossRef] [PubMed]

58. Wang, L.; Jacobson, O.; Avdic, D.; Rotstein, B.H.; Weiss, I.D.; Collier, L.; Chen, X.; Vasdev, N.; Liang, S.H. Ortho-Stabilized (18) F-Azido Click Agents and their Application in PET Imaging with Single-Stranded DNA Aptamers. *Angew. Chem. Int. Ed. Engl.* **2015**, *54*, 12777–12781. [CrossRef] [PubMed]

59. Kim, D.; Jeong, Y.Y.; Jon, S. A drug-loaded aptamer-gold nanoparticle bioconjugate for combined CT imaging and therapy of prostate cancer. *ACS Nano* **2010**, *4*, 3689–3696. [CrossRef] [PubMed]

60. Li, C.H.; Kuo, T.R.; Su, H.J.; Lai, W.Y.; Yang, P.C.; Chen, J.S.; Wang, D.Y.; Wu, Y.C.; Chen, C.C. Fluorescence-Guided Probes of Aptamer-Targeted Gold Nanoparticles with Computed Tomography Imaging Accesses for in Vivo Tumor Resection. *Sci. Rep.* **2015**, *5*, 15675. [CrossRef] [PubMed]

61. Ma, J.; Shen, M.; Xu, C.S.; Sun, Y.; Duan, Y.R.; Du, L.F. Biodegradable double-targeted PTX-mPEG-PLGA nanoparticles for ultrasound contrast enhanced imaging and antitumor therapy in vitro. *Oncotarget* **2016**, *7*, 80008–80018. [CrossRef] [PubMed]

62. Wu, M.; Wang, Y.; Wang, Y.; Zhang, M.; Luo, Y.; Tang, J.; Wang, Z.; Wang, D.; Hao, L.; Wang, Z. Paclitaxel-loaded and A10-3.2 aptamer-targeted poly(lactide-*co*-glycolic acid) nanobubbles for ultrasound imaging and therapy of prostate cancer. *Int. J. Nanomed.* **2017**, *12*, 5313–5330. [CrossRef] [PubMed]

63. Zhang, J.; Smaga, L.P.; Satyavolu, N.S.R.; Chan, J.; Lu, Y. DNA Aptamer-Based Activatable Probes for Photoacoustic Imaging in Living Mice. *J. Am. Chem. Soc.* **2017**, *139*, 17225–17228. [CrossRef] [PubMed]

64. Kang, W.J.; Lee, J.; Lee, Y.S.; Cho, S.; Ali, B.A.; Al-Khedhairy, A.A.; Heo, H.; Kim, S. Multimodal imaging probe for targeting cancer cells using uMUC-1 aptamer. *Colloids Surf. B Biointerfaces* **2015**, *136*, 134–140. [CrossRef] [PubMed]

65. Ni, S.; Yao, H.; Wang, L.; Lu, J.; Jiang, F.; Lu, A.; Zhang, G. Chemical Modifications of Nucleic Acid Aptamers for Therapeutic Purposes. *Int. J. Mol. Sci.* **2017**, *18*, 1683. [CrossRef] [PubMed]

66. Roy, K.; Kanwar, R.K.; Kanwar, J.R. LNA aptamer based multi-modal, Fe_3O_4-saturated lactoferrin (Fe_3O_4-bLf) nanocarriers for triple positive (EpCAM, CD133, CD44) colon tumor targeting and NIR, MRI and CT imaging. *Biomaterials* **2015**, *71*, 84–99. [CrossRef] [PubMed]

5

Clopidogrel Pharmacokinetics in Malaysian Population Groups: The Impact of Inter-Ethnic Variability

Zaril H. Zakaria [1,2] (iD), **Alan Y. Y. Fong** [1,3,4] (iD) and **Raj K. S. Badhan** [2,5,]* (iD)

[1] Ministry of Health Malaysia, Block E1, E3, E6, E7 & E10, Parcel E, Federal Government Administration Centre, Putrajaya 62590, Malaysia; zakariz1@aston.ac.uk (Z.H.Z.); alanfong@crc.gov.my (A.Y.Y.F.)

[2] Applied Health Research Group, School of Life and Health Sciences, Aston University, Birmingham B4 7ET, UK

[3] Sarawak Heart Centre, Kota Samarahan 94300, Malaysia

[4] Clinical Research Centre, Sarawak General Hospital, Kuching 93586, Malaysia

[5] Aston Pharmacy School, Aston University, Birmingham B4 7ET, UK

* Correspondence: r.k.s.badhan@aston.ac.uk

Abstract: Malaysia is a multi-ethnic society whereby the impact of pharmacogenetic differences between ethnic groups may contribute significantly to variability in clinical therapy. One of the leading causes of mortality in Malaysia is cardiovascular disease (CVD), which accounts for up to 26% of all hospital deaths annually. Clopidogrel is used as an adjunct treatment in the secondary prevention of cardiovascular events. CYP2C19 plays an integral part in the metabolism of clopidogrel to the active metabolite clopi-H4. However, CYP2C19 genetic polymorphism, prominent in Malaysians, could influence target clopi-H4 plasma concentrations for clinical efficacy. This study addresses how inter-ethnicity variability within the Malaysian population impacts the attainment of clopi-H4 target plasma concentration under different CYP2C19 polymorphisms through pharmacokinetic (PK) modelling. We illustrated a statistically significant difference ($P < 0.001$) in the clopi-H4 C_{max} between the extensive metabolisers (EM) and poor metabolisers (PM) phenotypes with either Malay or Malaysian Chinese population groups. Furthermore, the number of PM individuals with peak clopi-H4 concentrations below the minimum therapeutic level was partially recovered using a high-dose strategy (600 mg loading dose followed by a 150 mg maintenance dose), which resulted in an approximate 50% increase in subjects attaining the minimum clopi-H4 plasma concentration for a therapeutic effect.

Keywords: PBPK; pharmacokinetics; clopidogrel; CVD; Malaysian

1. Introduction

Malaysia is a multi-ethnic society with a population of over 32 million that is comprised of three predominant ethic groups, namely Malays (50.1%), Chinese (20.8%) and Indians (6.2%) [1]. In a recent report by the Malaysian National Centre for Adverse Drug Reaction, 13,789 adverse drug reactions were reported during the period from 2015 to 2016 [2]. Given the mixed ethnicity of Malaysia, the impact of pharmacogenetic differences amongst ethnic groups may contribute significantly to the prevalence of toxicity and ineffective clinical therapy [3–5].

One of the leading causes of mortality in Malaysia is cardiovascular disease (CVD), which accounts for 22.6% and 26.4% of all hospital deaths annually in Ministry of Health Malaysia hospitals and Malaysian private hospitals, respectively [6]. Among those deaths, ischaemic heart disease accounts for the majority of all reported cardiovascular mortality, followed by acute myocardial infarction.

Furthermore, mortality rates have increased steadily since 1990 despite improvements in health services [6].

Clopidogrel is a second generation thienopyridine antiplatelet drug and a prodrug that is metabolised through two pathways: initially by CYP2B6, CYP1A2 and CYP2C19 leading to the inactive carboxylic acid derivative (2-oxo-clopidogrel), and subsequently by CYP2C19, CYP2C9, CYP2B6 and CYP3A4, leading to its active metabolite (clopi-H4) [7] (Figure 1). The active metabolite confers clopidogrel its therapeutic response by inhibition of adenosine diphosphate-induced aggregation, which in turn activates the irreversible binding of the platelet P2Y12 receptor [8]. The contribution of CYP2C19 towards the formation of clopi-H4 has been further confirmed by several studies [9–11] and contributes 45% of the first step and 20% of the second step of total hepatic biotransformation [12,13]. Since CYP2C19 plays an integral part in the metabolism of clopidogrel, any disruption or modification in CYP2C19 expression could potentially affect the pharmacokinetic profiles of clopi-H4, hence leading to effects on its therapeutic response [14].

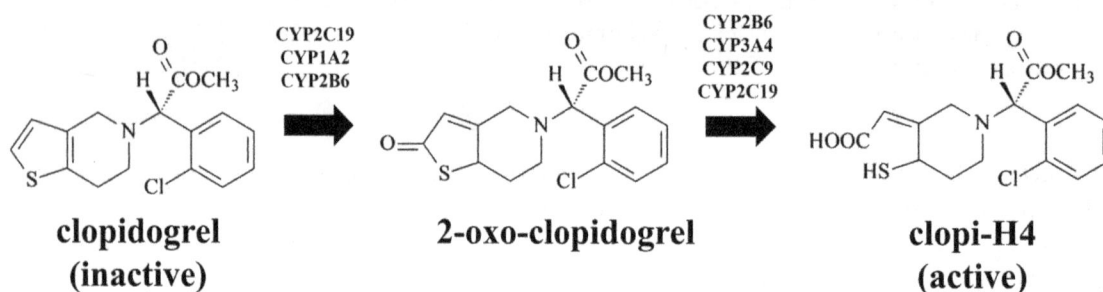

Figure 1. Biotransformation of clopidogrel to the active (H4) metabolite.

Clinically, approximately one-fourth of individuals who are treated with clopidogrel exhibit a sub-therapeutic response [15], with the loss-of-function genotype reducing platelet inhibition by clopidogrel [16,17] as a result of reduced clopi-H4 levels [12,18].

More than 50 genetic variants have been identified for CYP2C19 [19]. The wild-type CYP2C19*1 allele is related to functional CYP2C19 metabolism, with CYP2C19*2 and *3 being associated with a lost-of-function (LOF) [20]. Gain-of-function (GOF) variants have also been identified and are primarily related to the CYP2C19*17 variant, which results in higher catalytic activity of CYP2C19 [21]. Thus, individuals presenting with the homozygote and heterozygote allelic variants *2/*2, *3/*3, or *2/*3 are considered to be representative of poor metaboliser (PM) phenotypes; those with variants *1/*2 or *1/*3 (and possibly *2/*17 or *3/*17) are considered intermediate metaboliser (IM) phenotypes; those with *1/*1 are considered wild-type or extensive metaboliser (EM) phenotypes and those with *17/*17 or *1/*17 are considered ultra-rapid metabolisers (UM) [22]. Significant inter-ethnic differences exist in the prevalence of these allelic frequencies, with the CYP2C19*2 [23] and CYP2C19*3 [24] alleles in the broader Asian populations being significantly higher compared to other racial groups [3,25]. This would suggest that Asian population groups would be more likely to be resistant to clopidogrel therapy. In European population groups, EM phenotypes predominate with approximately 30% EM and 2% presenting as PM [26–28]. Within the Malaysian population group, Chinese and Malays have broadly similar prevalence of the *1/*1 genotype, 31.6% and 34.5%, respectively [26–29]. Furthermore, *1/*17 genotypes were broadly similar (3.5% and 3.5% for Chinese and Malays respectively). However, some differences were noted in the prevalence of genotypes, for example, *1/*2 was greater for Chinese (43.9%) compared to Malay (31%) and *1/*3 was higher for Malay (17.2%) compared to Chinese (3.5%) [29].

LOF genotypes can often result in reduced active metabolite plasma concentrations. For example, in a clinical study by Brandt et al. [18], the maximum clopi-H4 plasma concentration (C_{max}) for wild-type CYP2C19 subjects ($n = 56$) was 58.4 ± 9.2 ng/mL, compared to CYP2C19*2 carriers, for whom the mean C_{max} was reported to be 35.3 ± 4.3 ng/mL, a 40% decrease in C_{max}. Furthermore, pharmacogenetic studies have utilised dose optimisation to counter this reduced clopi-H4 C_{max}, whereby a loading dose of 600 mg followed by a maintenance dose of 150 mg could partially restore clopi-H4 to levels observed with a lower loading dose of 300 mg and the standard 75 mg maintenance dose [9].

The advent of personalised medicine has allowed the clinicians to better respond to the impact of genetic variability on clopidogrel therapy. However, such genotyping techniques have met with some contrasting views in relation to their clinic usefulness [30,31]. The impact of anthropometric difference within a diverse patient population group can further confound the understanding of the impact of CYP2C19 genetic variability within mixed populations, and these factored together may significantly alter the pharmacokinetics of drugs. Examples of these factors may include differences within patient demographics (body weight, age, glomerular filtration rate (GFR)), blood biochemistry (plasma proteins, haematocrit) and drug metabolism enzyme abundances (CYP abundance and polymorphism).

Precision medicine allows an individual's unique physiological characteristics to be incorporated into treatment options, whereby treatments are tailored to individual patients based on their individual genetic, biomarker, phenotypic, and psychosocial characteristics [32,33]. To assist in the process of integrating such a diverse range of anthropometric and genetic factors into clinical decision-making, the application of pharmacokinetic modelling and simulation has emerged as techniques to better individualise drug therapy. In particular, the field of population-based physiologically based pharmacokinetic (PBPK) modelling has rapidly gained traction by drug regulatory authorities and the wider pharmaceutical industry as a viable means to 'simulate' clinical trials and the pharmacokinetics of drug compounds within virtual population groups representative of individual population groups [34–39]. Furthermore, the application of PBPK modelling can allow for the use of population-specific anthropometric variability within virtual subjects, and this was recently demonstrated by our group when considering the optimisation of anti-malarial therapy in sub-Saharan African population groups using PBPK-based virtual clinical trials, where the population groups incorporated anthropometric and biochemical alterations from standard 'healthy volunteer' clinical trials subjects [40,41].

To our knowledge, we present here the first application of PBPK modelling to develop a Malaysian population group for the specific purpose of understating the impact of genotype drug therapy within this mixed-ethnicity population. The study directly addresses this inter-ethnicity variability and provides a research tool that brings together the complexity (at a cellular level) of systems-biology with the ease-of-use applicability of pharmacokinetic modelling to provide a robust predictive platform that can easily be adapted and developed as required within the Malaysian population. The objectives of the present study were two-fold: (i) to predict clopidogrel pharmacokinetics in the Malay and Malaysian Chinese adult population groups and (ii) to address the impact of the *1/*1, *2/*2, *1/*2 and *1/*17 CYP2C19 genotype on clopidogrel pharmacokinetic.

2. Results

2.1. Step 1: Malaysian Population Group Development

2.1.1. The National Cardiovascular Disease Database

The three largest population groups were selected for analysis and identified as Malay, Chinese and Indian, with Malay comprising the largest ethnic group contained within the National Cardiovascular Disease (NCVD) database (Table 1). The mean age, weight and BMI were significantly different between Malay and Malaysian Chinese ($p < 0.0001$) and Malaysian Chinese and Malaysian Indian ($p < 0.0001$), whereas mean height was relatively consistent across all population groups (1.63 m) and is not statistically significantly different (Table 1).

Table 1. Summary demographic data from the NCVD database.

Ethnicity		Age (years)	Height (m)	Weight (kg)	BMI (kg/m^2)
Malay	Mean	57.75	1.63	69.79	26.19
	Median	57.6	1.63	69.5	25.78
	N	23114	10250	12193	10170
	SD	11.62	0.08	14.24	4.35
Malaysian Chinese	Mean	62.89	1.63	67.17	25.11
	Median	63.1	1.63	66	24.79
	N	9929	4111	5259	4086
	SD	12.04	0.08	13.18	3.84
Malaysian Indian	Mean	57.7	1.63	69.61	25.95
	Median	57.3	1.64	69	25.52
	N	9167	4257	4809	4229
	SD	11.91	0.09	13.91	4.25

N: total number of recorded metrics; SD: standard deviation.

2.1.2. Development of Age–Weight Relationships for Malaysian Populations

Malaysian population groups were subsequently developed for the Malay and Malaysian Chinese groups. Polynomial mathematical relationship for gender-specific age–weight relationships for the Malay population group are described in Equations (1) and (2) for 20–65 year olds:

$$\text{Malay male body weight} = -786.757075 + (-105.598305 \times \text{age}) + 9.79604022 \times \text{age}^{1.5} + (-0.33871491 \times \text{age}^2) + 498.1612119 \times \text{age}^{0.5}, \tag{1}$$

$$\text{Malay female body weight} = -3348.57622 + 2424.271248 \times \text{age}^{0.5} + (-676.182360 \times \text{age}) + 92.98417478 \times \text{age}^{1.5} + (-6.31405170 \times \text{age}^2) + 0.169288237 \times \text{age}^{2.5}. \tag{2}$$

Visual predictive checks confirmed that model predicted age–weight relationships retained the same distribution across age ranges when compared to the NCVD for Malay males (Figure 2A) and females (Figure 2B).

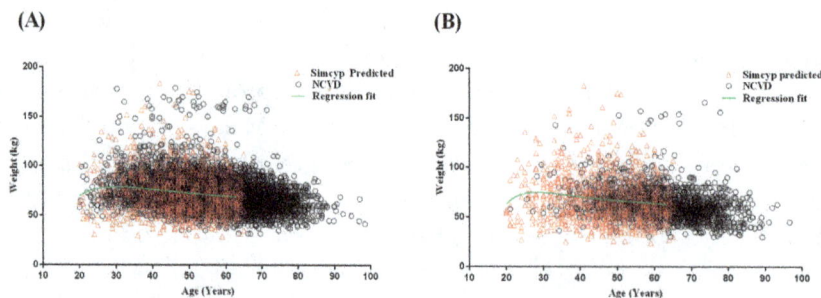

Figure 2. Visual predictive checks for the comparison between predicted and observed (NCVD) age–weight relationship for Malay male ($n = 18,601$) (**A**) and female ($n = 4513$) (**B**) populations. Red outlined triangles represent the Simcyp predicted population age–weight relationships. Black outlined circles represent the observed population age–weight relationships from the NCVD database. Green lines represent the fitted trend-line from the polynomial mathematical relationship.

The polynomial mathematical relationship for gender-specific age–weight relationships for the Malaysian Chinese population group is described in Equations (3) and (4) for 20–65 year olds:

$$\text{Malaysian Chinese male body weight} = (75.50929026 + (-3.86906581 \times \text{age}) + 0.034908233 \times \text{age}^2 + 0.001047109 \times \text{age}^3)/(1 + (-0.04452164 \times \text{age}) + 0.0000141817 \times \text{age}^2 + 0.0000206378 \times \text{age}^3), \tag{3}$$

$$\text{Malaysian Chinese female body weight} = 67.51927661 + (-0.00194867 \times age^2) + \\ 0.0000000434656 \times age^4. \tag{4}$$

Visual predictive checks were performed to assess the graphical qualification between the polynomial mathematical relationship for age and weight relationships of the software and the observed Malaysian Chinese male and female populations (Figure 3), and confirmed that model predicted age–weight relationships retained the same distribution across age ranges when compared to the NCVD (Figure 3).

(A)   **(B)**

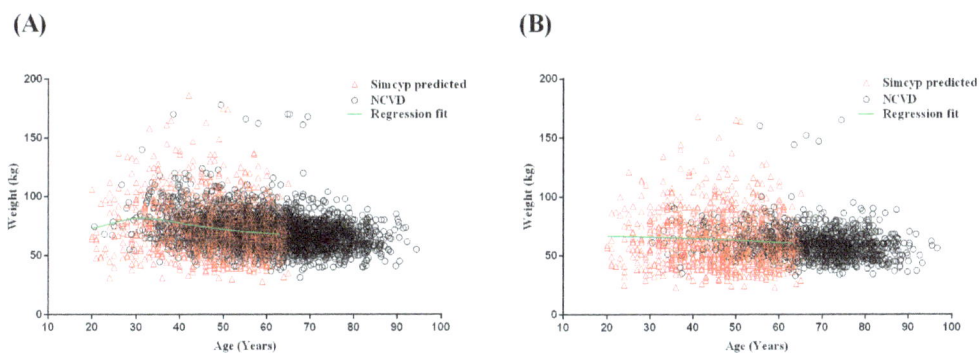

Figure 3. Visual predictive checks on the comparison between predicted and observed (NCVD) age–weight relationship for Chinese male ($n = 7445$) (**A**) and female ($n = 2484$) (**B**) population. Red outlined triangles represent the Simcyp predicted population age–weight relationships. Black outlined circles represent the observed population age–weight relationships from the NCVD database. Green lines represent the fitted trend-line from the polynomial mathematical relationship.

2.2. Step 2: Adult Simulations: Validation with Repaglinide, Tramadol and Rosuvastatin

2.2.1. Repaglinide

The repaglinide compound file within the Simcyp library was used in conjunction with the Simcyp 'Healthy Volunteer' population group to predict the plasma concentration–time profile for a single 2 mg oral dose of repaglinide in healthy Caucasian subjects. The resultant predictions were within the range of observed reported values (Figure 4) with model predicted t_{max} and C_{max} within two-fold of that reported and AUC within 2.15-fold of the reported (Table 2).

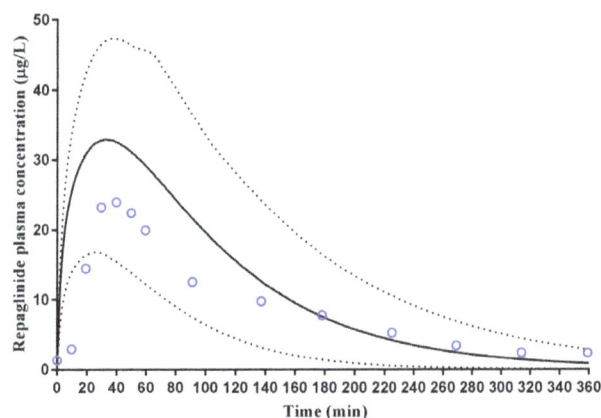

Figure 4. Simulated plasma concentration–time profile of repaglinide in healthy adults. A 2 mg oral dose of repaglinide was administered once daily to healthy adult volunteers ($n = 24$). Solid lines represent mean population prediction with dotted lines representing 5th and 95th percentile ranges. Open circles represent data for the observed study [42].

Subsequently, to further validate model simulations, the ability to predict repaglinide plasma concentrations following single and multiple dosing was assessed using a healthy volunteer population group. Predicted plasma concentrations following a single dose (day 1) and multiple doses (day 9) were within the range reported [43] (Figure 5), with model predicted t_{max}, C_{max} and AUC within two-fold of those reported [43] (Table 2). However, the terminal elimination phase was poorly predicted.

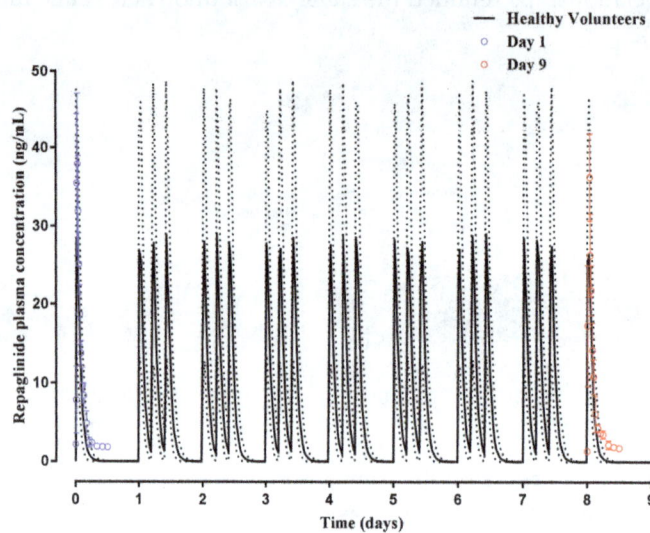

Figure 5. Simulated plasma concentration–time profile of repaglinide following single and multiple doses in healthy adults. An oral dose of 2 mg was administered once daily on day 1, and thereafter daily for nine days to healthy adult volunteers ($n = 12$). Solid lines represent mean predictions with dotted lines representing the 5th and 95th percentile ranges. Open circles represent data for the observed study at day 1 (single dose) and day 9 (multiple-dosing) [43].

The model was then extended to assess its application within Malay and Malaysian Chinese population groups. For the Malaysian Chinese population, we utilised the customised Malaysian Chinese population group in the model to predict repaglinide plasma concentrations following a single 2 mg oral dose (Figure 6). The predicted repaglinide plasma concentration was within the range reported with model predicted t_{max}, C_{max} and AUC within two-fold of those reported [43] (Table 2).

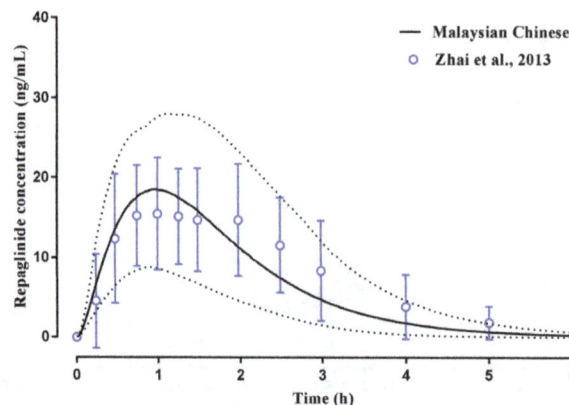

Figure 6. Simulated plasma concentration–time profile of repaglinide in healthy Malaysian Chinese adults. A 2 mg oral dose of repaglinide was administered once daily to adult healthy Chinese volunteers ($n = 22$) using the Malaysian Chinese population group. Solid lines represent mean predictions with dotted lines representing the 5th and 95th percentile ranges. Open circles represent data for the observed study [44].

For the Malay population group, model predicted C_{max} and t_{max} were within the range reported (Figure 7) with clearance (CL) predictions within two-fold of that reported and AUC 2.25-fold of that reported [45] (Table 2).

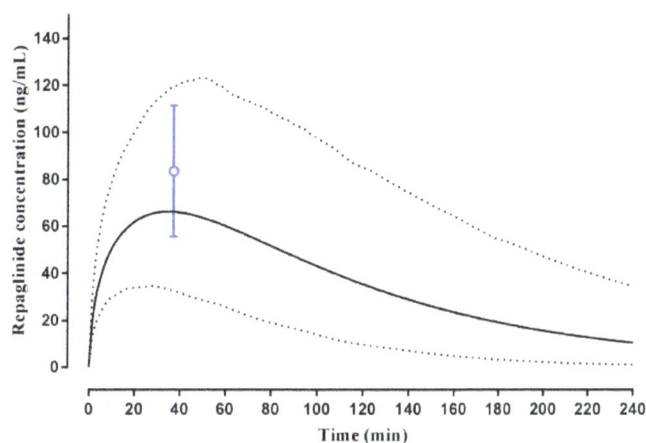

Figure 7. Simulated plasma concentration–time profile of repaglinide in healthy Malay adults. A 4 mg oral dose of repaglinide was administered once daily to adult healthy Malay volunteers ($n = 121$) using the custom Malay Simcyp population group. Solid lines represent mean predictions with dotted lines representing the 5th and 95th percentile ranges. Open circles represent data for the observed study [45].

2.2.2. Tramadol

Tramadol pharmacokinetics have been reported in mixed Malaysian subjects following an IV bolus dose [46]. Furthermore, T'jollyn et al. [47] have developed and validated a tramadol compound within Simcyp, and these studies were used as the basis for predicting tramadol pharmacokinetics in the Malay and Malaysian Chinese populations. Following a 100 mg IV-bolus dose of tramadol, simulated plasma concentrations for Malays and Malaysian Chinese were within the range reported by Gan et al. [46] (Figure 8) with model predicted CL and AUC within two-fold of that reported (Table 2).

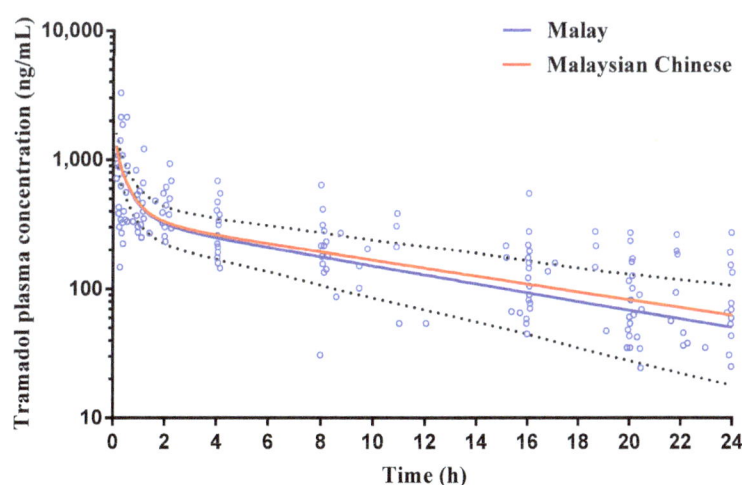

Figure 8. Simulated plasma concentration–time profile of tramadol intravenous bolus dosing in Malay and Malaysian Chinse subjects. An IV-bolus dose of 100 mg tramadol was administered to adult healthy mixed Malaysian volunteers ($n = 100$) using the custom Malaysian (Malay and Malaysian Chinese) Simcyp population group. Solid lines represent mean predictions with dotted lines represent the 5th and 95th percentile ranges. Open circles represent data for the observed study [46].

2.2.3. Rosuvastatin

Rosuvastatin pharmacokinetics have been reported in Caucasian and Asian (Chinese and Malay) subjects following a 40 mg oral dose [48]. Using the rosuvastatin compound within the Simcyp library, simulated plasma concentration–time profiles for all subjects were within the range reported by Lee et al. [48] (Figure 9), with model predicted C_{max}, t_{max} and AUC within two-fold of that reported (Table 2).

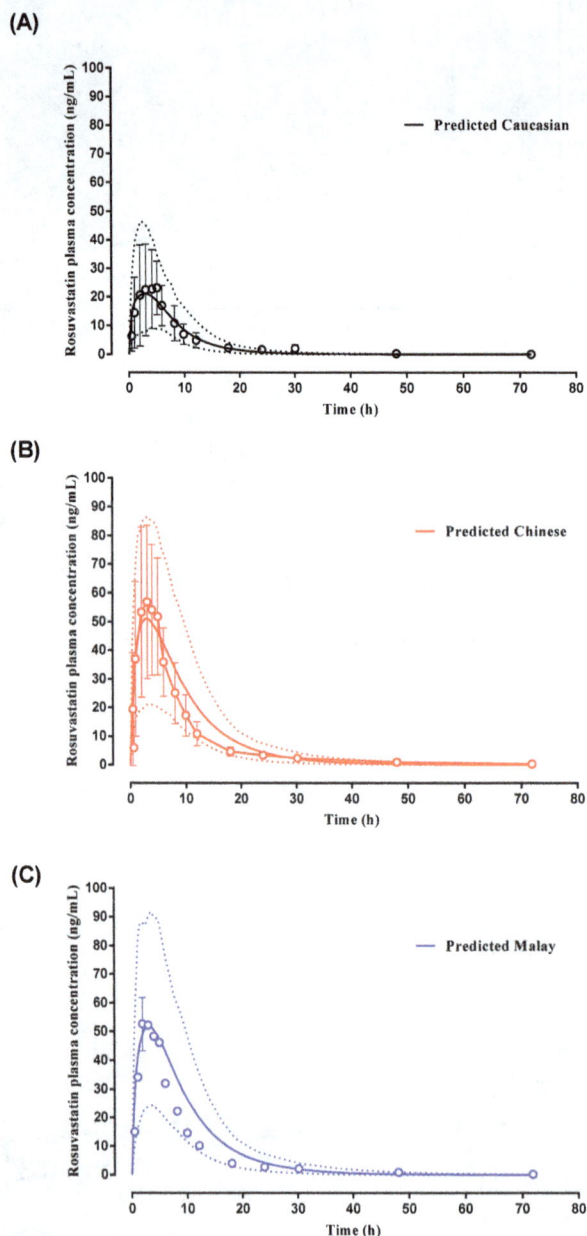

Figure 9. Simulated plasma concentration–time profile of rosuvastatin in (**A**) Caucasian, (**B**) Chinese and (**C**) Malay subjects. A single 40 mg oral dose was administered to adult population groups ($n = 36$ for each population group, matching the reported study recruitment for each population group) using the Simcyp Heathy Volunteer (Caucasian), Simcyp Healthy Chinese (Chinese) and custom Malay population groups. Solid lines represent mean predictions with dotted lines representing the 5th and 95th percentile ranges. Open circles represent mean data for the observed study with error bars indicating standard deviation where reported by Lee et al. [48] (and largely missing in results presented by Lee et al. for Malay subjects).

Table 2. Summary of predicted and observed pharmacokinetic parameters of repaglinide, tramadol and rosuvastatin.

Compound	Validation	CL (L/h) Observed	CL (L/h) Predicted	C_{max} (ng/mL) Observed	C_{max} (ng/mL) Predicted	t_{max} (h) Observed	t_{max} (h) Predicted	AUC (ng/mL·h) Observed	AUC (ng/mL·h) Predicted
Repaglinide	Hatorp et al., (2002) (Healthy volunteers)	-	12.17 (10.03–14.77)	26.0 µg/L	32.9 (16.4–47.0) µg/L	0.83 (0.31–1.35)	0.54 (0.18–0.91)	152.4 (62.8–242.0) µg/L·h	70.89 (15.51–73.82) µg/L·h
	Hatorp et al., (1999) (Single dose) (Healthy volunteers)	-	13.9 (10.33–18.70)	47.9 (15.9–79.9)	26.2 (19.61–35.0)	0.8 (0.2–1.4)	0.47 (0.31–0.60)	69.0 (61.2–76.8)	54.87 (21.57–106.1)
	Hatorp et al., (1999) (Multiple doses) (Healthy volunteers)	-	15.32 (12.24–20.57)	58.5 (8.1–108.9)	26.39 (11.53–46.85)	0.6 (0.5–0.7)	0.48 (0.32–0.61)	98.1 (84.54–111.66)	56.8 (22.59–109.1)
	Zhai et al. (2013) [1] (Chinese)	-	56.66 (21.10–146.00) (Malaysian Chinese)	20.0 (14.9–25.1)	18.5 (8.79–28.0) (Malaysian Chinese)	1.2 (0.5–1.9)	0.93 (0.82–1.08) (Malaysian Chinese)	46.3 (31.2–61.4)	39.51 (16.21–74.56) (Malaysian Chinese)
	Ruzilawati et al., (2010) (Malay)	11.82 (7.86–15.78)	10.41 (5.29–15.53)	83.56 (55.63–111.49)	67.5 (34.4–118)	0.62 (0.24–1.00)	0.58 (0.20–0.96)	340.66 (226.14–455.18)	151 (33.61–196)
Tramadol	Gan et al., (2002) [2] (Malaysian)	19.3 (13.1–25.5)	19.24 (13.31–33.11) (Malay); 18.36 (11.73–30.19) (Malaysian Chinese)	-	-	-	-	5078.4 (3117.3–7039.5)	4389 (2915–6128) (Malay); 4716 (3201–6658) (Malaysian Chinese)
Rosuvastatin	Lee et al., (2005) (Malay, Chinese, Healthy volunteers Caucasians)	-	21.87 (19.49–24.53) (Malay)	50.0 (42.2–59.3) (Malay)	49.91 (42.68–58.36) (Malay)	3.00 (0.50–5.00) (Malay)	3.01 (2.51–3.61) (Malay)	413 (354–482) (Malay)	552.84 (473.51–645.46) (Malay)
			21.28 (19.17–23.63) (Chinese)	59.1 (49.8–70.1) (Chinese)	53.83 (42.01–57.35) (Chinese)	3.00 (0.50–5.00) (Chinese)	2.90 (2.43–3.45) (Chinese)	500 (428–583) (Chinese)	553.18 (475.13–644.05) (Chinese)
			23.99 (22.40–25.70) (Healthy volunteers)	25.0 (21.1–29.6)	13.49 (10.55–14.28)	5.00 (1.00–8.00)	2.99 (2.15–3.16)	216 (186–252)	116.15 (98.70–136.68)

Data presented as mean (range). [1] Validation study was performed within a Malaysian Chinese group for comparison; Simulations were performed within a Malaysian Chinese population group for comparison. [2] Validation study was reported within a Malaysian population group without demarking ethnicities. Simulations were performed in Malay and Malaysian Chinese for comparison. CL: Oral clearance; C_{max}: maximum plasma concentration; t_{max}: time to maximum plasma concentration; AUC: area under the plasma concentration–time curve.

2.3. Step 3: Prediction of the Impact of CYP2C19 Polymorphisms on Clopidogrel Pharmacokinetics in Malaysians

To assess the impact of CYP2C19 SNPs on target clopi-H4 plasma concentrations (0.81–13.45 ng/mL) [49] simulations were conducted in Malay and Malaysian Chinese populations to assess the number of subjects within this therapeutic window. For these simulations, the lowest range of 0.81 ng/mL was used as a cut-off value to depict patients who were unresponsive to clopidogrel treatment. A loading dose of 300 mg was administered on day 1 and a maintenance dose of 75 mg once daily commenced from day 2 to day 5 and was administered to 400 subjects, each possessing either *1/*1, *2/*2, *1/*2 or *1/*17 genotypes (40 × 10 trials, 100 subjects per genotypes). This was conducted for both the Malay and the Malaysian Chinese population groups.

Within the Malay population, three subjects of *1/*1 genotype did not reach the target concentration, followed by 27 subjects with the *2/*2 genotype, 7 subjects with the *1/*2 genotype and three subjects with the *1/*17 genotype (Figure 10). In the Malaysian Chinese population, the number of subjects who did not reach the target concentration followed a similar pattern to that of the Malay population, with three subjects for the *1/*1 genotype, 28 subjects for the *2/*2 genotype, seven subjects for the *1/*2 genotype and four subjects for the *1/*17 genotype (Figure 10).

There were no statistically significant differences between Malay and Malaysian Chinese when comparing clopi-H4 C_{max} or C_{min} concentrations in each phenotype (Figure 10). However, as expected, in both Malay and Malaysian Chinese populations, the *2/*2 (PM) phenotype resulted in a statistically significant difference in mean clopi-H4 C_{max} when compared to all other phenotypes ($p < 0.001$).

(A)

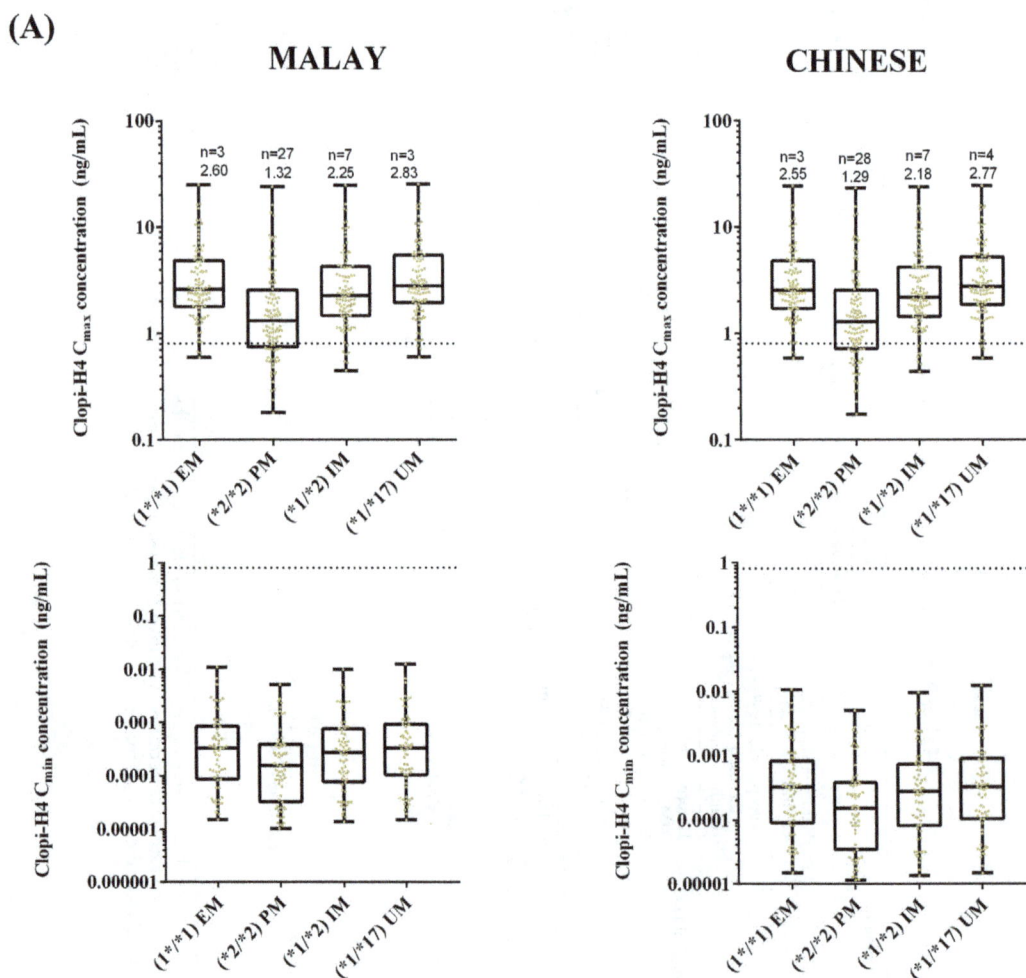

Figure 10. *Cont.*

(B)

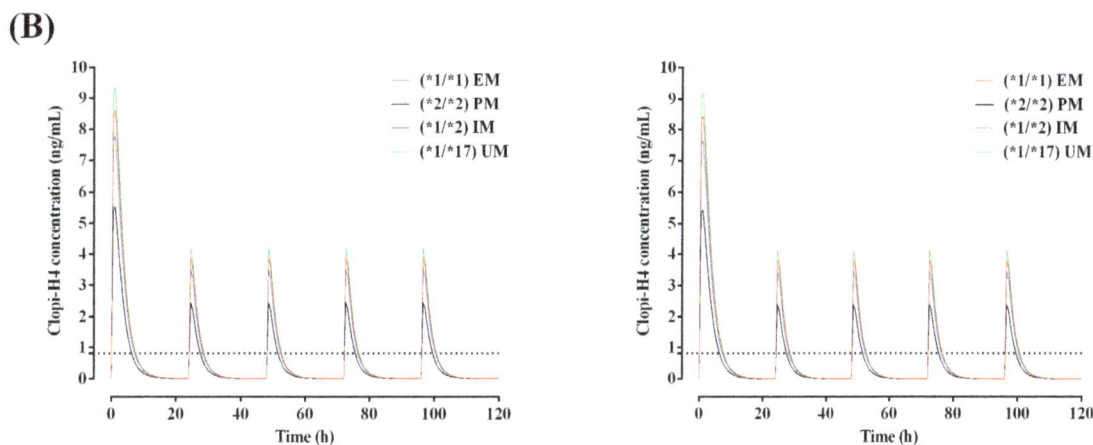

Figure 10. (**A**) impact of clopidogrel standard dose regimens on final dose clopi-H4 plasma C_{max} (upper panels) and C_{min} (lower panels) in Malay (left panels) and Malaysian Chinese (right panels) subjects, demarked for all EM, PM, IM or UM populations. Box and whisker plots represent maximum, 75th percentile, median, 25th percentile and minimum clopi-H4 C_{max}; (**B**) simulated mean plasma concentration–time profile of clopi-H4 in Malay (left panel) and Malaysian Chinese (right panel) subjects demarked for all EM, PM, IM or UM populations. All subjects ($n = 100$ for each phenotype) received a loading dose of 300 mg on day 1, followed by daily doses of 75 mg for four days. Solid lines represent mean plasma concentration–time predictions. Dashed horizontal lines represent the lower therapeutic limit for clopi-H4.

2.4. Step 4: Sensitivity Analysis for CYP2C19 Hepatic Abundances

Considering the lack of literature on reported CYP2C19 hepatic abundance data for Malays, the sensitivity of model predictions to changes in CYP2C19 hepatic abundance (assuming they varied from the default assumption that Chinese and Malay CYP2C19 abundances were similar) was assessed through simulating the number of subjects attaining target clopi-H4 concentrations when the hepatic mean enzyme abundances were increased or decreased by 30%. In the Malay population, a 30% increase in mean abundance values resulted in 2, 27, 6 and 1 subjects failing to reach the target concentration for the *1/*1, *2/*2, *1/*2 and *1/*17 genotypes, respectively (Figure 11). Furthermore, a 30% decrease of mean abundance values resulted in 6, 27, 8 and 6 subjects failing to reach the target concentration for the *1/*1, *2/*2, *1/*2 and *1/*17 genotypes, respectively (Figure 11).

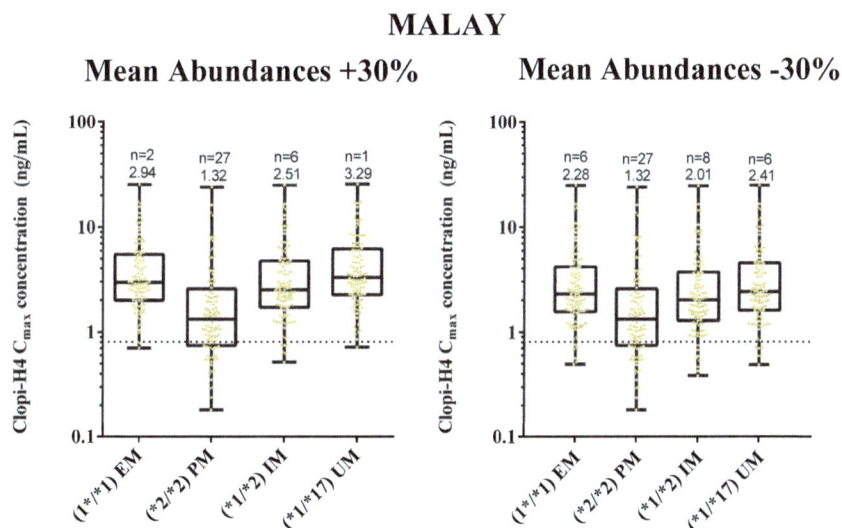

Figure 11. *Cont.*

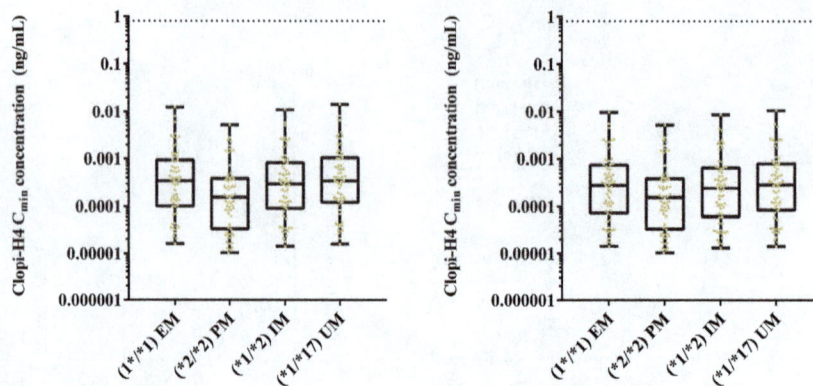

Figure 11. Impact of clopidogrel standard dose regimens on final dose clopi-H4 plasma C_{max} (upper panels) and C_{min} (lower panels) in Malay subjects under scenarios where mean hepatic CYP2C19 abundance is increased (left panels) or decreased (right panels) by 30%. All subjects are demarked for either all EM, PM, IM or UM populations. Box and whisker plots represent maximum, 75th percentile, median, 25th percentile and minimum clopi-H4 C_{max}. All subjects ($n = 100$ for each phenotype) received a loading dose of 300 mg on day 1, followed by daily doses of 75 mg for four days. Dashed horizontal lines represent the lower therapeutic limit for clopi-H4.

For the Malaysian Chinese population, a 30% increase in the mean abundances values resulted in 3, 27, 6 and 1 subjects failing to reach the target concentration for the *1/*1, *2/*2, *1/*2 and *1/*17 genotypes, respectively (Figure 12). Furthermore, a 30% decrease in the mean abundance values resulted in 6, 27, 8 and 6 subjects failing to reach the target concentration for the *1/*1, *2/*2, *1/*2 and *1/*17 genotypes, respectively (Figure 12). There were also no statistically significant inter-ethnic differences between the clopi-H4 peak and trough concentrations for each genotype.

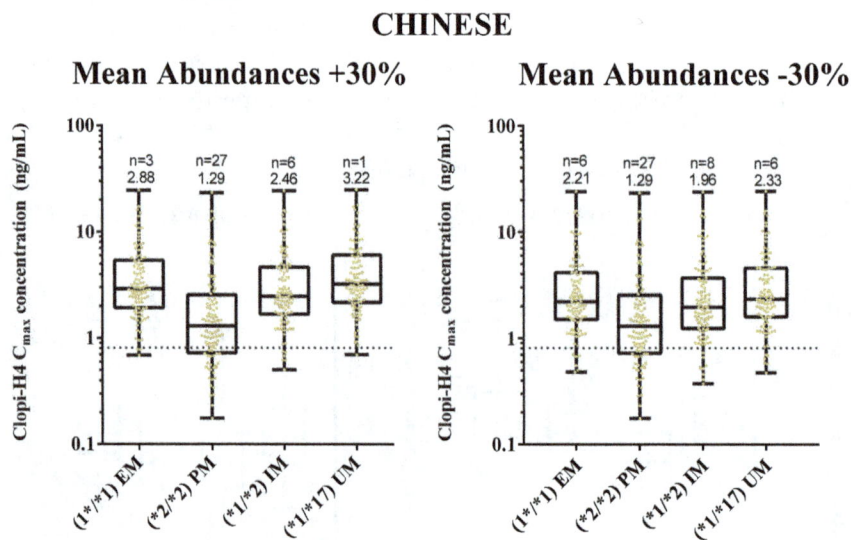

Figure 12. *Cont.*

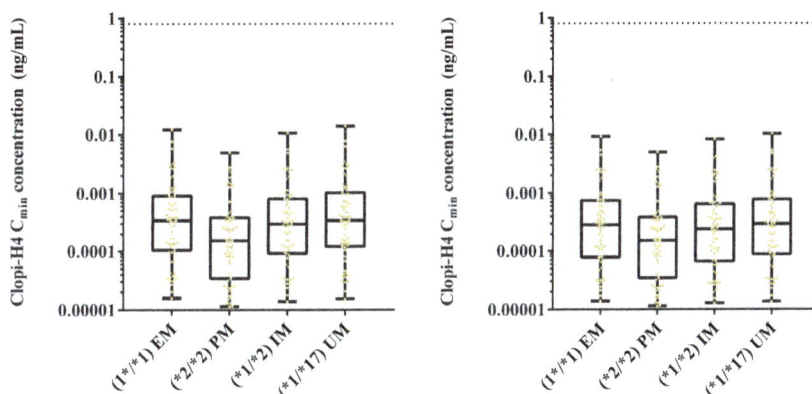

Figure 12. Impact of clopidogrel standard dose regimens on final dose clopi-H4 plasma C_{max} (upper panels) and C_{min} (lower panels) in Chinese subjects under scenarios where mean hepatic CYP2C19 abundance is increased (left panels) or decreased (right panels) by 30%. All subjects are demarked for either all EM, PM, IM or UM populations. Box and whisker plots represent maximum, 75th percentile, median, 25th percentile and minimum clopi-H4 C_{max}. All subjects ($n = 100$ for each phenotype) received a loading dose of 300 mg on day 1, followed by daily doses of 75 mg for four days. Dashed horizontal lines represent the lower therapeutic limit for clopi-H4.

2.5. Step 5: Dose Optimization in CYP2C19 Poor Metabolisers

Given the high number of subjects identified with clopi-H4 concentrations below the target threshold (Figure 10) in the PM phenotype group, the dosing regimen for clopidogrel was increased to a 'high-dose' scenario with a 600 mg loading dose followed by a four-day regimen of 150 mg daily (Figure 13). For a standard dose, 27 Malay and 28 Malaysian Chinese subjects had a clopi-H4 plasma concentration below the target minimum therapeutic concentration (Figure 10), which decreased to 12 (Malay) and 14 (Malaysian Chinese) for the high dose regimen (Figure 13A). No statistically significant differences were determined between Malay and Malaysian Chinese clopi-H4 C_{max} (Figure 13B).

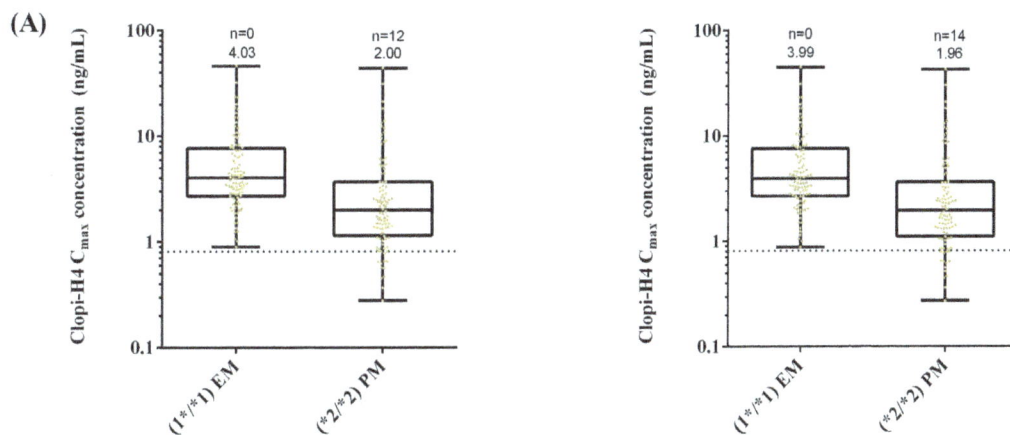

Figure 13. *Cont.*

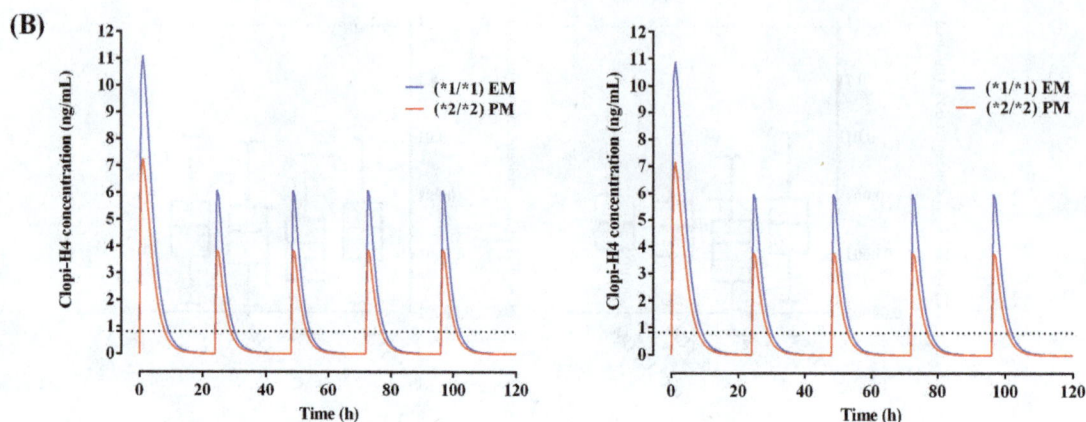

Figure 13. (**A**) impact of clopidogrel high dose regimen on clopi-H4 plasma C_{max} in Malay (left panel) and Malaysian Chinese (right panel) subjects; (**B**) simulated mean plasma concentration–time profile of clopi-H4 in Malay (left panel) and Malaysian Chinese (right panel) subjects. An oral loading dose of 600 mg was administered on day 1, followed by daily doses of 150 mg for four days using the custom Malaysian (Malay and Malaysian Chinese) Simcyp population group ($n = 100$), with dosing to populations of either all PM or all EM phenotypes. Solid plasma concentration lines represent mean predictions. Dashed horizontal lines represent the lower therapeutic limit for clopi-H4. Box and whisker plots represent maximum, 75th percentile, median, 25th percentile and minimum clopi-H4 C_{max}.

3. Discussion

Cardiovascular disease (CVD) is a leading global cause of mortality with recent reports highlighting that approximately 85% of CVD cases occur in low- to middle-income countries [50,51]. A primary cause of this increase is related to changes in economic development and lifestyle with reduced incidences of infectious diseases, all of which has led to a marked improvement in the life expectancy of low- to middle-income countries from 61.7 years in 1980 to 71.8 years in 2015 [50]. Furthermore, the higher incidences of non-communicable disease, such as diabetes mellitus, hypertension and dyslipidaemia, have all contributed to an overall increase in the incidence of CVD in low- to middle-income countries.

Despite these risks, the Ministry of Health (MOH) Malaysia has a proactive stance in relation to CVD and has maintained a long-standing database of cardiovascular disease in Malaysia, which is utilised to evaluate risk factors and treatment within Malaysia. The National Cardiovascular Database (NCVD) Registry [6] ensures the ongoing systematic collection, analysis and interpretation of cardiovascular disease data essential, which is essential and core to planning, implementation and evaluation of clinical and public health services within Malaysia. The NCVD was officially launched in 2006 by Dr. Ghani Mohamed Din (Deputy Director General of Health Malaysia) during the 10th Annual Scientific Meeting (ASM) of the National Heart Association of Malaysia (NHAM). To date, the NCVD register consists of 33,043 anonymised and voluntary patient records for patients undergoing acute coronary syndrome and percutaneous coronary intervention, spanning the years 2006–2015.

Although aspirin remains a primary treatment option for many CVD related disorders due to its cost-effectiveness [52], a key reason for clinicians moving towards a second-line therapy is often hypersensitivity of patients towards aspirin. In Malaysia, clopidogrel is recommended as a second-line therapy for ischemic cardiovascular events and also secondary prevention of ischemic stroke [53,54]. Clopidogrel is an antiplatelet agent, being predominantly metabolised into the active metabolite clopi-H4, primarily mediated by CYP2C19 [9–11]. However, CYP2C19 is highly polymorphic [55], with the PM phenotypes (*2/*2) known to be of higher prevalence in Asian populations when compared to Caucasians [56,57].

Outside of Southeast Asia, the use of predictive pharmacokinetics modelling to aid in both drug discovery and development along with clinical optimisation of drug therapy has exponentially increased over the past decade and has become a routine aspect of all clinical trials phases to both extrapolate dose to optimal therapy in population groups and to also identify covariates that may contribute to the variability in clinical response to drugs [58–60]. However, within Malaysia, the use of pharmacokinetic modelling to conduct such beneficial models' approaches is lacking.

Recently, we demonstrated the ability of physiologically-based pharmacokinetic modelling to optimise dosing of antimalarial drugs in special population groups from sub-Saharan African nations [40,41,61], where the unique physiological and anthropometric differences of African subjects (when compared to Caucasians) were incorporated into simulations. We have adapted this approach to now develop, for the first time, an appropriate virtual population group of the Malaysian population group for use in mechanistic pharmacokinetic modelling, with a focus on predicting the impact of CYP2C19 SNPs on clopidogrel and the active metabolite, clopi-H4, pharmacokinetic in the Malay and Malaysian Chinese population groups.

We adopted a robust 5-stage modelling approach that incorporated key data from the Malaysian NCVD database to develop virtual population groups, following validation of the modelling approaches using repaglinide, tramadol and rosuvastatin within healthy volunteers (Caucasian), Chinese and Malay population (Steps 1 and 2), followed by the simulation of clopidogrel and its active metabolite, clopi-H4 in the Malay and Malaysian Chinese population groups (Step 3). Next, the impact of CYP2C19 SNPs on the active metabolite, clopi-H4 in the Malay and Malaysian Chinese population groups were assessed with predictions of potential exposure to the clopidogrel therapy (Step 4). Finally, simulations were conducted to predict the potential impact of dosage optimisation in the CYP2C19 PM population (Step 5).

3.1. Step 1: Malaysian Population Development

In Step 1, we attempted to develop a representative Malaysian population by extracting relevant data such as gender, weight, age and ethnicity from the NCVD database [6], with which to develop the populations. For the Malay, Chinese and Indian population, the mean age, weight and BMI were significantly different between Malay and Chinese ($p < 0.0001$) and Chinese and Indian ($p < 0.0001$), whereas mean height was relatively consistent across all population group at 1.63 m and not statistically significantly different (Table 1). Since there was no significant difference between the heights of all the three populations, the default age–height relationship for the 'Chinese Volunteer' population group within Simcyp was used to represent these populations. Using the customised age–weight relationships for the two populations, the predicted distribution of body-weight with age for both the Malay (Figure 2) and Malaysian Chinese (Figure 3) populations was predicted well and in good agreement with individual subject data extracted from the NCVD data over the range of 20 to 65 years of age. This supports the development of appropriate population groups possessing suitable anthropometric age–weight relationship within the Malaysian population. In addition, this step incorporated appropriate blood biochemistry metrics to describe Malay and Malaysian Chinese population groups, something which is critical for driving unbound drug fraction within plasma and essential as clopidogrel, and its metabolites are extensively protein bound (see Section 4.1.1 Table 3) [62,63].

Table 3. Malay and Malaysian Chinese blood biochemistry.

Biochemistry	Malay	Malaysian Chinese
Haematocrit (%)	M: 43 [b] F: 38 [c]	M: 45.3 F: 40.5
AAG (g/L)	M: 0.65 [a] F: 0.64 [a]	M: 0.65 F: 0.64
HSA (g/L)	M: 47.3 [b] F: 46.3 [b]	M: 50.34 F: 49.38

AAG: α1-acidic glycoprotein; HSA: human serum albumin M: male; F: female; [a] Simcyp default values; [b] Hamzah et al. [64]; [c] Khor et al. [65].

3.2. Step 2: Adult Simulations: Validation with Repaglinide, Tramadol and Rosuvastatin

Having established a Malaysian virtual population group for use in predictive pharmacokinetic modelling, we subsequently assessed the ability of the customized population groups to predict repaglinide and tramadol plasma concentrations and pharmacokinetics in the Malay (Figure 7), Chinese (Figure 6) and Caucasian Healthy Volunteers (Figures 4 and 5) populations. In these simulations, model predictions were successfully predicted to within two-to-three-fold, C_{max}, t_{max}, CL and AUC was reported (Table 2) [44,45], and an appropriate population distribution was recapitulated. It was noted, however, that in Caucasians the model predicted a poorer terminal elimination phase of the plasma concentration–time profile when multi-dosing (Figure 5). This may, in part, be a result of the original study reporting plasma concentration–time profiles without using a log-linear scale, making precise determination of terminal points difficult. However, it should be noted that the AUC was predicted to within two-fold of that reported [43].

Subsequently, the customised Malay and Malaysian Chinese population group were further validated against a study whereby an IV bolus dose of tramadol was dosed to Malaysian subjects [46]. Model prediction AUC and Clearance were within two-fold of that reported (Table 2) with model predicted plasma concentration–time profiles spanning an appropriate range for the simulated population group when compared to the observed data (Figure 8). Finally, model validation was further confirmed through successful prediction of rosuvastatin plasma concentrations and pharmacokinetics in Caucasian, Chinese and Malays (Figure 9) with predicted C_{max}, t_{max}, and AUC to within two-fold of that reported [48] (Table 2).

3.3. Step 3: Prediction of the Impact of CYP2C19 Polymorphisms on Clopidogrel Pharmacokinetics in Malaysians

Having successfully validated the predicting capability of the customised population groups within pharmacokinetic models for repaglinide and tramadol, the model was expanded to assess its application to predict clopidogrel and its active metabolite, clopi-H4, pharmacokinetics in Malaysian subjects. In an attempt to establish the potential impact of CYP2C19 SNPs on clopi-H4 plasma concentration in Malay and Malaysian Chinese populations, we conducted simulations stratified across EM, PM, IM, and UM phenotypes. A statistically significant difference in the clopi-H4 C_{max} was predicted between the EM and PM groups within the Malay and Malaysian Chinese population (Figure 10), with clopi-H4 C_{max} decreasing by approximately 50% in the PM population groups compared to the EM population group in both Malay and Malaysian Chinese (Figure 10).

In a study by Simon et al. [9], clopi-H4 plasma concentrations were quantified for each phenotype in European subjects. Following a standard dose (300 mg loading dose followed by 4 days of 75 mg once daily), the last dose mean C_{max} was 13 ± 7.33 ng/mL for EM and 3.93 ± 1.93 ng/mL for PM. In both Malay and Chinese subjects, the median last dose C_{max} was significantly lower for EM (2.60 ng/mL and 2.55 ng/mL) (Figure 10A). However, the overall range of predicted C_{max} was similar to those reported [9]. This difference, however, may be attributed to the anthropometric differences between Southeast Asian/Far East Asian population groups and European (Caucasian) populations [66] in addition to differences in the prevalence of each genotype [23–28].

Similar reports for Malaysians subjects are currently lacking. However, in mainland Chinese subjects, clopi-H4 C_{max} for the study duration (i.e., first dose) was reported to be 18.9 ng/mL $\pm$ 11.8 ng/mL in EM (*1/*1) and 11.8 ng/mL $\pm$ 5.1 ng/mL in PM (*1/*2 or *2/*2) [67], within three-fold of the simulated mean C_{max} for EM (8.62 ng/mL $\pm$ 11.4 ng/mL) and PM (5.59 ng/mL $\pm$ 3.92 ng/mL) (Figure 10B) whilst also being within a similar range of observed concentrations, when taking into account the standard deviations reported for C_{max} [67].

No significant differences were observed in clopi-H4 plasma concentrations between the Malaysian Chinese and Malay populations when comparing CYP2C19-genotyped groups (Figure 10). This finding is consistent with reports of a similar frequency of CYP2C19 metaboliser groups between the Malay and Malaysian Chinese in a cohort of Malaysian patients taking clopidogrel [29,68,69]. Thus, although the impact of the CYP2C19 polymorphism on clopidogrel pharmacokinetic may lead to treatment failure in PM within the Malay and Malaysian Chinese population, due to the attenuation of clopi-H4 plasma concentration, the magnitude of this impact between these populations is largely minimal, with insignificant differences observed between them (Figure 10).

3.4. Step 4: Sensitivity Analysis for CYP2C19 Hepatic Abundances

Despite CYP2C19 polymorphisms having been previously characterised for Malaysians, the hepatic abundance of CYP2C19, and how it varies from Caucasian subjects, is currently lacking. Within the context of pharmacokinetic modelling, this is an important quantitative metric, allowing both the prediction of in vivo clearance (from in vitro hepatocyte/microsomal incubations) and, when combined with appropriate phenotype/genotype data, the ability to model the impact of polymorphisms on resultant drug pharmacokinetics. However, for the Chinese population group, hepatic CYP2C19 abundance has been quantified along with phenotype-specific abundances (8, 0, 6 and 10 pmol/mg protein for EM, PM, IM and UM, respectively), and these have been incorporated into the Simcyp population database and characterised/validated by Simcyp and other researchers [70,71].

However, comparisons to other Asian population groups (e.g., Japanese) show variations in the hepatic abundance for EM phenotypes (14 pmol/mg for Caucasians; 9 pmol/mg for Chinese; 1 pmol/mg for Japanese) [71]. Given this variation, it was prudent to simulate the impact of variation in CYP2C19 EM and PM phenotype abundance, and this was accomplished through applying a 30% increase and 30% decrease of mean abundance values for all CYP2C19-phenotyped groups in the Malay (Figure 11) and Chinese population (Figure 12).

With a 30% increase in mean abundances, there was a slight increase in patient's response towards clopidogrel treatment based on the clopi-H4 minimum limit of 0.81 ng/mL, ranging from 10% to 20% of the CYP2C19-phenotyped group in both populations. Similarly, with the 30% decrease of mean abundances, a slight decrease of patient's response can be observed varying between 10% and 30% of the CYP2C19-phenotyped group in both populations. Clearly, these observations are not novel, given that clopi-H4 plasma concentrations are related to the functional status of CYP2C19 within Asian populations [72]. However, of note was the fact that there was also no significant difference in the clopi-H4 C_{max} between the Malay and Malaysian Chinese population groups in relation to the CYP2C19-phenotyped group with the $\pm30\%$ mean abundance values (Figures 11 and 12), further confirming our earlier findings.

3.5. Step 5: Dose Optimisation in CYP2C19 Poor Metabolisers

In the final step, given the high percentage of subjects with a clopi-H4 C_{max} below the minimum therapeutic concentration under standard dosing procedures (300 mg loading dose followed by 75 mg for four days), we assessed the impact of a high-dose regimen on clopi-H4 C_{max}. Under these revised dosing conditions, the percentage of subjects with a clopi-H4 C_{max} below the minimum therapeutic concentration decreased to 12% (Malay) and 14% (Malaysian Chinese) (Figure 13). A number of previous clinical studies have considered the high dose versus standard dose clopidogrel treatment regimens, particularly for CYP2C19 PM, and identified no significant clinical concerns, with improved inhibition of platelet aggregation and clinical outcomes [73–76], and our simulations further agreed with these published findings. Thus, a 600 mg loading dose followed by a 150 mg maintenance dose may be appropriate for confirmed CYP2C19 PM Malay and Malaysian Chinese patients, particularly where platelet response is poor.

3.6. Study Limitations and Future Directions for Clopidogrel Use in Malaysia

It is important to address several limitations of the present study. Firstly, although we were able to develop robust pharmacokinetic models, the limited availability of hepatic CYP2C19 abundance data and phenotype/genotype specific abundance data in Malay or Malaysian Chinese was a primary limitation. We utilised existing data from the Chinese population group, which had been previously validated by Simcyp, as a surrogate for both Malay and Malaysian Chinese. It could be possible that inter-ethnic differences exist between Malay and Malaysian Chinese, which may alter the resultant simulations, although no significant differences in clopi-H4 C_{max} were noted in Step 4 (Section 2.4) of our modelling approach.

The focus of this study has been on LOF alleles (e.g., the PM phenotype). However, other SNPs have been reported to contribute towards the overall wide inter-individual variability associated with clopidogrel anti-platelet activity, such as the GOF variant CYP2C19*17 (rs12248560) that defines the ultra-rapid metaboliser phenotype. Whilst the importance of the LOF alleles are well characterised, the GOF variants are less well characterised and their impact of antiplatelet activity is contradictory, as highlighted by a number of meta-analysis studies [77–79]. Further modelling studies should investigate the relevance of the UM phenotype on clopi-H4 levels to identify whether the GOF alleles are important for overall clinical efficacy and clopi-H4 plasma concentrations.

Furthermore, there was a lack of published and robust genotyped pharmacokinetic data in Malaysian subjects, primarily plasma concentration–time profiles, which may have aided in model validation of the clopidogrel predictions. However, this has been completed by a prior group in Caucasian subjects [14]. Despite this, further investment in research and development infrastructure is required to ensure that pharmacokinetic modelling approaches are better integrated into clinical research to optimise study design and better utilise the clinical data obtained to provide evidence-based optimised therapy [80].

4. Materials and Methods

Population-based PBPK modelling was conducted using the virtual clinical trials simulator Simcyp (Simcyp Ltd., a Certara company, Sheffield, UK, Version 16). Simulations were performed for an exclusive CYP2C19 extensive metaboliser (EM) (CYP2C19*1/*1), poor metaboliser (PM) (CYP2C19*2/*2), intermediate metaboliser (IM) (CYP2C19*1/*2) and ultrarapid metaboliser (UM) (CYP2C19*1/*17) population groups. For all simulations, dosing occurred under fasted-conditions unless otherwise indicated. A detailed list of haplotypes associated with GOF or LOF alleles are detailed within the PharmGKB database (Accession number: PA124) [19].

4.1. Model Development

A five-stage stepwise approach was implemented for model development, validation and model refinement (Figure 14), which is fully described below.

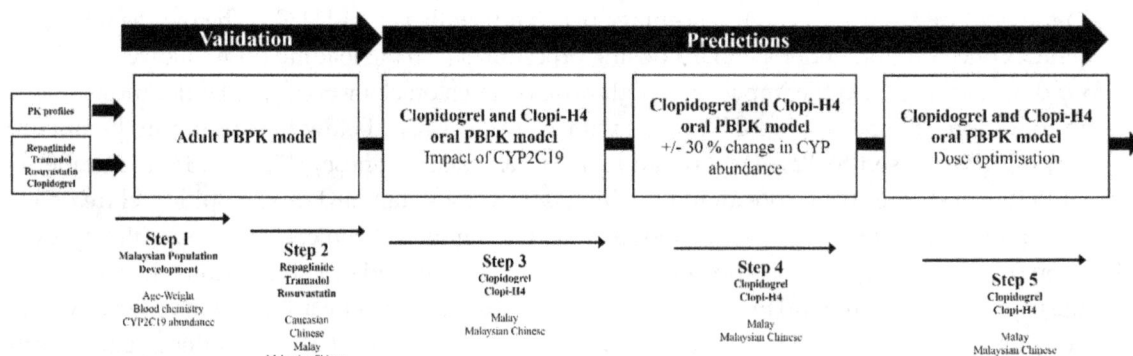

Figure 14. Model development strategy. The five-stage workflow approach implemented to study pharmacokinetics within Malaysian population groups.

Phenotype frequencies for CYP2C19 were incorporated for Caucasian (EM: 97.6%; PM: 2.4%) and Chinese (EM: 87%; PM: 13%) populations using the default frequencies recorded within Simcyp. Literature reported frequencies were utilised for Malay (EM: 51%; PM: 7%; IM: 38%; UM: 4%) [81].

4.1.1. Step 1: Malaysian Population Development

To develop a Malaysian population group for use in pharmacokinetic modelling, the National Cardiovascular Database (NCVD) Registry [6] was analysed for relevant population-level anthropometric data relevant to each ethnic group. The NCVD register is a Malaysian nationwide registry consisting of 33,043 anonymized and voluntary patient records for patients undergoing acute coronary syndrome and percutaneous coronary intervention, spanning the years 2006–2015. The NCVD is supported by the Ministry of Health Malaysia and co-sponsored by National Heart Association of Malaysia, with the aim to gather information about cardiovascular diseases in Malaysia. Within this database, relevant physiological parameters were limited to only (i) gender; (ii) age; (iii) weight and (iv) ethnicity.

To develop the Malaysian population group the two largest ethnic groups, Malays and Malaysian Chinese were considered, as they constitute 50.1% and 22.6% of the total Malaysian population, respectively [1]. Appropriate anthropometric age–body weight distributions were generated and used to establish mathematical (polynomial regression) relationships to predict body weight from age, using TableCurve2D (version, Systat Software, San Jose, CA, USA). The resultant polynomial regression equations were then applied within the population 'Demographics' section of Simcyp to create user-defined age–weight relationships for each population. Furthermore, blood chemistry was revised to match report haematocrit and plasma protein concentrations within the Malay and Malaysian Chinese population groups, as reported in the literature (Table 3).

In the absence of literature reported CYP2C19 hepatic abundance in the Malay and Malaysian Chinese subjects, the EM, PM, IM and UM phenotypes were allocated a hepatic abundance of 8, 0, 6 and 10 pmol/mg protein, respectively, based upon adaptations detailed within a validated Chinese population group developed by Simcyp, and which is available from the population library repository of Simcyp software. These abundances were assumed to be the same for both Malay and Malaysian Chinese population groups.

Compound Selection and Clinical Studies

A literature search for published clinical studies reporting plasma concentration–time profiles for ethnicity-specific Malaysian patients (Malay and Chinese) was able to identify repaglinide, tramadol, rosuvastatin and clopidogrel as therapeutic drugs where pharmacokinetic clinical data was available for population groups of interest. These studies were used for model development and validation. The three compounds of interest had previously been developed and validated within Simcyp and are available within the Simcyp library compound database, with repaglinide developed and pre-validated by Simcyp [82], tramadol developed and validated by T'jollyn et al. [47] and clopidogrel and its' primary metabolite (2-oxo-clopidogrel) and secondary metabolite (clopi-H4) previously developed and validated by Djebli et al. [14].

4.1.2. Step 2: Adult Simulations: Validation with Repaglinide, Tramadol and Rosuvastatin

To confirm the validity of the modelling approaches and the appropriateness of the customised Malaysian population groups, validation of the population group was conducted using repaglinide, tramadol and rosuvastatin from six published clinical studies: (i) a single 2 mg oral dose of repaglinide to healthy adult volunteers [42]; (ii) a single 2 mg oral dose of repaglinide on day 1 and subsequently 2 mg multiple doses orally on day 2 to day 9 in healthy young adults [43]; (iii) a single 2 mg oral dose of repaglinide dosed to healthy native Han Chinese adult volunteers [44]; (iv) a single 4 mg oral dose of repaglinide dosed to healthy adult Malay volunteers [45]; (v) a single dose of 100 mg tramadol given intravenously to adult mixed Malaysian volunteers [46] and (vi) a single oral dose of 40 mg rosuvastatin given Caucasian, Han Chinese and Malays [48] with appropriate hepatic uptake clearances incorporated as reported by Bae et al. [83]. All simulations replicated the study design reported by the clinical studies cited above.

4.1.3. Step 3: Prediction of the Impact of CYP2C19 Polymorphisms on Clopidogrel Pharmacokinetics in Malaysians

This step simulated the potential impact of SNPs CYP2C19 on the resultant clopi-H4 target plasma concentration range for patients known to result in a clinical response, namely 0.81 to 13.45 ng/mL [49], within the Malay and Malaysian Chinese population groups. For all simulation, clopi-H4 concentration of below 0.81 ng/mL was used as a cut-off value to depict patients who were unresponsive to clopidogrel treatment. Simulations were stratified across EM, PM, IM and UM phenotypes, and performed using a validated clopidogrel compound (18) using a trial design of 63 adult subjects who were administered a 300-mg loading dose (LD) and a 75-mg/day maintenance dose (MD) for four days.

4.1.4. Step 4: Sensitivity Analysis for CYP2C19 Hepatic Abundances

To address the absence of literature reported CYP2C19 hepatic abundances in the Malaysian population groups, two further scenarios were simulated whereby the mean abundances for the Malay and Malaysian Chinese population were set at 30% greater/less than that used as default (see Step 1). This allowed for the analysis of the sensitivity of model predictions to changes in abundance to be simulated through assessing the resulting impact on the number of subjects attaining clopi-H4 target concentrations.

4.1.5. Step 5: Dose Optimisation in CYP2C19 Poor Metabolisers

This step attempted to predict the potential impact of dosage optimisation in the CYP2C19 poor metabolisers' population, with an aim to recapitulate subjects into the clopi-H4 therapeutic window range. Simulations were run using the Malay and Malaysian Chinese population groups. Furthermore, based on the study by Simon et al. [32], the dosing regimen for clopidogrel was increased to a 'high-dose' scenario with a 600 mg loading dose followed by a four-day regimen of 150 mg daily.

4.2. Data Analysis

Clinical plasma concentration–time data points from studies identified in Step 1 (Section 4.1.1) were extracted using the WebPlotDigitizer v.3.10 (http://arohatgi.info/WebPlotDigitizer/). All simulations of plasma concentration–time profiles were presented in 5th to 95th percentiles and either in mean or median unless otherwise specified. For all adult simulations, age ranges and subject gender ratios were matched, where possible, to reported clinical studies. Where this information was not cited in clinical studies, a default age range of 40 to 65 years and gender ratio of 50% was selected. For simulations employing genotypes stratification, unless otherwise stated, a 100-subject simulation was run in a 10×10 trial (10 subjects per trial with 10 trials) per genotype to ensure that reasonable inter-/intra individual variability is captured within the model simulations.

4.3. Predictive Performance

In all simulations, a prediction to within two-fold of the observed data was generally accepted as part of the 'optimal' predictive performances range despite there being no uniform standard of acceptance to determine this criterion [84–86]. This acceptance criterion was used in our C_{max} and AUC comparisons with the published clinical data reported. However, this was not used as the sole determinate for model performance (see Section 4.4).

For the clopidogrel simulations, the target clopi-H4 plasma concentration was set at the lowest value of 0.81 ng/mL from the range of 0.81–13.45 ng/mL obtained from literature [49] and used to determine the impact of SNPs CYP2C19 on Malay and Malaysian Chinese population pharmacokinetics.

4.4. Visual Predictive Checks

To further validate model predictions where comparison were made to existing clinical studies, a visual predictive checking (VPC) strategy was adopted. This approach was described at the 2012 FDA Pediatric Advisory Committee (US Food and Drug Administration, 2012) [87]. In this approach, to graphically validate the predictability of the model, the 5th and 95th percentiles (along with mean or median) of predicted concentration–time profiles (generated from Simcyp) were graphically displayed along with the observed data for any validation data sets to ensure predicted data points largely overlapped with those from the observed data sets, which should contain (where possible) some measure of spread of observed plasma concentration data (e.g., a standard deviation for each mean concentration point).

5. Conclusions

Cardiovascular disease (CVD) is a leading cause of mortality and is increasingly prevalent in Malaysia, which places the Malaysian healthcare system at ever increasing risks and cost-burdens for treatment of patients. Given the unique ethnic diversity of the Malaysian population group, evidence-based approaches should account for the individual characteristics of patients rather than focusing on an average patient from a carefully selected patient population. Pharmacokinetic modelling can provide this approach through carefully developed and validated population models which can be applied to study a drug's pharmacokinetics in different geographical regions. This approach was applied to clopidogrel and illustrated the impact of a PM phenotype on reducing clopi-H4 C_{max}, which could be partially recovered using a high-dose strategy (600 mg loading dose followed by 150 mg maintenance dose), which resulted in an approximate 50% increase in subjects attaining the minimum clopi-H4 plasma concentration for a therapeutic effect. Furthermore, we illustrated limited variation clopi-H4 pharmacokinetics between the two key ethnic groups, Malays and Malaysian Chinese, suggesting that inter-ethnic differences within Malaysia may not impact upon clopidogrel therapy. It should be noted, however, that the current lack of existing clopidogrel pharmacokinetics data in multi-ethnic population groups is lacking within Malaysian populations, and this data would be valuable to support the work presented within this manuscript and to also aid in validating the outcomes presented.

This study has illustrated the benefit of the application of pharmacokinetic modelling, which incorporates pharmacogenetics information, to mixed ethnic population groups. The current lack of an integrated approach within Malaysia, in addition to the sparse routine application of pharmacokinetic modelling to clinical data, should be addressed to support better clinical drug decision-making.

Author Contributions: Conceptualization, R.K.S.B. and Z.H.Z.; Methodology, R.K.S.B. and Z.H.Z.; Software, Z.H.Z.; Validation, Z.H.Z.; Formal Analysis, R.K.S.B., Z.H.Z. and A.Y.Y.F.; Investigation, Z.H.Z. and R.K.S.B.; Writing—Original Draft Preparation, R.K.S.B. and Z.H.Z.; Writing—Review and Editing, R.K.S.B., Z.H.Z. and A.Y.Y.F.; Supervision, R.K.S.B. and A.Y.Y.F.

Funding: This research was funded by the Ministry of Health Malaysia, Grant No. KKM510-4/4/3/3 Jld. 4 (138).

Acknowledgments: The authors would like to thank the Director General of Health Malaysia for permission to publish this manuscript. The authors would like to record their thanks to the National Heart Association of Malaysia, the staff and institutions, who contributed to the NCVD registry.

References

1. Ho, M. *Current Population Estimates, Malaysia, 2014–2016*; The Office of Chief Statistician Malaysia, Department of Statistics Malaysia: Putrajaya, Malaysia, 2016.
2. National Pharmaceutical Regulatory Agency, Ministry of Health Malaysia. *National Centre for Adverse Drug Reaction Monitoring Annual Report*; National Pharmaceutical Regulatory Agency: Putrajaya, Malaysia, 2018.
3. Xie, H.G.; Kim, R.B.; Wood, A.J.; Michael Stein, C.M. Molecular basis of ethnic differences in drug disposition and response. *Annu. Rev. Pharmacol. Toxicol.* **2001**, *41*, 815–850. [CrossRef] [PubMed]

4.   Yusoff, N.; Saleem, M.; Nagaya, D.; Yahaya, B.; Rasmaizatul Akma, R.; Moosa, N.; Ismail, R.; Tan, C. Cross-ethnic distribution of clinically relevant Cyp2c19 genotypes and haplotypes. *J. Pharm. Pharmacoproteomics* **2015**, *6*, 147. [CrossRef]

5.   Yang, Y.; Wong, L.; Lee, T.; Mustafa, A.; Mohamed, Z.; Lang, C.C. Genetic polymorphism of cytochrome P450 2C19 in healthy Malaysian subjects. *Br. J. Clin. Pharmacol.* **2004**, *58*, 332–335. [CrossRef] [PubMed]

6.   Health Facts 2017, Ministry of Health Malaysia, Putrajaya, Malaysia. Available online: http://www.moh.gov.my/english.php/pages/view/56 (accessed on 9 July 2018).

7.   Cattaneo, M. Response variability to clopidogrel: Is tailored treatment, based on laboratory testing, the right solution? *J. Thromb. Haemost.* **2012**, *10*, 327–336. [CrossRef] [PubMed]

8.   Bhatt, D.L.; Topol, E.J. Scientific and therapeutic advances in antiplatelet therapy. *Nat. Rev. Drug Discov.* **2003**, *2*, 15–28. [CrossRef] [PubMed]

9.   Simon, T.; Bhatt, D.L.; Bergougnan, L.; Farenc, C.; Pearson, K.; Perrin, L.; Vicaut, E.; Lacreta, F.; Hurbin, F.; Dubar, M. Genetic polymorphisms and the impact of a higher clopidogrel dose regimen on active metabolite exposure and antiplatelet response in healthy subjects. *Clin. Pharmacol. Ther.* **2011**, *90*, 287–295. [CrossRef] [PubMed]

10.   Mega, J.L.; Close, S.L.; Wiviott, S.D.; Shen, L.; Hockett, R.D.; Brandt, J.T.; Walker, J.R.; Antman, E.M.; Macias, W.; Braunwald, E. Cytochrome p-450 polymorphisms and response to clopidogrel. *N. Engl. J. Med.* **2009**, *360*, 354–362. [CrossRef] [PubMed]

11.   Kim, K.; Park, P.; Hong, S.; Park, J.Y. The effect of CYP2C19 polymorphism on the pharmacokinetics and pharmacodynamics of clopidogrel: A possible mechanism for clopidogrel resistance. *Clin. Pharmacol. Ther.* **2008**, *84*, 236–242. [CrossRef] [PubMed]

12.   Holmes, D.R., Jr.; Dehmer, G.J.; Kaul, S.; Leifer, D.; O'Gara, P.T.; Stein, C.M. ACCF/AHA clopidogrel clinical alert: Approaches to the fda "boxed warning": A report of the american college of cardiology foundation task force on clinical expert consensus documents and the american heart association endorsed by the society for cardiovascular angiography and interventions and the society of thoracic surgeons. *J. Am. Coll. Cardiol.* **2010**, *56*, 321–341. [PubMed]

13.   Kazui, M.; Nishiya, Y.; Ishizuka, T.; Hagihara, K.; Farid, N.A.; Okazaki, O.; Ikeda, T.; Kurihara, A. Identification of the human cytochrome p450 enzymes involved in the two oxidative steps in the bioactivation of clopidogrel to its pharmacologically active metabolite. *Drug Metab. Dispos. Biol. Fate Chem.* **2010**, *38*, 92–99. [CrossRef] [PubMed]

14.   Djebli, N.; Fabre, D.; Boulenc, X.; Fabre, G.; Sultan, E.; Hurbin, F. Physiologically-based pharmacokinetic modeling for sequential metabolism: Effect of CYP2C19 genetic polymorphism on clopidogrel and clopidogrel active metabolite pharmacokinetics. *Drug Metab. Dispos.* **2015**, *43*, 510–522. [CrossRef] [PubMed]

15.   Cappola, T.P.; Margulies, K.B. Functional genomics applied to cardiovascular medicine. *Circulation* **2011**, *124*, 87–94. [CrossRef] [PubMed]

16.   Wei, Y.Q.; Wang, D.G.; Yang, H.; Cao, H. Cytochrome P450 CYP 2C19*2 associated with adverse 1-year cardiovascular events in patients with acute coronary syndrome. *PLoS ONE* **2015**, *10*, e0132561. [CrossRef] [PubMed]

17.   Shuldiner, A.R.; O'Connell, J.R.; Bliden, K.P.; Gandhi, A.; Ryan, K.; Horenstein, R.B.; Damcott, C.M.; Pakyz, R.; Tantry, U.S.; Gibson, Q.; et al. Association of cytochrome P450 2C19 genotype with the antiplatelet effect and clinical efficacy of clopidogrel therapy. *JAMA* **2009**, *302*, 849–857. [CrossRef] [PubMed]

18.   Brandt, J.T.; Close, S.L.; Iturria, S.J.; Payne, C.D.; Farid, N.A.; Ernest, C.S., 2nd; Lachno, D.R.; Salazar, D.; Winters, K.J. Common polymorphisms of CYP2C19 and CYP2C9 affect the pharmacokinetic and pharmacodynamic response to clopidogrel but not prasugrel. *J. Thromb. Haemost.* **2007**, *5*, 2429–2436. [CrossRef] [PubMed]

19.   Home Page of the Pharmacogene Variation (Pharmvar) Consortium. Available online: https://www.pharmvar.org/gene/CYP2C19 (accessed on 9 July 2018).

20.   Yin, T.; Miyata, T. Pharmacogenomics of clopidogrel: Evidence and perspectives. *Thromb. Res.* **2011**, *128*, 307–316. [CrossRef] [PubMed]

21.   Amin, A.M.; Sheau Chin, L.; Azri Mohamed Noor, D.; Sk Abdul Kader, M.A.; Kah Hay, Y.; Ibrahim, B. The personalization of clopidogrel antiplatelet therapy: The role of integrative pharmacogenetics and pharmacometabolomics. *Cardiol. Res. Pract.* **2017**, *2017*, 8062796. [CrossRef] [PubMed]

22.	Scott, S.A.; Sangkuhl, K.; Stein, C.M.; Hulot, J.S.; Mega, J.L.; Roden, D.M.; Klein, T.E.; Sabatine, M.S.; Johnson, J.A.; Shuldiner, A.R. Clinical pharmacogenetics implementation consortium guidelines for cyp2c19 genotype and clopidogrel therapy: 2013 update. *Clin. Pharmacol. Ther.* **2013**, *94*, 317–323. [CrossRef] [PubMed]

23.	De Morais, S.; Wilkinson, G.R.; Blaisdell, J.; Nakamura, K.; Meyer, U.A.; Goldstein, J.A. The major genetic defect responsible for the polymorphism of s-mephenytoin metabolism in humans. *J. Biol. Chem.* **1994**, *269*, 15419–15422. [PubMed]

24.	De Morais, S.; Wilkinson, G.R.; Blaisdell, J.; Meyer, U.A.; Nakamura, K.; Goldstein, J.A. Identification of a new genetic defect responsible for the polymorphism of (s)-mephenytoin metabolism in Japanese. *Mol. Pharmacol.* **1994**, *46*, 594–598. [PubMed]

25.	Desta, Z.; Zhao, X.; Shin, J.-G.; Flockhart, D.A. Clinical significance of the cytochrome P450 2C19 genetic polymorphism. *Clin. Pharmacokinet.* **2002**, *41*, 913–958. [CrossRef] [PubMed]

26.	Cacabelos, R.; Martinez-Bouza, R.; Carril, J.C.; Fernandez-Novoa, L.; Lombardi, V.; Carrera, I.; Corzo, L.; McKay, A. Genomics and pharmacogenomics of brain disorders. *Curr. Pharm. Biotechnol.* **2012**, *13*, 674–725. [CrossRef] [PubMed]

27.	Cacabelos, R.; Martinez, R.; Fernandez-Novoa, L.; Carril, J.C.; Lombardi, V.; Carrera, I.; Corzo, L.; Tellado, I.; Leszek, J.; McKay, A.; et al. Genomics of dementia: Apoe- and CYP2D6-related pharmacogenetics. *Int. J. Alzheimer's Dis.* **2012**, *2012*, 518901.

28.	Mega, J.L.; Simon, T.; Collet, J.P.; Anderson, J.L.; Antman, E.M.; Bliden, K.; Cannon, C.P.; Danchin, N.; Giusti, B.; Gurbel, P.; et al. Reduced-function CYP2C19 genotype and risk of adverse clinical outcomes among patients treated with clopidogrel predominantly for PCI: A meta-analysis. *JAMA* **2010**, *304*, 1821–1830. [CrossRef] [PubMed]

29.	Mejin, M.; Tiong, W.N.; Lai, L.Y.; Tiong, L.L.; Bujang, A.M.; Hwang, S.S.; Ong, T.K.; Fong, A.Y. CYP2C19 genotypes and their impact on clopidogrel responsiveness in percutaneous coronary intervention. *Int. J. Clin. Pharm.* **2013**, *35*, 621–628. [CrossRef] [PubMed]

30.	Gurbel, P.A.; Tantry, U.S. Do platelet function testing and genotyping improve outcome in patients treated with antithrombotic agents?: Platelet function testing and genotyping improve outcome in patients treated with antithrombotic agents. *Circulation* **2012**, *125*, 1276–1287. [CrossRef] [PubMed]

31.	Krishna, V.; Diamond, G.A.; Kaul, S. Do platelet function testing and genotyping improve outcome in patients treated with antithrombotic agents?: The role of platelet reactivity and genotype testing in the prevention of atherothrombotic cardiovascular events remains unproven. *Circulation* **2012**, *125*, 1288–1303. [CrossRef] [PubMed]

32.	Collins, F.S.; Varmus, H. A new initiative on precision medicine. *N. Engl. J. Med.* **2015**, *372*, 793–795. [CrossRef] [PubMed]

33.	Jameson, J.L.; Longo, D.L. Precision medicine—personalized, problematic, and promising. *N. Engl. J. Med.* **2015**, *372*, 2229–2234. [CrossRef] [PubMed]

34.	U.S. Food and Drug Administration. *Advancing Regulatory Science for Public Health—A Framework for FDA'S Regulatory Science Initiative*; U.S. Food and Drug Administration: Silver Spring, MD, USA, 2010.

35.	U.S. Food and Drug Administration. Guidance for industry clinical lactation studies—Study design, data analysis, and recommendations for labeling. *Fed. Regist.* **2005**, *70*, 6697.

36.	Zhang, L.; Reynolds, K.S.; Zhao, P.; Huang, S.-M. Drug interactions evaluation: An integrated part of risk assessment of therapeutics. *Toxicol. Appl. Pharmacol.* **2010**, *243*, 134–145. [CrossRef] [PubMed]

37.	Huang, W.; Lee, S.L.; Lawrence, X.Y. Mechanistic approaches to predicting oral drug absorption. *AAPS J.* **2009**, *11*, 217–224. [CrossRef] [PubMed]

38.	U.S. Food and Drug Administration. *Drug Development and Drug Interactions*; U.S. Food and Drug Administration: Silver Spring, MD, USA, 2011.

39.	U.S. Food and Drug Administration. *Physiologically Based Pharmacokinetic Analyses—Format and Content. Guidance for Industry*; U.S. Food and Drug Administration: Silver Spring, MD, USA, 2016.

40.	Olafuyi, O.; Coleman, M.; Badhan, R.K.S. The application of physiologically based pharmacokinetic modelling to assess the impact of antiretroviral-mediated drug-drug interactions on piperaquine antimalarial therapy during pregnancy. *Biopharm. Drug Dispos.* **2017**, *38*, 464–478. [CrossRef] [PubMed]

41. Olafuyi, O.; Coleman, M.; Badhan, R.K.S. Development of a paediatric physiologically based pharmacokinetic model to assess the impact of drug-drug interactions in tuberculosis co-infected malaria subjects: A case study with artemether-lumefantrine and the CYP3A4-inducer rifampicin. *Eur. J. Pharm. Sci.* **2017**, *106*, 20–33. [CrossRef] [PubMed]

42. Hatorp, V. Clinical pharmacokinetics and pharmacodynamics of repaglinide. *Clin. Pharmacokinet.* **2002**, *41*, 471–483. [CrossRef] [PubMed]

43. Hatorp, V.; Huang, W.-C.; Strange, P. Repaglinide pharmacokinetics in healthy young adult and elderly subjects. *Clin. Ther.* **1999**, *21*, 702–710. [CrossRef]

44. Zhai, X.-J.; Hu, K.; Chen, F.; Lu, Y.-N. Comparative bioavailability and tolerability of a single 2-mg dose of 2 repaglinide tablet formulations in fasting, healthy chinese male volunteers: An open-label, randomized-sequence, 2-period crossover study. *Curr. Ther. Res.* **2013**, *75*, 48–52. [CrossRef] [PubMed]

45. Ruzilawati, A.; Gan, S. CYP3A4 genetic polymorphism influences repaglinide's pharmacokinetics. *Pharmacology* **2010**, *85*, 357–364. [CrossRef] [PubMed]

46. Gan, S.; Ismail, R.; Adnan, W.W.; Wan, Z. Correlation of tramadol pharmacokinetics and CYP2D6* 10 genotype in malaysian subjects. *J. Pharm. Biomed. Anal.* **2002**, *30*, 189–195. [CrossRef]

47. T'jollyn, H.; Snoeys, J.; Vermeulen, A.; Michelet, R.; Cuyckens, F.; Mannens, G.; Van Peer, A.; Annaert, P.; Allegaert, K.; Van Bocxlaer, J. Physiologically based pharmacokinetic predictions of tramadol exposure throughout pediatric life: An analysis of the different clearance contributors with emphasis on CYP2D6 maturation. *AAPS J.* **2015**, *17*, 1376–1387. [CrossRef] [PubMed]

48. Lee, E.; Ryan, S.; Birmingham, B.; Zalikowski, J.; March, R.; Ambrose, H.; Moore, R.; Lee, C.; Chen, Y.; Schneck, D. Rosuvastatin pharmacokinetics and pharmacogenetics in white and asian subjects residing in the same environment. *Clin. Pharmacol. Ther.* **2005**, *78*, 330–341. [CrossRef] [PubMed]

49. Karaźniewicz-Łada, M.; Danielak, D.; Burchardt, P.; Kruszyna, Ł.; Komosa, A.; Lesiak, M.; Główka, F. Clinical pharmacokinetics of clopidogrel and its metabolites in patients with cardiovascular diseases. *Clin. Pharmacokinet.* **2014**, *53*, 155–164. [CrossRef] [PubMed]

50. Wang, H.; Naghavi, M.; Allen, C.; Barber, R.M.; Bhutta, Z.A.; Carter, A.; Casey, D.C.; Charlson, F.J.; Chen, A.Z.; Coates, M.M.; et al. Global, regional, and national life expectancy, all-cause mortality, and cause-specific mortality for 249 causes of death, 1980–2015: A systematic analysis for the global burden of disease study 2015. *Lancet* **2016**, *388*, 1459–1544. [CrossRef]

51. Reddy, K.S.; Yusuf, S. Emerging epidemic of cardiovascular disease in developing countries. *Circulation* **1998**, *97*, 596–601. [CrossRef] [PubMed]

52. Greving, J.P.; Buskens, E.; Koffijberg, H.; Algra, A. Cost-effectiveness of aspirin treatment in the primary prevention of cardiovascular disease events in subgroups based on age, gender, and varying cardiovascular risk. *Circulation* **2008**, *117*, 2875–2883. [CrossRef] [PubMed]

53. Luk, H.H.; Pang, J.; Li, L.S.W.; Ng, M. Use of antiplatelet drugs in the stroke unit of a hong kong hospital. *Pharm. World Sci.* **2005**, *27*, 258–262. [CrossRef] [PubMed]

54. Uchiyama, S.; Fukuuchi, Y.; Yamaguchi, T. The safety and efficacy of clopidogrel versus ticlopidine in japanese stroke patients: Combined results of two phase iii, multicenter, randomized clinical trials. *J. Neurol.* **2009**, *256*, 888–897. [CrossRef] [PubMed]

55. Lee, J.B.; Lee, K.A.; Lee, K.Y. Cytochrome P450 2C19 polymorphism is associated with reduced clopidogrel response in cerebrovascular disease. *Yonsei Med. J.* **2011**, *52*, 734–738. [CrossRef] [PubMed]

56. Man, M.; Farmen, M.; Dumaual, C.; Teng, C.H.; Moser, B.; Irie, S.; Noh, G.J.; Njau, R.; Close, S.; Wise, S. Genetic variation in metabolizing enzyme and transporter genes: Comprehensive assessment in 3 major East Asian subpopulations with comparison to Caucasians and Africans. *J. Clin. Pharmacol.* **2010**, *50*, 929–940. [CrossRef] [PubMed]

57. Gaedigk, A. Interethnic differences of drug-metabolizing enzymes. *Int. J. Clin. Pharmacol. Ther.* **2000**, *38*, 61–68. [CrossRef] [PubMed]

58. Chen, Y.; Jin, J.Y.; Mukadam, S.; Malhi, V.; Kenny, J.R. Application of IVIVE and PBPK modeling in prospective prediction of clinical pharmacokinetics: Strategy and approach during the drug discovery phase with four case studies. *Biopharm. Drug Dispos.* **2012**, *33*, 85–98. [CrossRef] [PubMed]

59. Budha, N.R.; Leabman, M.; Jin, J.Y.; Wada, D.R.; Baruch, A.; Peng, K.; Tingley, W.G.; Davis, J.D. Modeling and simulation to support phase 2 dose selection for RG7652, a fully human monoclonal antibody against proprotein convertase subtilisin/kexin type 9. *AAPS J.* **2015**, *17*, 881–890. [CrossRef] [PubMed]

60. Cecchelli, R.; Berezowski, V.; Lundquist, S.; Culot, M.; Renftel, M.; Dehouck, M.-P.; Fenart, L. Modelling of the blood-brain barrier in drug discovery and development. *Nat. Rev. Drug Discov.* **2007**, *6*, 650–661. [CrossRef] [PubMed]

61. Zakaria, Z.; Badhan, R.K. The impact of CYP2B6 polymorphisms on the interactions of efavirenz with lumefantrine: Implications for paediatric antimalarial therapy. *Eur. J. Pharm. Sci.* **2018**, *119*, 90–101. [CrossRef] [PubMed]

62. Bhindi, R.; Ormerod, O.; Newton, J.; Banning, A.; Testa, L. Interaction between statins and clopidogrel: Is there anything clinically relevant? *QJM* **2008**, *101*, 915–925. [CrossRef] [PubMed]

63. Rolan, P. Plasma protein binding displacement interactions—Why are they still regarded as clinically important? *Br. J. Clin. Pharmacol.* **1994**, *37*, 125–128. [CrossRef] [PubMed]

64. Hamzah, A.A.; Bakar, Z.; Sani, N.A.; Tan, J.; Damanhuri, M.A.; Aripin, K.; Rani, M.M.; Noh, N.; Razali, R.; Mohamad, M. Relationship between education and cognitive performance among healthy malay adults. *Sains Malays.* **2016**, *45*, 1371–1379.

65. Khor, G.; Duraisamy, G.; Loh, S.; Green, T.; Skeaff, C. Dietary and blood folate status of malaysian women of childbearing age. *Asia Pac. J. Clin. Nutr.* **2006**, *15*, 341–349. [PubMed]

66. Lim, K.G. A review of adult obesity research in malaysia. *Med. J. Malays.* **2016**, *71*, 1–19.

67. Wang, X.-Q.; Shen, C.-L.; Wang, B.-N.; Huang, X.-H.; Hu, Z.-L.; Li, J. Genetic polymorphisms of CYP2C19*2 and ABCB1 C3435T affect the pharmacokinetic and pharmacodynamic responses to clopidogrel in 401 patients with acute coronary syndrome. *Gene* **2015**, *558*, 200–207. [CrossRef] [PubMed]

68. Chan, M.Y.; Tan, K.; Tan, H.-C.; Huan, P.-T.; Li, B.; Phua, Q.-H.; Lee, H.-K.; Lee, C.-H.; Low, A.; Becker, R.C. CYP2C19 and PON1 polymorphisms regulating clopidogrel bioactivation in chinese, malay and indian subjects. *Pharmacogenomics* **2012**, *13*, 533–542. [CrossRef] [PubMed]

69. Rosdi, R.A.; Yusoff, N.M.; Ismail, R.; Choon, T.S.; Musa, N.; Yusoff, S. A minireview of CYP2C9 and CYP2C19 single nucleotide polymorphisms (SNPS) among malaysian populations. *J. Biomed. Clin. Sci.* **2017**, *2*, 47–52.

70. Wang, H.-Y.; Chen, X.; Jiang, J.; Shi, J.; Hu, P. Evaluating a physiologically based pharmacokinetic model for predicting the pharmacokinetics of midazolam in chinese after oral administration. *Acta Pharmacol. Sin.* **2016**, *37*, 276–284. [CrossRef] [PubMed]

71. Feng, S.; Cleary, Y.; Parrott, N.; Hu, P.; Weber, C.; Wang, Y.; Yin, O.Q.; Shi, J. Evaluating a physiologically based pharmacokinetic model for prediction of omeprazole clearance and assessing ethnic sensitivity in CYP2C19 metabolic pathway. *Eur. J. Clin. Pharmacol.* **2015**, *71*, 617–624. [CrossRef] [PubMed]

72. Hasan, M.S.; Basri, H.B.; Hin, L.P.; Stanslas, J. Genetic polymorphisms and drug interactions leading to clopidogrel resistance: Why the asian population requires special attention. *Int. J. Neurosci.* **2013**, *123*, 143–154. [CrossRef] [PubMed]

73. Tang, Y.D.; Wang, W.; Yang, M.; Zhang, K.; Chen, J.; Qiao, S.; Yan, H.; Wu, Y.; Huang, X.; Xu, B.; et al. Randomized comparisons of double-dose clopidogrel or adjunctive cilostazol versus standard dual antiplatelet in patients with high posttreatment platelet reactivity: Results of the creative trial. *Circulation* **2018**, *137*, 2231–2245. [CrossRef] [PubMed]

74. Bossard, M.; Granger, C.B.; Tanguay, J.F.; Montalescot, G.; Faxon, D.P.; Jolly, S.S.; Widimsky, P.; Niemela, K.; Steg, P.G.; Natarajan, M.K.; et al. Double-dose versus standard-dose clopidogrel according to smoking status among patients with acute coronary syndromes undergoing percutaneous coronary intervention. *J. Am. Heart Assoc.* **2017**, *6*. [CrossRef] [PubMed]

75. Chen, S.; Zhang, Y.; Wang, L.; Geng, Y.; Gu, J.; Hao, Q.; Wang, H.; Qi, P. Effects of dual-dose clopidogrel, clopidogrel combined with tongxinluo capsule, and ticagrelor on patients with coronary heart disease and CYP2C19*2 gene mutation after percutaneous coronary interventions (PCI). *Med. Sci. Monit.* **2017**, *23*, 3824–3830. [CrossRef] [PubMed]

76. Collet, J.-P.; Hulot, J.-S.; Anzaha, G.; Pena, A.; Chastre, T.; Caron, C.; Silvain, J.; Cayla, G.; Bellemain-Appaix, A.; Vignalou, J.-B.; et al. High doses of clopidogrel to overcome genetic resistance. *JACC Cardiovasc. Interv.* **2011**, *4*, 392–402. [CrossRef] [PubMed]

77. Li, Y.; Tang, H.L.; Hu, Y.F.; Xie, H.G. The gain-of-function variant allele CYP2C19*17: A double-edged sword between thrombosis and bleeding in clopidogrel-treated patients. *J. Thromb. Haemost.* **2012**, *10*, 199–206. [CrossRef] [PubMed]

78. Zabalza, M.; Subirana, I.; Sala, J.; Lluis-Ganella, C.; Lucas, G.; Tomas, M.; Masia, R.; Marrugat, J.; Brugada, R.; Elosua, R. Meta-analyses of the association between cytochrome CYP2C19 loss- and gain-of-function polymorphisms and cardiovascular outcomes in patients with coronary artery disease treated with clopidogrel. *Heart* **2012**, *98*, 100–108. [CrossRef] [PubMed]

79. Bauer, T.; Bouman, H.J.; van Werkum, J.W.; Ford, N.F.; ten Berg, J.M.; Taubert, D. Impact of CYP2C19 variant genotypes on clinical efficacy of antiplatelet treatment with clopidogrel: Systematic review and meta-analysis. *BMJ* **2011**, *343*, d4588. [CrossRef] [PubMed]

80. Wilffert, B.; Swen, J.; Mulder, H.; Touw, D.; Maitland-Van der Zee, A.-H.; Deneer, V.; KNMP Working Group Pharmacogenetics. From evidence based medicine to mechanism based medicine. Reviewing the role of pharmacogenetics. *Int. J. Clin. Pharm.* **2013**, *35*, 369–375. [CrossRef] [PubMed]

81. Goh, L.L.; Lim, C.W.; Sim, W.C.; Toh, L.X.; Leong, K.P. Analysis of genetic variation in CYP450 genes for clinical implementation. *PLoS ONE* **2017**, *12*, e0169233. [CrossRef] [PubMed]

82. Varma, M.V.S.; Lai, Y.; Kimoto, E.; Goosen, T.C.; El-Kattan, A.F.; Kumar, V. Mechanistic modeling to predict the transporter- and enzyme-mediated drug-drug interactions of repaglinide. *Pharm. Res.* **2013**, *30*, 1188–1199. [CrossRef] [PubMed]

83. Bae, S.H.; Park, W.S.; Han, S.; Park, G.J.; Lee, J.; Hong, T.; Jeon, S.; Yim, D.S. Physiologically-based pharmacokinetic predictions of intestinal BCRP-mediated drug interactions of rosuvastatin in Koreans. *Korean J. Physiol. Pharmacol.* **2018**, *22*, 321–329. [CrossRef] [PubMed]

84. Edginton, A.N.; Schmitt, W.; Willmann, S. Development and evaluation of a generic physiologically based pharmacokinetic model for children. *Clin. Pharmacokinet.* **2006**, *45*, 1013–1034. [CrossRef] [PubMed]

85. Ginsberg, G.; Hattis, D.; Russ, A.; Sonawane, B. Physiologically based pharmacokinetic (PBPK) modeling of caffeine and theophylline in neonates and adults: Implications for assessing children's risks from environmental agents. *J. Toxicol. Environ. Health Part A* **2004**, *67*, 297–329. [CrossRef] [PubMed]

86. Parrott, N.; Davies, B.; Hoffmann, G.; Koerner, A.; Lave, T.; Prinssen, E.; Theogaraj, E.; Singer, T. Development of a physiologically based model for oseltamivir and simulation of pharmacokinetics in neonates and infants. *Clin. Pharmacokinet.* **2011**, *50*, 613–623. [CrossRef] [PubMed]

87. U.S. Food and Drug Administration. Summary Minutes of the Advisory Committee for Pharmaceutical Science and Clinical Pharmacology. Available online: https://wayback.archive-it.org/7993/20170403224110/https://www.fda.gov/AdvisoryCommittees/CommitteesMeetingMaterials/Drugs/AdvisoryCommitteeforPharmaceuticalScienceandClinicalPharmacology/ucm286697.htm (accessed on 29 May 2018).

6

Mitoxantrone is more Toxic than Doxorubicin in SH-SY5Y Human Cells: A 'Chemobrain' In Vitro Study

Daniela Almeida [1,†], Rita Pinho [1,†], Verónica Correia [1], Jorge Soares [1], Maria de Lourdes Bastos [1], Félix Carvalho [1], João Paulo Capela [1,2] and Vera Marisa Costa [1,*]

[1] UCIBIO, REQUIMTE, Laboratory of Toxicology, Faculty of Pharmacy, University of Porto, Rua de Jorge Viterbo Ferreira, 228, 4050-313 Porto, Portugal; anadaniela_16@hotmail.com (D.A.); rita.pinho94@gmail.com (R.P.); vero_correi@hotmail.com (V.C.); jorge.emt.soares@gmail.com (J.S.); mlbastos@ff.up.pt (M.d.L.B.); felixdc@ff.up.pt (F.C.); joaoc@ufp.edu.pt (J.P.C.)

[2] FP-ENAS (Unidade de Investigação UFP em Energia, Ambiente e Saúde), CEBIMED (Centro de Estudos em Biomedicina), Faculdade de Ciências da Saúde, Universidade Fernando Pessoa, 4249-004 Porto, Portugal

* Correspondence: veramcosta@ff.up.pt

† Both authors contributed equally to this work.

Abstract: The potential neurotoxic effects of anticancer drugs, like doxorubicin (DOX) and mitoxantrone (MTX; also used in multiple sclerosis), are presently important reasons for concern, following epidemiological data indicating that cancer survivors submitted to chemotherapy may suffer cognitive deficits. We evaluated the in vitro neurotoxicity of two commonly used chemotherapeutic drugs, DOX and MTX, and study their underlying mechanisms in the SH-SY5Y human neuronal cell model. Undifferentiated human SH-SY5Y cells were exposed to DOX or MTX (0.13, 0.2 and 0.5 μM) for 48 h and two cytotoxicity assays were performed, the 3-(4,5-dimethylthiazol-2-yl)-2,5-diphenyltetrazolium (MTT) reduction and the neutral red (NR) incorporation assays. Phase contrast microphotographs, Hoechst, and acridine orange/ethidium bromide stains were performed. Mitochondrial membrane potential was also assessed. Moreover, putative protective drugs, namely the antioxidants N-acetyl-L-cysteine (NAC; 1 mM) and 100 μM tiron, the inhibitor of caspase-3/7, Ac-DEVD-CHO (100 μM), and a protein synthesis inhibitor, cycloheximide (CHX; 10 nM), were tested to prevent DOX- or MTX-induced toxicity. The MTT reduction assay was also done in differentiated SH-SY5Y cells following exposure to 0.2 μM DOX or MTX. MTX was more toxic than DOX in both cytotoxicity assays and according to the morphological analyses. MTX also evoked a higher number of apoptotic nuclei than DOX. Both drugs, at the 0.13 μM concentration, caused mitochondrial membrane potential depolarization after a 48-h exposure. Regarding the putative neuroprotectors, 1 mM NAC was not able to prevent the cytotoxicity caused by either drug. Notwithstanding, 100 μM tiron was capable of partially reverting MTX-induced cytotoxicity in the NR uptake assay. One hundred μM Ac-DEVD-CHO and 10 nM cycloheximide (CHX) also partially prevented the toxicity induced by DOX in the NR uptake assay. MTX was more toxic than DOX in differentiated SH-SY5Y cells, while MTX had similar toxicity in differentiated and undifferentiated SH-SY5Y cells. In fact, MTX was the most neurotoxic drug tested and the mechanisms involved seem dissimilar among drugs. Thus, its toxicity mechanisms need to be further investigated as to determine the putative neurotoxicity for multiple sclerosis and cancer patients.

Keywords: mitoxantrone; doxorubicin; neurotoxicity; SH-SY5Y cells

1. Introduction

Deaths after neoplasms have been increasing globally, rising from 7.58 million deaths in 2006 to 8.93 million deaths in 2016 [1]. Although new treatments have emerged recently, chemotherapy is still the most common treatment for most cancers [2,3]. Mitoxantrone (MTX) is an anticancer drug used in the treatment of metastatic breast cancer, non-Hodgkin's lymphoma, and acute myeloid leukaemia in adults; while in combination regimens, it is indicated in the remission-induction treatment of blast crisis in chronic myeloid leukaemia, and in combination with corticosteroids for palliation (e.g., pain relief) related to advanced castrate-resistant prostate cancer [4]. Moreover, the U.S. Food and Drug Administration (FDA) approved its use in secondary progressive multiple sclerosis (SPMS), in progressive relapsing multiple sclerosis (MS), and for patients with worsening relapsing-remitting (RR) MS [5]. Various MTX dosage schedules can be used in cancer patients, although in adults with solid tumors, $12-14$ mg/m^2 every 3–4 weeks is usual [6]. MTX is given intravenously at a dose of 12 mg/m^2 every 3 months to MS patients. Although a maximum cumulative lifetime dose of 140 mg/m^2 should not be surpassed, recommendations exist of lower cumulative doses being given to MS patients as they seem more susceptible to cardiotoxicity [7]. Doxorubicin (DOX) is used in the treatment of the following cancers: metastatic breast cancer, advanced cancer of the ovary, Kaposi's sarcoma and multiple myeloma [8]. DOX and MTX are both topoisomerase II inhibitors and exert their antineoplastic action by intercalating into DNA and producing both DNA strand-breaks and interstrand cross-links; they also interfere with RNA synthesis [4,8]. New drugs are emerging for cancer treatments, but chemotherapy is still the most common and well-characterized option in several cancers [3,9].

Although life expectancy is largely increasing due to the chemotherapeutic regiments available, serious side effects emerge after chemotherapy. Mielossupression and cardiotoxicity of MTX (and also of its analog, DOX) are common concerns among cancer treated patients [2,10–12]. However, data have shown that brain tissue is also susceptible to the toxicity of chemotherapeutic agents, despite presumption of blood-brain barrier (BBB) protection [13]. "Chemobrain" is the term used to describe the cognitive decline associated with chemotherapy. Persistent changes in cognitive function, including memory loss, distractibility, and difficulty in performing multiple tasks, have been observed in breast cancer survivors after treatment with chemotherapeutic agents, including DOX [14]. Women with breast cancer and treated with four cycles of DOX and cyclophosphamide had significant decreases in visuospatial skill and total cognitive scores, following chemotherapy [15]. In a broader study by the same authors, cognitive impairment was found in 23% of women prior to chemotherapy. Thereafter, they received the combination of DOX and cyclophosphamide or followed by a taxane. Significant decreases in the cognitive domains of visuospatial skill, attention, delayed memory, and motor function were observed after receiving chemotherapy, but improvements followed 6 months after the completion of chemotherapy [16]. The authors stated that having a breast cancer diagnosis can result in cognitive impairment and that chemotherapy may have a negative acute impact on cognitive function [16]. However, other data support long-term neurotoxic effects of chemotherapy. Long-term survivors of breast cancer or lymphoma, who had been treated with systemic chemotherapy (DOX being present in several of the systemic regimens taken), scored significantly lower on several neuropsychological tests compared to those treated with local therapy only, particularly in the domains of verbal memory, and psychomotor functioning; also they were in the lower quartile on the Neuropsychological Performance Index, and self-reported greater problems with working memory on the Squire Memory Self-Rating Questionnaire [17]. Some in vitro data demonstrate that both apoptosis and oxidative stress can be involved in DOX-induced neurotoxicity [18,19]. Moreover, treatment with DOX increases circulating level of tumor necrosis factor-alpha and leads to decline in mitochondrial respiration and mitochondrial protein nitration, being nitric oxide an important mediator of those effects in mice [20]. Regarding MTX, little data is available about its putative neurotoxicity, although some questions were placed in the past whether increased incidence of central nervous system (CNS) hemorrhages in patients with secondary acute promyelocytic leukemia were a consequence of MTX treatment [21]. As far as local neurological side effects are concerned, the administration of MTX caused very short-lived partial Jacksonian motor seizures; momentary light headache lasting 1–2 h and slight drowsiness lasting no more than 6 h in patients with recurrent glioblastomas enrolled for second tumor debulking with local positioning of a reservoir containing MTX [22]. In two patients, a hemorrhage occurred in the absence of any clinical deficits and vanished in both cases within a month [22]. Most importantly, the new use of MTX on MS may pose as an added risk for MTX-induced neurotoxicity, as dysregulation of the BBB is an early cerebrovascular abnormality seen in the MS patient brain [23], circumventing the important function of BBB as the retaining wall preventing drug passage into the CNS. In a work by Fulda et al. DOX and MTX were compared in neuroblastoma SK-N-SH cells and DOX was more toxic than MTX, according to monolayer proliferation assay [24]; however more studies are required. Therefore, our work aimed to determine the neurotoxicity profile of MTX and compare it with a known neurotoxic chemotherapeutic drug, DOX. SH-SY5Y cells are a frequent neuronal model used in neurotoxicity studies and are a subline of the parental line SK-N-SH. Those human cells were used herein as an in vitro neuronal model and several determinations were performed. Moreover, pharmacological active drugs were used as putative protectors, according to the data previously published on the putative DOX neurotoxic mechanisms [18,19,25–27].

2. Results

2.1. The Cytotoxicity of Mitoxantrone Was Significantly Higher Than That of Doxorubicin

At 24 h, in the 3-(4,5-dimethylthiazol-2-yl)-2,5-diphenyl tetrazolium bromide (MTT) reduction assay, all concentrations of either DOX or MTX caused significant cytotoxicity when compared to control (Figure 1A), MTX being more cytotoxic than DOX [31.5 ± 10.5% (MTX) versus 46.9 ± 15.4% (DOX) for the lowest concentration; 32.6 ± 12.2% (MTX) versus 51.2 ± 14.3% (DOX) for the 0.2 µM intermediate concentration; and 41.4 ± 10.5% (MTX) versus 58.5 ± 10.8% (DOX) for the highest concentration (0.5 µM)]. Of note that, in the MTT assay, we could not find a concentration-dependent toxicity for MTX at both time-points tested. Moreover, DOX 0.5 µM was less toxic than the lowest DOX concentration (0.13 µM) tested at 24 h.

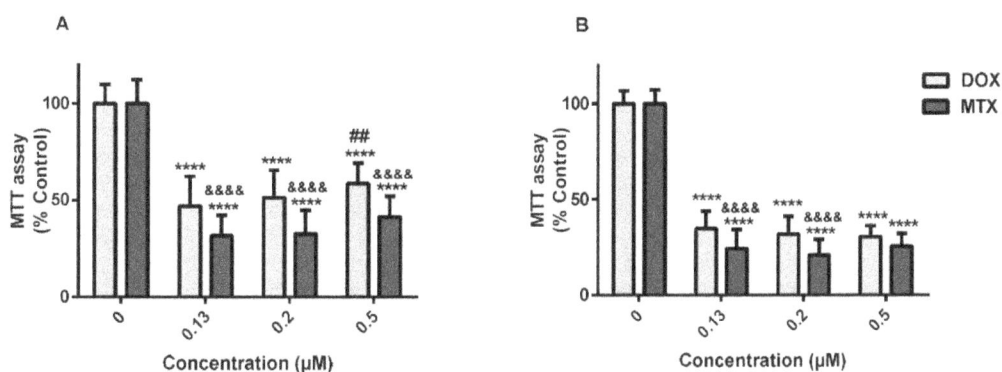

Figure 1. MTT reduction assay after exposure to 0.5, 0.2 and 0.13 µM DOX (light grey) or 0.5, 0.2 and 0.13 µM MTX (dark grey) after 24 h (**A**) or 48 h (**B**) in undifferentiated SH-SY5Y cells. Sterile PBS was used as control. Results are presented as mean ± SD of 23–35 wells, of 5–6 independent experiments. Statistical analyses were performed using two-way ANOVA followed by the Bonferroni *post-hoc* test(**** $p < 0.0001$ versus control; ## $p < 0.01$ versus the same drug at 0.13 µM; &&&& $p < 0.0001$ MTX versus the same DOX concentration).

At the 48 h time-point, MTX caused the highest toxicity at concentrations of 0.13 µM and 0.2 µM, when compared to DOX in the same concentrations (Figure 1B). At 24 h, significant differences were observed between the two molecules, in the neutral red (NR) uptake assay, MTX being more cytotoxic than DOX (Figure 2A). At 48 h, significant differences between DOX and MTX were only found at

0.5 µM (DOX: 47.2 ± 13.3%; MTX: 35.6 ± 10.1%) (Figure 2B). Additionally, in the NR uptake assay and following a 24-h exposure, the lower concentration (0.13 µM) of both DOX and MTX was more toxic than the highest concentration tested (0.5 µM) (Figure 2A). Meanwhile, this difference was not verified at 48 h (Figure 2B).

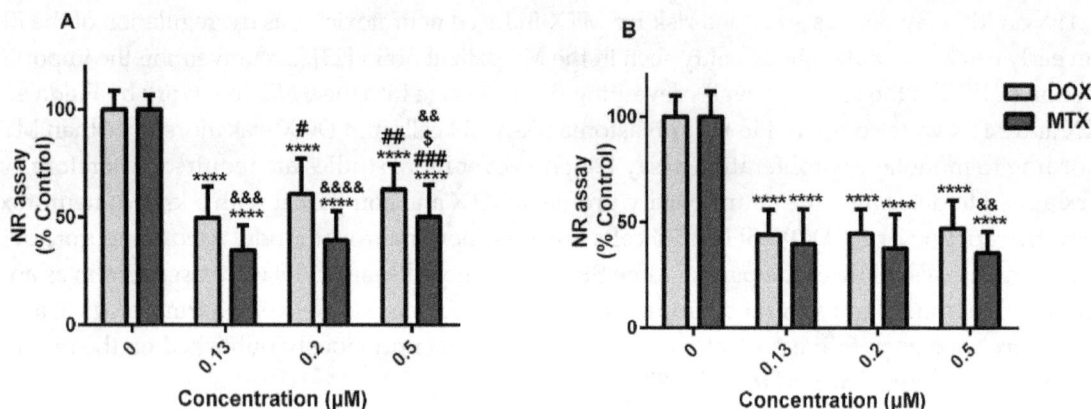

Figure 2. NR uptake assay after exposure to 0.5, 0.2 and 0.13 µM DOX (light grey) or 0.5, 0.2 and 0.13 µM MTX (dark grey) after 24 h (**A**) or 48 h (**B**) in undifferentiated SH-SY5Y cells. Sterile PBS was used as control. Results are presented as mean ± SD of 24–37 wells, of 5–7 independent experiments. Statistical analyses were performed using two-way ANOVA followed by the Bonferroni *post-hoc* test (**** $p < 0.0001$ versus control; # $p < 0.05$ versus the same drug at 0.13 µM; ## $p < 0.01$ versus the same drug at 0.13 µM; ### $p < 0.001$ versus the same drug at 0.13 µM; && $p < 0.01$ MTX versus 0.5 µM DOX; &&& $p < 0.001$ MTX versus 0.13 µM DOX; &&&& $p < 0.0001$ MTX versus 0.2 µM DOX; $ $p < 0.05$ versus same molecule at concentration 0.2 µM).

2.2. Mitoxantrone Led to Cellular Damage in SH-SY5Y Cells, with Signs of Apoptosis Most Evident at the Lowest Concentration after a 48-h Exposure

A decrease in cell density was observed in all MTX-treated cells with a typical loss of shape and loss of neurites, at 48 h (Figure 3). The neurotoxic phenomenon was more expressive than the one observed in cells incubated with MTX for 24 h (data not shown). Cell number was substantially decreased after MTX treatment, as seen in the Hoechst staining (Table 1). Additionally, the lower concentration of MTX (0.13 µM) had a higher number of cells with apoptotic nuclear morphology, namely nuclear fragmentation, as well as chromatin condensation than the other MTX concentrations tested (Figure 3 and Table 1).

Table 1. Number of cells and condensed nuclei after the Hoescht staining at 48 h.

Parameters				
MTX	Control	0.13 µM	0.2 µM	0.5 µM
Condensed nuclei	4 ± 4	205 ± 111	130 ± 29	117 ± 29
Number of cells	439 ± 102	357 ± 95	259 ± 19	212 ± 15
Ratio of condensed nuclei/number of cells	0.89 ± 0.76	57.04 ± 24.98 *	50.09 ± 9.30	54.87 ± 9.54
DOX	Control	0.13 µM	0.2 µM	0.5 µM
Condensed nuclei	2 ± 1	43 ± 8	26 ± 12	84 ± 14
Number of cells	436 ± 98	263 ± 29	186 ± 59	170 ± 18
Ratio of condensed nuclei/number of cells	0.39 ± 0.27	16.20 ± 2.05	13.53 ± 2.57	49.00 ± 4.00 **

Results are presented as mean ± SD of two independent experiments and two different fields each. Each field was counted manually and the microphotographs were taken with the magnification of 200×. Statistical analyses were performed on the ratio of condensed nuclei/number of cells using the Kruskal-Wallis test, followed by the Dunn's *post-hoc* test. (* $p < 0.05$; ** $p < 0.01$ versus control).

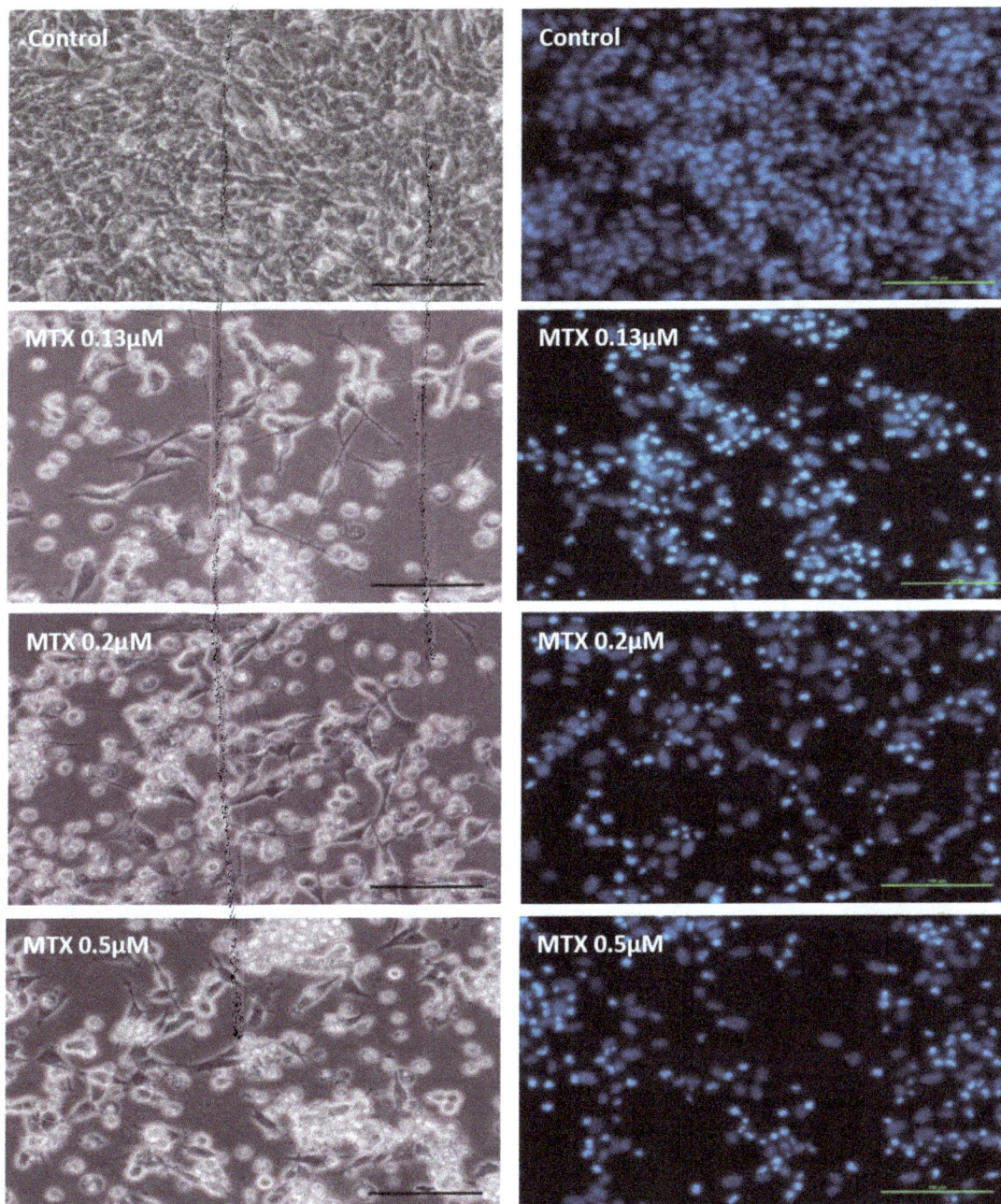

Figure 3. Phase-contrast microphotographs (left column) of undifferentiated SH-SY5Y cells exposed to PBS (control) or 0.13 μM MTX, 0.2 μM MTX and 0.5 μM MTX. Right side, fluorescence microscopy (Hoechst 33258 staining) of undifferentiated SH-SY5Y cells incubated with PBS (control) or 0.13 μM, 0.2 μM and 0.5 μM MTX. The microphotographs were taken after a 48-h exposure to the various conditions. Images are representative of two independent experiments with at least two wells (scale bar represents 100 μm).

The toxicity observed at 48 h (Figure 4) was higher after DOX exposure than at 24 h at the same concentrations (data not shown). At 48 h, DOX caused a substantial decrease in cell density when compared to control and many cells treated with DOX had rounded appearance without neuritis (Figure 4). In the fluorescence microscopy photographs, nuclear fragmentation and chromatin condensation were observed after a 48-h exposure to DOX, with a higher number of apoptotic cells at the highest concentration tested (0.5 μM) (Figure 4 and Table 1).

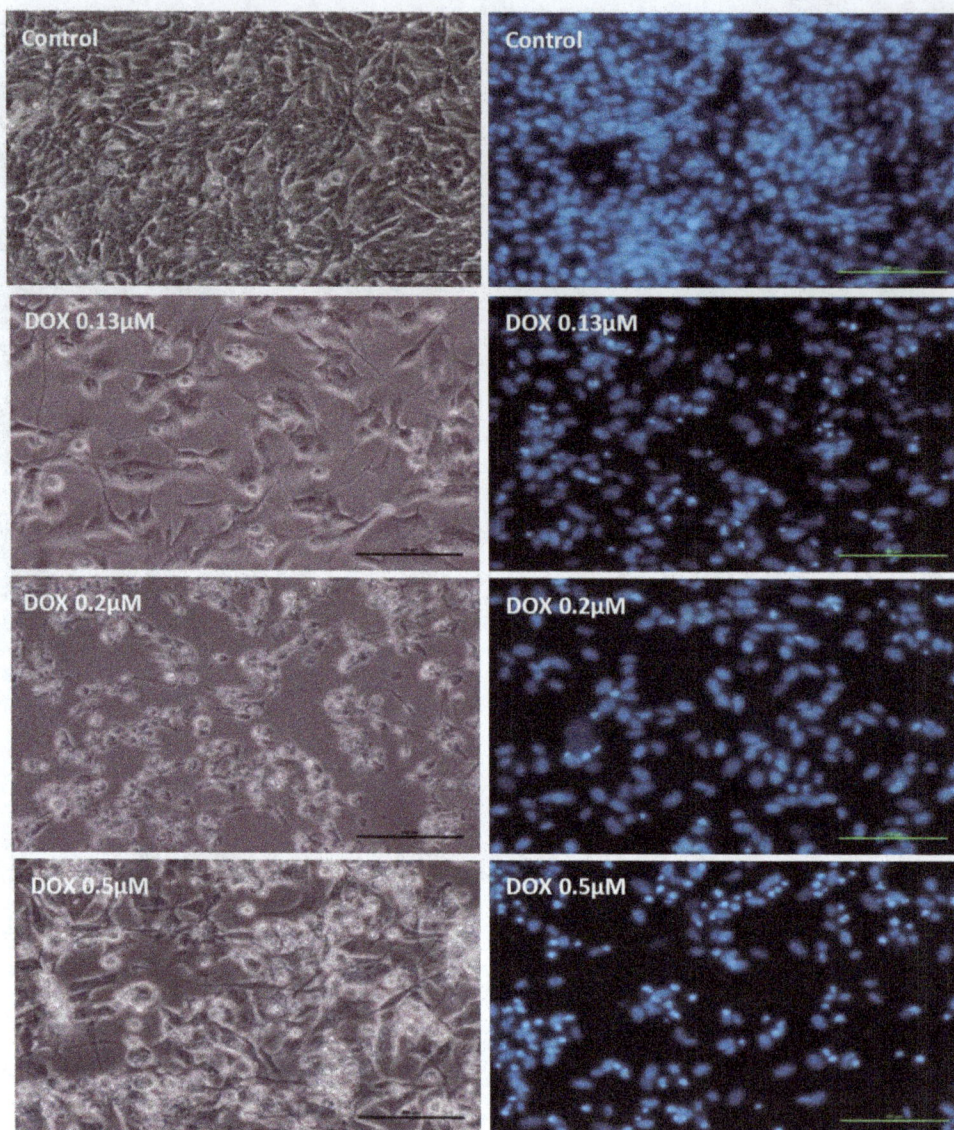

Figure 4. Phase-contrast microphotographs (left column) of undifferentiated SH-SY5Y cells incubated with PBS (control) or 0.13 μM, 0.2 μM and 0.5 μM DOX. Right side, fluorescence microscopy (Hoechst 33258 staining) of undifferentiated SH-SY5Y cells incubated with PBS (control) or 0.13 μM, 0.2 μM and 0.5 μM DOX. The microphotographs were taken after a 48-h exposure to the various conditions. Images are representative of two independent experiments with at least two wells (scale bar represents 100 μm).

2.3. Mitoxantrone and Doxorubicin Caused Apoptosis in Undifferentiated SH-SY5Y Cells

In Figures 5 and 6, cells with well-colored green and large nuclei (white arrow) were seen in the control living cells. In SH-SY5Y cells exposed to MTX for 48 h, cells with condensed green nucleus (pink arrows), indicative of early apoptotic cells, were observed with very few adherent cells in the field (Figure 5). After exposure to 0.5 μM MTX, the lack of neurites was evident, when compared to the two lower concentrations (Figure 5). In Figure 6, cells incubated with DOX for 48 h are shown, and several red dots of nuclear condensation within the cells or condensed nuclei, both signs of apoptosis (pink arrows) were noteworthy in all concentrations. At 48 h, a higher number of cells per field was observed in DOX-exposed cells when compared with MTX-incubated SH-SY5Y cells, in the same concentrations.

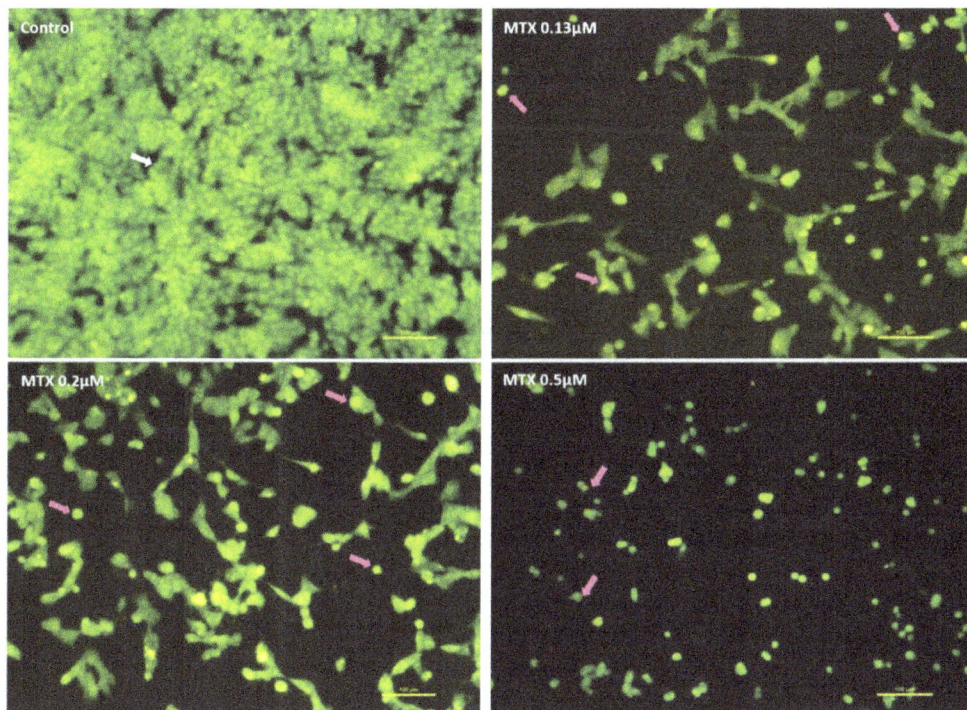

Figure 5. Representative fluorescence microscopic photos following acridine orange/ethidium bromide staining in undifferentiated SH-SY5Y cells after a 48-h incubation with MTX (0.13 μM; 0.2 μM; 0.5 μM) and control cells. White arrow: viable cells; pink arrows: cells with signs of apoptosis. Images are representative of two independent experiments with at least two wells. Scale bar represents 100 μm.

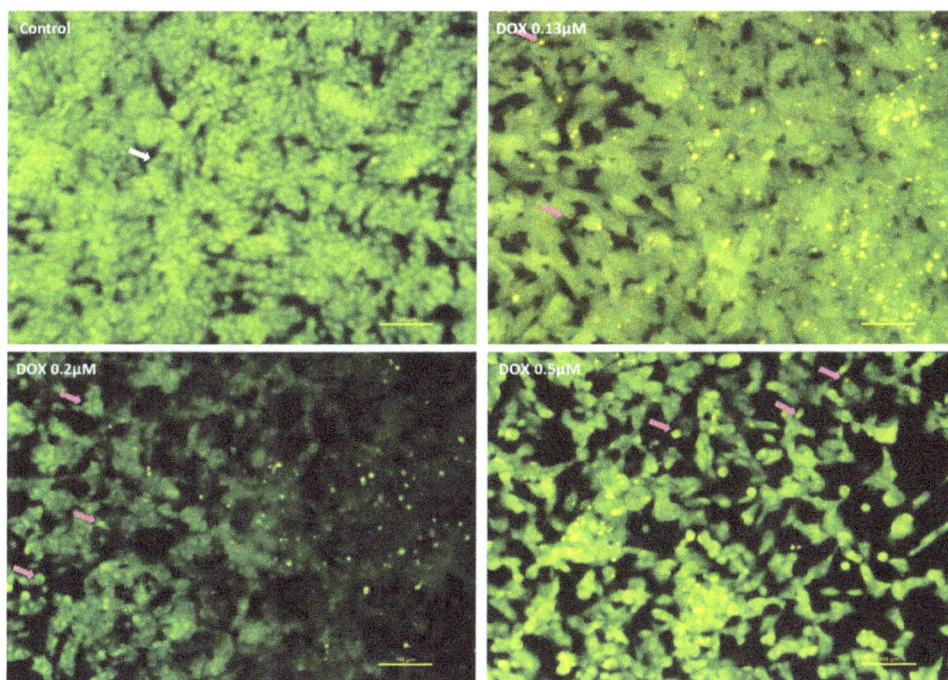

Figure 6. Representative fluorescence microscopic photos following acridine orange/ethidium bromide staining in undifferentiated SH-SY5Y cells after a 48-h incubation with DOX (0.13 μM; 0.2 μM; 0.5 μM) and control cells. White arrow: viable cells; pink arrows: cells with signs of apoptosis. Images are representative of two independent experiments with at least two wells. Scale bar represents 100 μm.

2.4. Both Doxorubicin and Mitoxantrone Caused a Decrease in the Mitochondria Potential of Neuronal Cells at 0.13 μM

The transmembrane mitochondrial potential of undifferentiated SH-SY5Y cells following a 48-h exposure can be seen in Figure 7. Control cells were bright green. The lower concentration of MTX (0.13 μM) led to a total depolarization of the mitochondria, when compared to the control cells. Meanwhile, 0.13 μM DOX also caused evident depolarization of cells after a 48-h exposure.

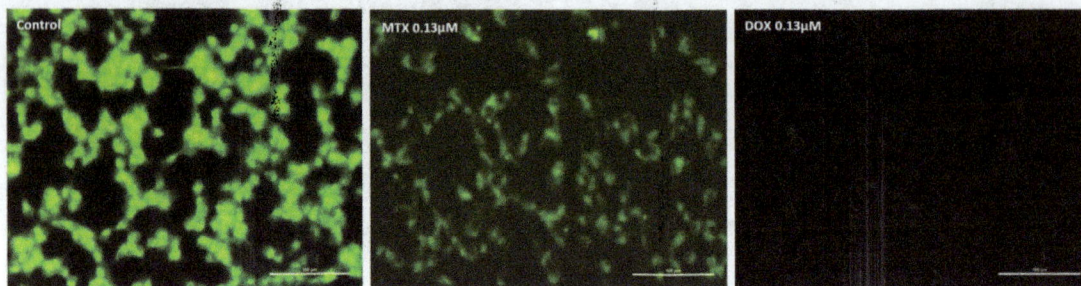

Figure 7. Microphotographs showing the mitochondrial transmembrane potential of undifferentiated SH-SY5Y control cells, and cells incubated with 0.13 μM MTX or 0.13 μM DOX for 48 h. Images are representative of two independent experiments with at least two wells. Scale bar represents 100 μm.

2.5. Tiron, an Antioxidant, was the Only Drug That Partially Prevented the Cytotoxicity of Mitoxantrone in the Neutral Red Uptake Assay

Tiron was able to partially prevent the MTX-induced cytotoxicity in undifferentiated SH-SY5Y cells in the NR uptake assay, but not in the MTT reduction assay at 48 h (data not shown). In the MTT reduction assay, the values obtained after exposure to 0.2 μM MTX, either alone or in combination with 100 μM tiron, were always lower than control and not different between themselves (data not shown). Moreover, 100 μM tiron alone did not cause any cellular cytotoxicity. The MTX 0.2 μM exposed cells (29.0 ± 7.6%) had lower levels of NR uptake than the control cells (100.0 ± 8.4%), which revealed its neurotoxic nature (Figure 8A). However, when compared with MTX + tiron (41.1 ± 11.3%), 100 μM tiron revealed to be protective (Figure 8A). Moreover, there was no significant difference between the 100 μM tiron condition (96.2 ± 11.6%) and control cells (100.0 ± 8.4%) (Figure 8A). *N*-acetyl-L-cysteine (NAC, 1 mM), also an antioxidant, was not able to avoid the cytotoxicity induced by 0.2 μM MTX at 48 h in undifferentiated SH-SY5Y cells, neither in the MTT reduction assay nor in the NR uptake assay (data not shown). Also, neither 10 nM CHX nor 100 μM Ac-DEVD-CHO, an inhibitor of caspase-3/7, were able to prevent the cytotoxicity observed after exposure to 0.2 μM MTX in the MTT reduction assay or in the NR uptake assay (data not shown).

2.6. Cycloheximide, a Protein Synthesis Inhibitor, and Ac-DEVD-CHO, an Inhibitor of Caspase-3, Partially Counteracted the Doxorubicin-Induced Toxicity

CHX was able to partially prevent DOX-induced cytotoxicity in undifferentiated SH-SY5Y cells in the NR uptake assay (Figure 8B), but not in the MTT assay at 48 h (data not shown). In the NR uptake assay, the values after exposure to 0.2 μM DOX (32.9 ± 8.4%) were lower than the control (100.0 ± 8.2%, Figure 8B). The DOX + CHX (40.2 ± 9.5%) condition had also lower values than those of control, but significantly higher than that obtained after exposure to 0.2 μM DOX alone, revealing the neuroprotective action of CHX. In the NR uptake assay, 10 nM CHX exposed cells (93.8 ± 8.1%) did not differ to the respective control (Figure 8B: 100.0 ± 8.2%).

The caspase-3 inhibitor was able to provide partial neuroprotection against 0.2 μM DOX toxicity in undifferentiated SH-SY5Y cells in the NR uptake assay (Figure 8C). DOX + Ac-DEVD-CHO had significantly higher NR uptake values (40.1 ± 5.0%) than those of 0.2 μM DOX alone (32.3 ± 7.2%), demonstrating that the inhibitor had a partial neuroprotective action against the anticancer drug toxicity. Of note, 100 µM Ac-DEVD-CHO (89.3 ± 10.8%) caused some toxicity *per se* when compared to control cells (100.0 ± 6.7%). In the MTT reduction assay, 0.2 µM DOX and DOX + Ac-DEVD-CHO conditions had similar values (data not shown).

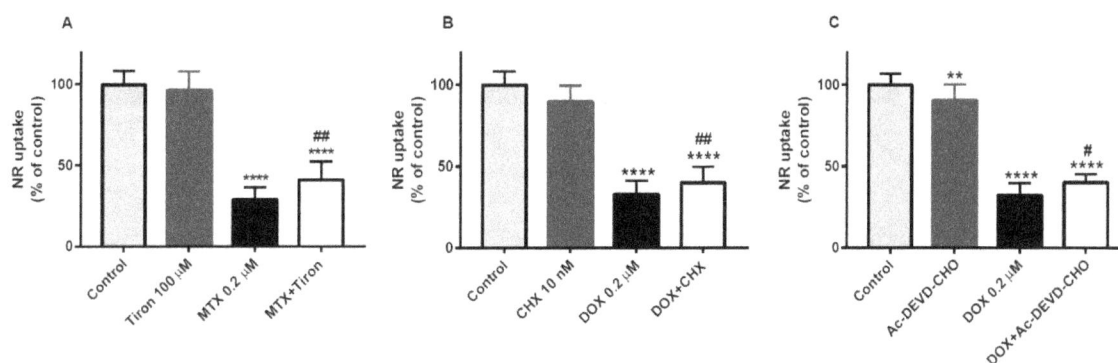

Figure 8. (**A**) NR uptake assay in undifferentiated SH-SY5Y cells proving the protective effect of tiron against MTX neurotoxicity. Four conditions were tested: control (with PBS); 100 µM tiron; 0.2 µM MTX; 0.2 µM MTX + 100 µM tiron. Results are presented as mean ± SD of 17–24 wells of 3–4 independent experiments. Statistical analyses were performed using the one-way ANOVA, followed by the Tukey's *post hoc* test (**** $p < 0.0001$ versus control; ## $p < 0.01$ versus 0.2 µM MTX). (**B**) NR uptake assay in undifferentiated SH-SY5Y cells showing the protective effect of cycloheximide (CHX) against DOX neurotoxicity. Four conditions were tested: control (with PBS); 10 nM CHX; 0.2 µM DOX; 0.2 µM DOX + 10 nM CHX. Results are presented as mean ± SD of 14–18 wells of 3 independent experiments. Statistical analyses were performed using the Kruskal–Wallis test, followed by the Dunn's *post hoc* test (**** $p < 0.0001$ versus control; ## $p < 0.01$ versus 0.2 µM DOX). (**C**) NR uptake assay in undifferentiated SH-SY5Y cells proving the protective effect of Ac-DEVD-CHO against DOX neurotoxicity. Four conditions were tested: control (with PBS); 100 µM Ac-DEVD-CHO; 0.2 µM DOX; 0.2 µM DOX + 100 µM Ac-DEVD-CHO. Results are presented as mean ± SD of 15–18 wells of 3 independent experiments. Statistical analyses were performed using the one-way ANOVA, followed by the Tukey's *post hoc* test (** $p < 0.01$, **** $p < 0.0001$ versus control; # $p < 0.05$ versus 0.2 µM DOX).

One mM NAC was not able to counteract the cytotoxicity induced by 0.2 µM DOX at 48 h in undifferentiated SH-SY5Y cells, neither in the MTT reduction assay nor in the NR uptake assay (data not shown). Moreover, tiron was not protective against DOX-induced neurotoxicity, in both cytotoxicity assays performed, as the 0.2 µM DOX and DOX + tiron conditions did not show significant differences among themselves (data not shown).

2.7. Doxorubicin Caused Greater Cytotoxicity in Undifferentiated SH-SY5Y Cells than in Differentiated Cells According to the MTT Reduction Assay

Following a 48-h exposure, differentiated SH-SY5Y cells exposed to 0.2 µM MTX presented slightly higher values in the MTT reduction test than undifferentiated cells, but with no statistical significance (differentiated cells: 29.0 ± 7.1%; undifferentiated cells: 22.6 ± 11.5%) (Figure 9A). At 48 h, the differentiated cells exposed to 0.2 µM DOX presented substantially higher MTT reduction values (66.2 ± 6.0%) than in undifferentiated cells at the same conditions (34.8 ± 6.8%) (Figure 9B).

2.8. Mitoxantrone is More Neurotoxic than Doxorubicin in Differentiated SH-SY5Y Cells in the MTT Reduction Assay

Both DOX and MTX caused neurotoxicity in differentiated SH-SY5Y cells after a 48-h exposure (Figure 9C). In the MTT reduction assay, 0.2 µM MTX (29.0 ± 7.1%) was more cytotoxic than 0.2 µM DOX (66.2 ± 6.0%) in differentiated SH-SY5Y cells (Figure 9C).

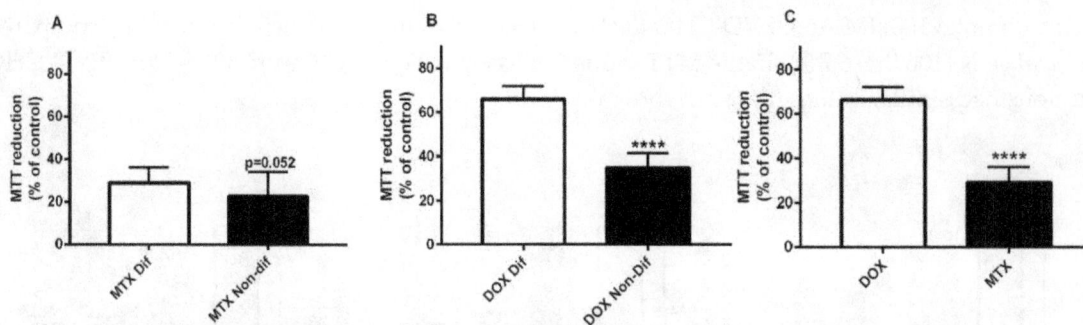

Figure 9. MTT reduction assay after exposure to 0.2 μM MTX (**A**) or 0.2 μM DOX (**B**) in differentiated or undifferentiated SH-SY5Y cells. Four conditions were tested: 0.2 μM MTX in differentiated cells, 0.2 μM MTX in undifferentiated cells, 0.2 μM DOX in differentiated cells and 0.2 μM DOX in undifferentiated cells. Values are expressed as percentage of control and are presented as mean ± SD. The results were obtained from 12–24 wells, from 2–4 independent experiments. Data were statistically analyzed using the unpaired t-test (**** $p < 0.0001$ versus differentiated cells treated with drug 0.2 μM). (**C**) MTT reduction assay after exposure to MTX or DOX in differentiated SH-SY5Y cells. Two conditions were tested: 0.2 μM DOX and 0.2 μM MTX. Values are expressed as percentage of control and are presented as mean ± SD. The results were obtained from 12 wells and 2 independent experiments. Data were statistically analyzed using the unpaired t-test (**** $p < 0.0001$ versus 0.2 μM DOX).

3. Discussion

This study revealed the following major findings: (1) MTX and DOX caused a time-dependent cytotoxicity in the NR uptake and in the MTT reduction assays, in undifferentiated SH-SY5Y cells; (2) MTX was shown to cause greater cytotoxicity at 24 h than DOX in undifferentiated SH-SY5Y cells; (3) MTX caused greater morphological damage, with lower cell density and neurites loss, when compared to DOX; (4) both drugs caused signs of apoptosis, in particular MTX, as both revealed by Hoechst and the ethidium bromide and acridine orange stains; (5) the lower concentration of DOX and MTX (0.13 μM) caused significant mitochondrial depolarization in undifferentiated SH-SY5Y cells; (6) tiron, an antioxidant, partially avoided the neurotoxicity exerted by MTX on undifferentiated SH-SY5Y cells in the NR uptake assay; (7) CHX and the caspase inhibitor, Ac-DEVD-CHO, were partially neuroprotective against the cytotoxicity caused by DOX on undifferentiated SH-SY5Y cells in the NR uptake assay; (8) in the MTT reduction assay, the cytotoxicity caused by MTX was similar, regardless of SH-SY5Y cells differentiation status, whereas DOX was more toxic in undifferentiated SH-SY5Y cells; and (9) in differentiated SH-SY5Y cells, MTX was shown to be more neurotoxic than DOX, according to the MTT reduction assay.

Drugs used in chemotherapy, such as DOX and MTX, may be responsible for neuronal damage with consequent neurotoxicity [22,28]. Persistent changes in cognitive function, including memory loss, distractibility, and difficulty in performing multiple tasks, have been observed in breast cancer survivors after chemotherapy, namely with DOX [15–17]. One could argue that BBB works as a protective barrier avoiding the entrance of several compounds and it is generally accepted that efflux transporters, namely P-glycoprotein and breast cancer resistance protein (BCRP) present in BBB, would extensively prevent the entrance of DOX and MTX to the CNS [29,30]. However, pharmacokinetic data obtained *post mortem* of treated patients show that both drugs are present in the brain [31,32]. Moreover, although MTX and DOX are given in very different doses to cancer patients, those doses are considered equivalent in the clinical practice [33]. In plasma of cancer-treated patients, DOX ranged between 0.04 to 1.16 μM and MTX levels were between 0.04 to 0.3 μM [34–39], while it is expected that the brain may be exposed to lower concentrations of those found in the plasma. We observed that both MTX and DOX, at clinically relevant concentrations, caused a high degree of cytotoxicity in undifferentiated SH-SY5Y cells in both the MTT reduction and NR uptake assays, MTX being more cytotoxic. The greater toxicity of MTX herein may be due to its superior lipophilicity [40], making this drug more easily permeable and accumulated inside the cells. A study published in 2005 also reported that MTX is also more cytotoxic than DOX in two immortalized cell lines (NIH 3T3 and B14), using the MTT reduction assay [41]. However, other authors reported that, in cardiac (H9c2) and breast cancer (MTLn3) cells, DOX was slightly more cytotoxic than MTX, according to the trypan blue exclusion technique [42]. Nevertheless, the trypan blue exclusion technique may present some subjectivity regarding the cell-counting operator and it does not allow counting the cells that completely disintegrated. Still, the toxicity of these two drugs seems to be dependent on the cellular model. Lopes et al. found in primary rat cortical neurons that DOX (0.1 and 0.5 μM) caused a substantial degree of toxicity (higher than toxic dose 50) when tested for 48 h according to the MTT reduction assay [19]. Meanwhile, in the same study, 10 μM DOX was less toxic than the lower concentrations tested (0.1 or 0.5 μM). That is in agreement with our results in undifferentiated SH-SY5Y cells, where 0.13 μM of DOX was more toxic than 0.5 μM both in the MTT and NR assays at 24 h. We used two cytotoxicity assays, the NR uptake and the MTT reduction assays, and several morphological evaluations or stains. Most authors agree that using several cytotoxicity tests, with different inherent mechanisms can help elucidate the underlying cytotoxicity of the drugs tested [19,43,44]. Nonetheless, herein there were no major differences between the two cytotoxicity tests performed in each drug; however, MTX is more toxic in both time points and concentrations and morphological evaluation corroborates the highest MTX cytotoxicity.

DOX and MTX kill cancer cells by intercalating their DNA and inhibiting topoisomerase II [4]. However, in non-target sites, such as the brain, these drugs also cause damage [14,15]. As neurons are post-mitotic cells, their injury can cause irreversible loss [14]. Regarding the mechanisms involved in the putative neurotoxicity of DOX or MTX, data are still scarce. In this work, undifferentiated SH-SY5Y cells were sensitive to DOX and MTX in a time-dependent manner and signs of apoptosis were confirmed by two stains. In Hoechst staining, MTX and DOX in all the conditions tested, caused signs of apoptosis, although more evident in 0.5 μM DOX and in 0.13 μM MTX, at 48 h. The acridine orange/ethidium bromide staining confirmed that both drugs caused apoptosis in the concentrations tested at 48 h. In primary cortical neurons, DOX caused signs of apoptosis, albeit dependent on DOX concentration. In those cells, only the lowest concentrations tested (0.1 and 0.5 μM) showed activation of caspase 3 and DNA fragmentation [19]. Loss of cell adhesion, loss of nuclear envelope, nuclear fragmentation and decrease in cell size are typical signs of apoptosis [45] and we observed those effects in the DOX and MTX-exposed undifferentiated SH-SY5Y cells. In mice, the oxidative damage caused by DOX was capable of enhancing the expression of pro-apoptotic factors, such as BAD protein, and decreasing the expression of Bcl-2 anti-apoptotic protein families, which would consequently lead to mitochondrial membrane loss of potential, promote the release of cytochrome c and apoptosis [46]. In the present study, the effects on mitochondrial membrane potential were evaluated at the lowest concentration (0.13 μM) and evident mitochondrial depolarization was observed, which agrees with the ability of both drugs to trigger mitochondrial damage. Rats treated with seven weekly injections of vehicle (subcutaneous, saline solution) or DOX (subcutaneous, 2 mg·kg^{-1}), and then sacrificed one week after the last administration had brain mitochondrial fractions isolated, and the authors found that DOX treatment induced an increase in thiobarbituric acid-reactive substances and vitamin E levels and a decrease in reduced glutathione content and aconitase activity, while potentiated the mitochondrial permeability transition pore opening induced by calcium [47]. Also, DOX-induced caspase-8 and -3 activity increases and decrease in mitochondrial potential in several types of primary neuronal cells, although DOX impact was dependent on the cells' development stage [26]. Those works demonstrated that DOX causes mitochondrial affection and oxidative stress. Lopes and colleagues also focused on neuronal oxidative stress caused by DOX, in primary cortical neurons, and found that it decreased glutathione and increased reactive species and quinoprotein levels [18]. The decrease of antioxidant defenses, such as glutathione, and increase of oxidative stress seem to contribute to neuronal damage [13], like it happens in the heart after DOX exposure [10]. Taking into account the ability of DOX to promote oxidative stress, we sought to prevent the neurotoxicity of DOX and MTX in undifferentiated SH-SY5Y cells using two antioxidants. NAC works as precursor in the synthesis of glutathione and acts as an antioxidant [48,49]; however, in this work it failed to provide any protection against 0.2 μM MTX or DOX toxicity. Rat cortical astrocytes were previously used to test the protective effect of NAC against DOX-induced toxicity [50]. NAC, when pre-incubated at a concentration of 5 mM, was able to reduce lipid peroxidation induced by DOX (10 mg/mL), and also partially counteracted DOX-induced cytotoxicity, when evaluated by the MTT reduction assay. The concentrations used, as well as the cellular model, may explain the differences observed in our work, where NAC showed no protective effect against DOX. Indeed, in rat cortical neurons, DOX only decreased glutathione cellular levels when cells were exposed to 0.5 μM for 24 h, not significantly altering this parameter at 0.1, 5 and 20 μM concentrations, possibly due to the overproduction of peroxynitrite seen in that concentration (0.5 μM) and not significantly seen in the others [18]. The putative protective action of KU-55933, an inhibitor of kinase ataxia-telangiectasia mutated (ATM), a protein engaged in DNA damage repair, was studied in SH-SY5Y cells exposed to DOX. KU-55933 inhibited the cell death induced by H_2O_2 [0.5 mM and 1 mM in undifferentiated and retinoic acid (RA)-differentiated SH-SY5Y cells, respectively] or DOX (0.25 and 1 μM in undifferentiated- and RA-differentiated SH-SY5Y cells, respectively) in undifferentiated and RA-differentiated SHSY5Y cells, with a more pronounced effect in the latter cell phenotype. Furthermore, this ATM inhibitor attenuated the DOX- but not H_2O_2-induced caspase-3 activity increase in both SH-SY5Y cells, showing that oxidative stress is not the unique mechanism of DOX-induced neurotoxicity [51]. Another antioxidant, tiron 100 μM, a superoxide anion radical scavenger, was tested here. Tiron was unable to prevent the toxicity of DOX, but it partially avoided the toxicity induced by MTX. Interestingly, oxidative stress appears to be involved in the cytotoxicity mechanism of MTX in our neuronal model; however, MTX, in other cellular models, namely H9c2 and MTLn3, did not led to reactive oxygen species increase, unlike DOX [42]. However, late formation of reactive species is observed after MTX incubation following mitochondrial affectation [52]. Our results advocate for MTX-induced toxicity to mitochondria in this model. Superoxide anion radical is mainly produced in mitochondria and MTX interferes in both the ATP levels and in ATP synthase expression and activity, leading to late reactive species formation [52,53]. Regarding DOX, other reactive oxygen or nitrogen species (not the superoxide anion radical), may be involved in the putative oxidative stress promoted by DOX. Truthfully, the activation of nitric oxide synthase has been reported in cortical neurons incubated with DOX, thus contributing to the formation of nitric oxide and subsequently reactive nitrogen species [18].

Herein, DOX and MTX caused apoptotic nuclei in undifferentiated SH-SY5Y cells. These results are in accordance to previous studies showing that MTX causes an increase in apoptotic cells at concentrations as low as 0.3 ng/mL in postmitotic sympathetic neurons after a 24-h exposure [54] and that DOX causes necrosis and apoptosis in rat cortical neurons at concentrations in the μM range [19]. We demonstrated that 10 nM CHX, a protein synthesis inhibitor, partially avoided the toxicity caused by 0.2 μM DOX, in line to a previous finding showing that CHX was able to totally revert the cell death caused by 0.5 μM DOX in cortical rat neurons [19]. Based on these data, even in different cellular models, it is possible to conclude that DOX-induced cytotoxicity is dependent on de novo protein synthesis. On the other hand, CHX was not able to lessen MTX-induced cytotoxicity in our neuronal model, indicating different toxicity mechanisms for DOX and MTX.

Programmed cell death may be dependent or independent of caspases. A caspase-3 inhibitor, Ac-DEVD-CHO, partially reverted the neurotoxicity of 0.2 μM DOX in undifferentiated SH-SY5Y cells. In rat cortical neurons, exposure for 24 h to 0.1 and 0.5 μM DOX was found to increase caspase-3 activity [19], and the caspase-3 inhibitor, Z-DEVD-fmk, inhibited this effect, although it did not prevent cell death [19]. In the case of MTX, the caspase-3 inhibitor had no protective effect on undifferentiated SH-5YSY cells, although MTX was shown to activate caspase-3 in H9c2 cells [52]. However, since MTX is more lipophilic than DOX [41] and led to a higher number of apoptotic nuclei in undifferentiated SH-SY5Y cells in our work, the concentration of the caspase inhibitor may have been insufficient to prevent the toxicity of MTX or a non-caspase mediated apoptosis may also have been triggered. Actually, in two immortalized cell lines (NIH 3T3 and B14 cells) both DOX and MTX activated caspase-3 and the inhibitor Ac-DEVD-CHO did not show any significant effect on drug cytotoxicity either [41]. Moreover, DOX has been shown to activate the apoptosis inducing factor (AIF), which leads to caspase-3 independent apoptosis [25].

To assess whether there would be significant differences in the cytotoxicity promoted by DOX and MTX in undifferentiated *versus* differentiated SH-SY5Y cells, the cytotoxicity of both 0.2 µM DOX and 0.2 µM MTX was assessed at 48 h using the MTT reduction test. The MTT reduction test has been the most described cytotoxicity assay in the literature and in our results with undifferentiated SH-SY5Y cells, it was the most sensitive assay towards both DOX and MTX neurotoxicity. In our work, DOX was more neurotoxic in undifferentiated SH-SY5Y cells than in differentiated cells, revealing that the cellular modifications following differentiation may be protective to differentiated SH-SY5Y cells. These results are in line with those published earlier by Jantas and coworkers, who reported that undifferentiated SH-SY5Y cells were more sensitive to DOX (concentration range 0.1 to 5 µM) cytotoxicity in the lactate dehydrogenase release assay, and that DOX increased caspase 3 activity in undifferentiated, but not in RA-differentiated SH-SY5Y cells (cells differentiated for 7 days with 10 µM RA) [27]. Accordingly, we saw that the caspase-3 inhibitor, Ac-DEVD-CHO, could attenuate DOX toxicity in undifferentiated SH-SY5Y cells. The same group published another report revealing that DOX-evoked cell death in the MTT test (cells exposed 24 h to 0.25 or 1 µM) was attenuated by specific activators of group III metabotropic glutamate receptors in undifferentiated, but not in RA-differentiated SH-SY5Y cells [25]. In fact, cells subjected to the differentiation protocol undergo several biochemical changes. In particular, our group has shown that SH-SY5Y cells gain dopaminergic characteristics and suffer a strong slowdown in cell division capacity [48,55]. At the biochemical level, an increase in the density of dopamine receptors D2 and D3 on the cell surface of differentiated cells, an increase in tyrosine hydroxylase expression and in the dopamine transporter, rendering them dopaminergic neuronal characteristics [48,55]. RA differentiated SH-SY5Y cells were shown to be more resistant to apoptosis via increasing the expression of Bcl-2 anti-apoptotic protein family (cells differentiated for 4 days with 10 µM RA) [56]. In another neuroblastoma cell line, SK-*N*-SH, cells differentiated with RA (3 µM) or 4b-phorbol 12-myristate 13-acetate (PMA, 20 nM), a compound chemically related to 12-O-tetradecanoylphorbol 13-acetate (TPA), were more resistant to apoptosis than undifferentiated cells. PMA treated cells had an increased expression of Bcl-2 and RA treatment increased Bcl-x$_L$, and these increases of anti-apoptotic proteins show how differentiation can render cells more resistant to apoptotic stimuli [57], namely those possibly caused by DOX herein. Additionally, RA differentiation induces a dramatic increase in the energy metabolism of SH-SY5Y cells, and shifts the dependence on energy production from glycolysis to oxidative phosphorylation [58,59] advocating that DOX causes energetic stress, and differentiated SH-SY5Y are more resilient cells possibly because they rely more on mitochondrial energy production. Actually, in murine cardiac HL-1 cells, ATP levels and glycolytic fluxes were significantly reduced after DOX treatment [60]. When comparing to MTX cytotoxicity in both undifferentiated and differentiated cells, no significant differences were seen but a tendency occurred towards a higher toxicity in undifferentiated cells. Neurons are very sensitive to mitochondrial toxins [61] and MTX is a mitochondrial toxin [43,52,53], even in mainly glycolytic cells [52]. This extensive neurotoxicity combined with its higher lipophilicity, make MTX a more dangerous drug to the brain than DOX. These data combined with its new use in MS, broadens MTX neurotoxic potential since BBB in MS patients is largely affected [23]. Thus, potential deleterious effects of MTX in the brain should not be overlooked or regarded as a natural path in the disabling and incurable MS and MTX neurotoxic effects should be further studied.

4. Materials and Methods

4.1. Materials

MTX, DOX, trypsin-EDTA solution, trypan blue solution 0.4% (w/v) and Dulbecco's modified Eagle medium (DMEM) high glucose, sodium bicarbonate, 3-(4,5-dimethylthiazol-2-yl)-2,5-diphenyl tetrazolium bromide (MTT), neutral red (NR) solution, Hoechst 33258 solution, 3,3'-dihexyloxacarbocyanine iodide (DiO6), dimethyl sulfoxide (DMSO), RA, TPA, NAC, tiron, CHX, Ac-DEVD-CHO, an inhibitor of caspase-3/7, and paraformaldehyde were obtained from Sigma-Aldrich (Taufkirchen, Germany). Human neuroblastoma SH-SY5Y cells were obtained from the European Collection of Cell Cultures (Sigma-Aldrich, Taufkirchen, Germany). All sterile plastic material was obtained from Corning Costar (Corning, NY, USA). Penicillin/streptomycin (10.000 units/mL/ 10.000 µg/mL) and the phosphate buffer solution (PBS) without calcium and magnesium were obtained from Biochrom (Berlin, Germany). Fetal bovine serum (FBS), PBS with calcium and magnesium and Hank's balanced salt solution (HBSS) were obtained from Gibco (Paisley, UK).

4.2. Cell Culture

Human SH-SY5Y neuroblastoma cells are a commonly used neuronal model for the study of neurotoxicity, as they maintain several neuron markers [55]. SH-SY5Y cells were grown in complete DMEM that consisted of DMEM supplemented with 10% (v/v) FBS and 1% (v/v) of penicillin/streptomycin. Cells were cultured and maintained at 37 °C in a 5% CO_2 incubator (Heraeus, Hanau, Germany) throughout all procedures. Stock cultures of SH-SY5Y cells were maintained in 25 cm^3 flasks and grown until confluence (80–90% confluence). Cells were washed with PBS, trypsinized (trypsin/EDTA) and counted following trypan blue staining using a Fuchs-Rosenthal counting chamber. The cell suspension was then seeded in multi-well plates at a density of 50,000 cells/cm^2. All experiments were done using cells from passage 25 to 40.

4.3. Undifferentiated SH-SY5Y Cells

After seeding the cells in plates, they were maintained for 24 h to allow them to attach, and then exposed to DOX or MTX (0.13; 0.2; 0.5 µM) for 24 or 48 h. NR uptake and MTT reduction assays, phase contrast microscopy, Hoechst stain, ethidium bromide and acridine orange stain, mitochondrial membrane potential evaluation were subsequently done.

For testing putative protectors against the toxicity of MTX or DOX, undifferentiated SH-SY5Y cells were pre-incubated with 1 mM NAC, 100 µM tiron, 10 nM CHX, or 100 µM of the caspase 3/7 inhibitor Ac-DEVD-CHO [43,49], for 30 min before exposure to 0.2 µM DOX or 0.2 µM MTX for 48 h. NR uptake and MTT reduction assays were performed after that exposure period.

4.4. Differentiated SH-SY5Y Cells

SH-SY5Y cells can be differentiated and a dopaminergic state is obtained after differentiation, while undifferentiated SH-SY5Y cell respond as catecholaminergic neurons [55]. For differentiating cells into a dopaminergic phenotype, cells (density 25,000 cells/cm^2) were seeded in complete DMEM medium containing 10 nM RA for three days. At the third day, cells were then exposed to 80 nM TPA on complete DMEM medium and kept for another three days [48,49]. After the 6-day differentiation protocol, the cells were exposed to 0.2 µM DOX or MTX for 48 h, and the MTT reduction test was performed.

4.5. Cytotoxicity Evaluation

To compare DOX and MTX cytotoxicity and to determine if putative protectors could prevent against DOX or MTX-induced toxicity, two assays were used: the NR lysosomal uptake and the MTT reduction assays. Both methods were performed 24 or 48 h after the cells' exposure to cytostatic drugs in 48-well plates.

4.6. MTT Reduction Assay

The MTT colorimetric assay is based on the mitochondrial reduction of the tetrazolium salt and formazan formation. At the selected time-point, the cellular medium was changed and 200 μL of complete medium and 20 μL of MTT (5 mg/mL) were added to each well. A 3-h incubation period at 37 °C was then necessary to allow the reduction of MTT in both differentiated and undifferentiated SH-SY5Y cells. The medium was then removed and 200 μL of DMSO were added. The plate was shacked for 15 min until total dissolution of the formazans. Spectrophotometric measurement of the formazans formed was then done at 550 nm in a multi-well plate reader (Biotech Synergy HT, Winooski, VT, USA). The percentage of MTT reduction of control cells was set to 100% and the values of each treatment are expressed as percentage of control cells.

4.7. Neutral Red Lysosomal Uptake Assay

The NR uptake assay is based on the ability of viable cells to uptake the supravitally dye that penetrates cell membranes and concentrates in lysosomes. After a 48-h exposure time, the medium was removed and warm NR (33 μg/mL) enriched medium was placed in each well (250 μL/well). Plates were kept at 37 °C for 3 h, protected from light. The medium was then removed and the wells were washed with 250 μL of warm HBSS solution with calcium and magnesium. Thereafter, the HBSS solution was rejected and 200 μL of the lysis solution (50% ethanol/1% acetic acid) were added. The plate was shaken for 15 min, protected from light, until a homogeneous solution was obtained. The absorbance was read at two wavelengths, 540 and 690 nm (reference), on a multi-well plate reader (Biotech Synergy HT, Winooski, VT, USA) and results are presented as percentage of control cells, whose mean values were set to 100%.

4.8. Microscopic Evaluation of the Cells

4.8.1. Phase Contrast Microscopy

In undifferentiated SH-SY5Y cells, phase-contrast microscopy morphological evaluation was performed in 12-well plates to determine the toxic effects of both cytostatic drugs after a 24- or 48-h exposure. An Nikon Eclipse TS100 inverted microscope equipped with a DS-Fi1 camera (Tokyo, Japan) was used.

4.8.2. Hoechst Staining

To evaluate the effects of MTX and DOX on the nuclear morphology of undifferentiated SH-SY5Y cells, the Hoechst staining was performed following a 24-h or a 48-h exposure to the drugs, as previously described [43]. Briefly, cells were fixed in 4% paraformaldehyde (10 min, 4 °C) and washed three times with PBS with calcium and magnesium. Cells were stained with the nuclear dye Hoechst 33258 (final concentration of 5 μg/mL) for 10 min at 37 °C (protected from light), and then washed three times, at room temperature, with PBS containing calcium and magnesium. Cells were examined in a Nikon Eclipse TS100 microscope equipped with a Nikon DS-Fi1 camera, using a standard fluorescein filter ($\lambda_{excitation}$ = 346 nm and $\lambda_{emission}$ = 460 nm) and then counted manually for total cells and condensed nucleuses.

4.8.3. Ethidium Bromide and Acridine Orange Staining

The fluorescent DNA-intercalating dyes ethidium bromide and acridine orange are used to discriminate between necrotic and apoptotic cell death. Ethidium bromide intercalates with nucleic acids if the outer cellular membrane is ruptured. Acridine orange diffuses through intact membranes of live cells and largely accumulates in acidic vesicles. After a 48-h incubation with MTX or DOX, the medium was removed and the protocol was done as previously described [49]. Cells were examined in a Nikon Eclipse TS100 microscope equipped with a Nikon DS-Fi1 camera, using a standard fluorescein filter ($\lambda_{excitation}$ = 485 nm and $\lambda_{emission}$ = 525 nm).

4.8.4. Evaluation of the Mitochondrial Membrane Potential

The evaluation of the mitochondrial membrane potential was also done as previously described [43]. Briefly, cells were incubated for 48 h with 0.13 µM MTX or 0.13 µM DOX and subsequently incubated for 30 min at 37 °C with DiO6 (35 nM/well). Each condition had a well without any DiO6 to evaluate whether any component of the medium or drugs tested emitted any residual fluorescence that could interfere with the readings. After the 30 min incubation time, cells were washed twice with warm PBS with calcium and magnesium and photographs were taken in a fluorescence microscope (Nikon Eclipse TS100 equipped with a Nikon DS-Fi1 camera), using a standard fluorescein filter ($\lambda_{excitation}$ = 485 nm and $\lambda_{emission}$ = 520 nm).

5. Statistical Analysis

The results are expressed as mean ± standard deviation. When the two molecules and several concentrations were compared at different concentrations, statistical analysis was performed using the two-way ANOVA test, followed by the Bonferroni *post-hoc* test, once a significant p value was reached. When dealing with three or more conditions, the D'Agostino & Pearson normality test was used to evaluate data distribution. A parametric analysis of variance (ANOVA) was performed when data distribution was normal, followed by the Tukey's *post hoc* test. When data did not follow a normal distribution, statistical analysis was performed using the Kruskal-Wallis test, followed by the Dunn's *post-hoc* test, once a significant p value was reached. Statistical significance was set at $p < 0.05$. All statistical analyses were performed using GraphPad Prism 7 software (GraphPad Software, La Jolla, CA, USA). All details of the statistical analyses can be found in the figure legends.

Author Contributions: D.A., R.P., V.C., J.S., J.P.C. and V.M.C. performed the experimental procedures. D.A., R.P., and V.M.C. organized the data. M.L.B., F.C. and J.P.C. contributed for data interpretation. All authors read, revised and approved the final manuscript. V.M.C. planned the experiments and drafted the paper.

Acknowledgments: V.M.C. thanks Fundação para a Ciência e Tecnologia (FCT) for her grant SFRH/BPD/110001/2015. JS received financial support from Universidade do Porto/FMUP through FSE-Fundo Social Europeu, NORTE 2020-Programa Operacional Regional do Norte (NORTE-08-5369-FSE-000011). This work was supported by FEDER funds through the Operational Programme for Competitiveness Factors—COMPETE and by national funds by FCT within the project "PTDC/DTP-FTO/1489/2014—POCI-01-0145-FEDER-016537".

Abbreviations

BBB	Blood-brain barrier
CHX	Cycloheximide
CNS	Central nervous system
DMEM	Dulbecco's modified Eagle medium
DOX	Doxorubicin
EMA	European Medicines Agency
HBSS	Hanks' balanced salt solution
MS	Multiple sclerosis
MTT	3-(4,5-Dimethylthiazol-2-yl)-2,5-diphenyl tetrazolium bromide
MTX	Mitoxantrone
NAC	*N*-Acetyl-L-cysteine
NR	Neutral Red
PBS	Phosphate buffered saline
RA	Retinoic acid
TPA	12-*O*-tetradecanoylphorbol 13-acetate

References

1. GBD. Global, regional, and national age-sex specific mortality for 264 causes of death, 1980–2016: A systematic analysis for the Global Burden of Disease Study 2016. *Lancet* **2017**, *390*, 1151–1210.

2. Hrynchak, I.; Sousa, E.; Pinto, M.; Costa, V.M. The importance of drug metabolites synthesis: The case-study of cardiotoxic anticancer drugs. *Drug Metab. Rev.* **2017**, *49*, 158–196. [CrossRef] [PubMed]

3. Shih, Y.-C.; Smieliauskas, F.; Geynisman, D.; Kelly, R.; Smith, T. Trends in the cost and use of targeted cancer therapies for the privately insured noneldery: 2001 to 2011. *J. Clin. Oncol.* **2015**, *33*, 2190–2199. [CrossRef] [PubMed]

4. European Medicines Agency (EMA). *Novantrone and Associated Names*; EMA: London, UK, 2016; Available online: http://www.ema.europa.eu/docs/en_GB/document_library/Referrals_document/Novantrone_30/WC500209683.pdf (accessed on 29 April 2018).

5. Goodin, D.S.; Arnason, B.G.; Coyle, P.K.; Frohman, E.M.; Paty, D.W. The use of mitoxantrone (Novantrone) for the treatment of multiple sclerosis: Report of the Therapeutics and Technology Assessment Subcommittee of the American Academy of Neurology. *Neurology* **2003**, *61*, 1332–1338. [CrossRef] [PubMed]

6. Evison, B.J.; Sleebs, B.E.; Watson, K.G.; Phillips, D.R.; Cutts, S.M. Mitoxantrone, More than Just Another Topoisomerase II Poison. *Med. Res. Rev.* **2016**, *36*, 248–299. [CrossRef] [PubMed]

7. Marriott, J.J.; Miyasaki, J.M.; Gronseth, G.; O'Connor, P.W. Evidence Report: The efficacy and safety of mitoxantrone (Novantrone) in the treatment of multiple sclerosis: Report of the Therapeutics and Technology Assessment Subcommittee of the American Academy of Neurology(CME). *Neurology* **2010**, *74*, 1463–1470. [CrossRef] [PubMed]

8. European Medicines Agency (EMA). *Recommendations on the Use of Caelyx (Doxorubicin Hydrochloride)*; EMA: London, UK, 2011; Available online: http://www.ema.europa.eu/docs/en_GB/document_library/Medicine_QA/2011/11/WC500117926.pdf (accessed on 29 April 2018).

9. Frei, E.I.; Eder, J.P. Combination chemotherapy. In *Holland-Frei Cancer Medicine.*, 6th ed.; Kufe, D.W., Pollock, R.E., Bast, R.C., Weichselbaum, R.R., Eds.; BC Decker: Hamilton, ON, USA, 2003. Available online: https://www.ncbi.nlm.nih.gov/books/NBK13955/ (accessed on 29 April 2018).

10. Costa, V.M.; Carvalho, F.; Duarte, J.A.; Bastos M., L.; Remiâo, F. The heart as a target for xenobiotic toxicity: The cardiac susceptibility to oxidative stress. *Chem. Res. Toxicol.* **2013**, *26*, 1285–1311. [CrossRef] [PubMed]

11. Mladenka, P.; Applova, L.; Patocka, J.; Costa, V.M.; Remiao, F.; Pourova, J.; Mladenka, A.; Karlickova, J.; Jahodar, L.; Voprsalova, M.; et al. Comprehensive review of cardiovascular toxicity of drugs and related agents. *Med. Res. Rev.* **2018**. [CrossRef] [PubMed]

12. Reis-Mendes, A.F.; Sousa, E.; de Lourdes Bastos, M.; Costa, V.M. The role of the metabolism of anticancer drugs in their induced-cardiotoxicity. *Curr. Drug Metab.* **2015**, *17*, 75–90. [CrossRef] [PubMed]

13. Ahles, T.A.; Saykin, A.J. Candidate mechanisms for chemotherapy-induced cognitive changes. *Nat. Rev. Cancer* **2007**, *7*, 192–201. [CrossRef] [PubMed]

14. Chen, Y.; Jungsuwadee, P.; Vore, M.; Butterfield, D.A.; St Clair, D.K. Collateral damage in cancer chemotherapy: Oxidative stress in nontargeted tissues. *Mol. Interv.* **2007**, *7*, 147–156. [CrossRef] [PubMed]

15. Jansen, C.E.; Dodd, M.J.; Miaskowski, C.A.; Dowling, G.A.; Kramer, J. Preliminary results of a longitudinal study of changes in cognitive function in breast cancer patients undergoing chemotherapy with doxorubicin and cyclophosphamide. *Psychooncology* **2008**, *17*, 1189–1195. [CrossRef] [PubMed]

16. Jansen, C.E.; Cooper, B.A.; Dodd, M.J.; Miaskowski, C.A. A prospective longitudinal study of chemotherapy-induced cognitive changes in breast cancer patients. *Support. Care Cancer* **2011**, *19*, 1647–1656. [CrossRef] [PubMed]

17. Ahles, T.A.; Saykin, A.J.; Furstenberg, C.T.; Cole, B.; Mott, L.A.; Skalla, K.; Whedon, M.B.; Bivens, S.; Mitchell, T.; Greenberg, E.R.; et al. Neuropsychologic impact of standard-dose systemic chemotherapy in long-term survivors of breast cancer and lymphoma. *J. Clin. Oncol.* **2002**, *20*, 485–493. [CrossRef] [PubMed]

18. Lopes, M.A.; Meisel, A.; Carvalho, F.D.; Bastos, M.L. Neuronal nitric oxide synthase is a key factor in doxorubicin-induced toxicity to rat-isolated cortical neurons. *Neurotox. Res.* **2011**, *19*, 14–22. [CrossRef] [PubMed]

19. Lopes, M.A.; Meisel, A.; Dirnagl, U.; Carvalho, F.D.; Bastos, M.L. Doxorubicin induces biphasic neurotoxicity to rat cortical neurons. *Neurotoxicology* **2008**, *29*, 286–293. [CrossRef] [PubMed]

20. Tangpong, J.; Cole, M.P.; Sultana, R.; Estus, S.; Vore, M.; St Clair, W.; Ratanachaiyavong, S.; St Clair, D.K.; Butterfield, D.A. Adriamycin-mediated nitration of manganese superoxide dismutase in the central nervous system: Insight into the mechanism of chemobrain. *J. Neurochem.* **2007**, *100*, 191–201. [CrossRef] [PubMed]

21. Taube, F.; Stölzel, F.; Thiede, C.; Ehninger, G.; Laniado, M.; Schaich, M. Increased incidence of central nervous system hemorrhages in patients with secondary acute promyelocytic leukemia after treatment of multiple sclerosis with mitoxantrone? *Haematologica* **2011**, *96*, e31–e32. [CrossRef] [PubMed]

22. Boiardi, A.; Eoli, M.; Salmaggi, A.; Lamperti, E.; Botturi, A.; Broggi, G.; Bissola, L.; Finocchiaro, G.; Silvani, A. Systemic temozolomide combined with loco-regional mitoxantrone in treating recurrent glioblastoma. *J. Neurooncol.* **2005**, *75*, 215–220. [CrossRef] [PubMed]

23. Minagar, A.; Alexander, J.S. Blood-brain barrier disruption in multiple sclerosis. *Mult. Scler.* **2003**, *9*, 540–549. [CrossRef] [PubMed]

24. Fulda, S.; Honer, M.; Menke-Moellers, I.; Berthold, F. Antiproliferative potential of cytostatic drugs on neuroblastoma cells in vitro. *Eur. J. Cancer* **1995**, *31*, 616–621. [CrossRef]

25. Jantas, D.; Greda, A.; Leskiewicz, M.; Grygier, B.; Pilc, A.; Lason, W. Neuroprotective effects of mGluR II and III activators against staurosporine- and doxorubicin-induced cellular injury in SH-SY5Y cells: New evidence for a mechanism involving inhibition of AIF translocation. *Neurochem. Int.* **2015**, *88*, 124–137. [CrossRef] [PubMed]

26. Jantas, D.; Lason, W. Protective effect of memantine against doxorubicin toxicity in primary neuronal cell cultures: Influence a development stage. *Neurotox. Res.* **2009**, *15*, 24–37. [CrossRef] [PubMed]

27. Jantas, D.; Pytel, M.; Mozrzymas, J.W.; Leskiewicz, M.; Regulska, M.; Antkiewicz-Michaluk, L.; Lason, W. The attenuating effect of memantine on staurosporine-, salsolinol- and doxorubicin-induced apoptosis in human neuroblastoma SH-SY5Y cells. *Neurochem. Int.* **2008**, *52*, 864–877. [CrossRef] [PubMed]

28. Gaman, A.M.; Uzoni, A.; Popa-Wagner, A.; Andrei, A.; Petcu, E.B. The role of oxidative stress in etiopathogenesis of chemotherapy induced cognitive impairment (CICI)-"Chemobrain". *Aging Dis.* **2016**, *7*, 307–317. [PubMed]

29. Silva, R.; Vilas-Boas, V.; Carmo, H.; Dinis-Oliveira, R.J.; Carvalho, F.; de Lourdes Bastos, M.; Remiao, F. Modulation of P-glycoprotein efflux pump: Induction and activation as a therapeutic strategy. *Pharmacol. Ther.* **2015**, *149*, 1–123. [CrossRef] [PubMed]

30. Homolya, L.; Orban, T.I.; Csanady, L.; Sarkadi, B. Mitoxantrone is expelled by the ABCG2 multidrug transporter directly from the plasma membrane. *Biochim. Biophys. Acta* **2011**, *1808*, 154–163. [CrossRef] [PubMed]

31. Stewart, D.J.; Grewaal, D.; Green, R.M.; Mikhael, N.; Goel, R.; Montpetit, V.A.; Redmond, M.D. Concentrations of doxorubicin and its metabolites in human autopsy heart and other tissues. *Anticancer Res.* **1993**, *13*, 1945–1952. [PubMed]

32. Green, R.M.; Stewart, D.J.; Hugenholtz, H.; Richard, M.T.; Thibault, M.; Montpetit, V. Human central nervous system and plasma pharmacology of mitoxantrone. *J. Neurooncol.* **1988**, *6*, 75–83. [CrossRef] [PubMed]

33. Pastore, A.; Geiger, S.; Baur, D.; Hausmann, A.; Tischer, J.; Horster, S.; Stemmler, H.J. Cardiotoxicity after anthracycline treatment in survivors of adult cancers: Monitoring by USCOM, Echocardiography and Serum Biomarkers. *World J. Oncol.* **2013**, *4*, 18–25. [CrossRef] [PubMed]

34. Frost, B.M.; Eksborg, S.; Björk, O.; Abrahamsson, J.; Behrendtz, M.; Castor, A.; Forestier, E.; Lönnerholm, G. Pharmacokinetics of doxorubicin in children with acute lymphoblastic leukemia: Multi-institutional collaborative study. *Med. Pediatr. Oncol.* **2002**, *38*, 329–337. [CrossRef] [PubMed]

35. Palle, J.; Frost, B.-M.; Peterson, C.; Gustafsson, G.; Hellebostad, M.; Kanerva, J.; Schmiegelow, K. Nordic Society for Pediatric Hematology and Oncology. Doxorubicin pharmacokinetics is correlated to the effect of induction therapy in children with acute myeloid leukemia. *Anticancer Drugs* **2006**, *17*, 385–392. [CrossRef] [PubMed]

36. Barpe, D.R.; Rosa, D.D.; Froehlich, P.E. Pharmacokinetic evaluation of doxorubicin plasma levels in normal and overweight patients with breast cancer and simulation of dose adjustment by different indexes of body mass. *Eur. J. Pharm. Sci.* **2010**, *41*, 458–463. [CrossRef] [PubMed]

37. Voon, P.J.; Yap, H.L.; Ma, C.Y.; Lu, F.; Wong, A.L.; Sapari, N.S.; Soong, R.; Soh, T.I.; Goh, B.C.; Lee, H.S.; et al. Correlation of aldo-ketoreductase (AKR) 1C3 genetic variant with doxorubicin pharmacodynamics in Asian breast cancer patients. *Br. J. Clin. Pharmacol.* **2013**, *75*, 1497–1505. [CrossRef] [PubMed]

38. Alberts, D.S.; Peng, Y.M.; Bowden, G.T.; Dalton, W.S.; Mackel, C. Pharmacology of mitoxantrone: Mode of action and pharmacokinetics. *Investig. New Drugs* **1985**, *3*, 101–107. [CrossRef]

39. Batra, V.K.; Morrison, J.A.; Woodward, D.L.; Siverd, N.S.; Yacobi, A. Pharmacokinetics of mitoxantrone in man and laboratory animals. *Drug Metab. Rev.* **1986**, *17*, 311–329. [CrossRef] [PubMed]

40. Andersson, B.S.; Eksborg, S.; Vidal, R.F.; Sundberg, M.; Carlberg, M. Anthraquinone-induced cell injury: Acute toxicity of carminomycin, epirubicin, idarubicin and mitoxantrone in isolated cardiomyocytes. *Toxicology* **1999**, *135*, 11–20. [CrossRef]

41. Koceva-Chyla, A.; Jedrzejczak, M.; Skierski, J.; Kania, K.; Jozwiak, Z. Mechanisms of induction of apoptosis by anthraquinone anticancer drugs aclarubicin and mitoxantrone in comparison with doxorubicin: Relation to drug cytotoxicity and caspase-3 activation. *Apoptosis* **2005**, *10*, 1497–1514. [CrossRef] [PubMed]

42. Kluza, J.; Marchetti, P.; Gallego, M.A.; Lancel, S.; Fournier, C.; Loyens, A.; Beauvillain, J.C.; Bailly, C. Mitochondrial proliferation during apoptosis induced by anticancer agents: Effects of doxorubicin and mitoxantrone on cancer and cardiac cells. *Oncogene* **2004**, *23*, 7018–7030. [CrossRef] [PubMed]

43. Reis-Mendes, A.; Gomes, A.S.; Carvalho, R.A.; Carvalho, F.; Remião, F.; Pinto, M.; Bastos, M.L.; Sousa, E.; Costa, V.M. Naphthoquinoxaline metabolite of mitoxantrone is less cardiotoxic than the parent compound and it can be a more cardiosafe drug in anticancer therapy. *Arch. Toxicol.* **2017**, *91*, 1871–1890. [CrossRef] [PubMed]

44. Soares, A.S.; Costa, V.M.; Diniz, C.; Fresco, P. Potentiation of cytotoxicity of paclitaxel in combination with Cl-IB-MECA in human C32 metastatic melanoma cells: A new possible therapeutic strategy for melanoma. *Biomed. Pharmacother.* **2013**, *67*, 777–789. [CrossRef] [PubMed]

45. Kwon, H.K.; Lee, J.H.; Shin, H.J.; Kim, J.H.; Choi, S. Structural and functional analysis of cell adhesion and nuclear envelope nano-topography in cell death. *Sci. Rep.* **2015**, *5*, 15623. [CrossRef] [PubMed]

46. Pal, S.; Ahir, M.; Sil, P.C. Doxorubicin-induced neurotoxicity is attenuated by a 43-kD protein from the leaves of *Cajanus indicus* L. via NF-kappaB and mitochondria dependent pathways. *Free Radic. Res.* **2012**, *46*, 785–798. [CrossRef] [PubMed]

47. Cardoso, S.; Santos, R.X.; Carvalho, C.; Correia, S.; Pereira, G.C.; Pereira, S.S.; Oliveira, P.J.; Santos, M.S.; Proenca, T.; Moreira, P.I. Doxorubicin increases the susceptibility of brain mitochondria to Ca^{2+}-induced permeability transition and oxidative damage. *Free Radic. Biol. Med.* **2008**, *45*, 1395–1402. [CrossRef] [PubMed]

48. Ferreira, P.S.; Nogueira, T.B.; Costa, V.M.; Branco, P.S.; Ferreira, L.M.; Fernandes, E.; Bastos, M.L.; Meisel, A.; Carvalho, F.; Capela, J.P. Neurotoxicity of "ecstasy" and its metabolites in human dopaminergic differentiated SH-SY5Y cells. *Toxicol. Lett.* **2013**, *216*, 159–170. [CrossRef] [PubMed]

49. Feio-Azevedo, R.; Costa, V.M.; Ferreira, L.M.; Branco, P.S.; Pereira, F.C.; Bastos, M.L.; Carvalho, F.; Capela, J.P. Toxicity of the amphetamine metabolites 4-hydroxyamphetamine and 4-hydroxynorephedrine in human dopaminergic differentiated SH-SY5Y cells. *Toxicol. Lett.* **2017**, *269*, 65–76. [CrossRef] [PubMed]

50. Park, E.S.; Kim, S.D.; Lee, M.H.; Lee, H.S.; Lee, I.S.; Sung, J.K.; Yoon, Y.S. Protective effects of *N*-acetylcysteine and selenium against doxorubicin toxicity in rats. *J. Vet. Sci.* **2003**, *4*, 129–136. [PubMed]

51. Chwastek, J.; Jantas, D.; Lason, W. The ATM kinase inhibitor KU-55933 provides neuroprotection against hydrogen peroxide-induced cell damage via a gammaH2AX/p-p53/caspase-3-independent mechanism: Inhibition of calpain and cathepsin D. *Int. J. Biochem. Cell Biol.* **2017**, *87*, 38–53. [CrossRef] [PubMed]

52. Rossato, L.G.; Costa, V.M.; Vilas-Boas, V.; de Lourdes Bastos, M.; Rolo, A.; Palmeira, C.; Remiao, F. Therapeutic concentrations of mitoxantrone elicit energetic imbalance in H9c2 cells as an earlier event. *Cardiovasc. Toxicol.* **2013**, *13*, 413–425. [CrossRef] [PubMed]

53. Rossato, L.G.; Costa, V.M.; Dallegrave, E.; Arbo, M.; Silva, R.; Ferreira, R.; Amado, F.; Dinis-Oliveira, R.J.; Duarte, J.A.; de Lourdes Bastos, M.; et al. Mitochondrial cumulative damage induced by mitoxantrone: Late onset cardiac energetic impairment. *Cardiovasc. Toxicol.* **2014**, *14*, 30–40. [CrossRef] [PubMed]

54. Tomkins, C.E.; Edwards, S.N.; Tolkovsky, A.M. Apoptosis is induced in post-mitotic rat sympathetic neurons by arabinosides and topoisomerase II inhibitors in the presence of NGF. *J. Cell. Sci.* **1994**, *107 Pt 6*, 1499–1507. [PubMed]

55. Barbosa, D.J.; Capela, J.P.; de Lourdes Bastos, M.; Carvalho, F. In vitro models for neurotoxicology research. *Toxicol. Res.* **2015**, *4*, 801–842. [CrossRef]

56. Wenker, S.D.; Chamorro, M.E.; Vota, D.M.; Callero, M.A.; Vittori, D.C.; Nesse, A.B. Differential antiapoptotic effect of erythropoietin on undifferentiated and retinoic acid-differentiated SH-SY5Y cells. *J. Cell. Biochem.* **2010**, *110*, 151–161. [CrossRef] [PubMed]

57. Lombet, A.; Zujovic, V.; Kandouz, M.; Billardon, C.; Carvajal-Gonzalez, S.; Gompel, A.; Rostene, W. Resistance
     to induced apoptosis in the human neuroblastoma cell line SK-*N*-SH in relation to neuronal differentiation.
     Role of Bcl-2 protein family. *Eur. J. Biochem.* **2001**, *268*, 1352–1362. [CrossRef] [PubMed]
58. Schneider, L.; Giordano, S.; Zelickson, B.R.; S Johnson, M.; A Benavides, G.; Ouyang, X.; Fineberg, N.;
     Darley-Usmar, V.M.; Zhang, J. Differentiation of SH-SY5Y cells to a neuronal phenotype changes cellular
     bioenergetics and the response to oxidative stress. *Free Radic. Biol. Med.* **2011**, *51*, 2007–2017. [CrossRef]
     [PubMed]
59. Xun, Z.; Lee, D.-Y.; Lim, J.; Canaria, C.A.; Barnebey, A.; Yanonne, S.M.; McMurray, C.T. Retinoic acid-induced
     differentiation increases the rate of oxygen consumption and enhances the spare respiratory capacity of
     mitochondria in SH-SY5Y cells. *Mech. Ageing Dev.* **2012**, *133*, 176–185. [CrossRef] [PubMed]
60. Strigun, A.; Wahrheit, J.; Niklas, J.; Heinzle, E.; Noor, F. Doxorubicin increases oxidative metabolism in
     HL-1 cardiomyocytes as shown by 13C metabolic flux analysis. *Toxicol. Sci.* **2012**, *125*, 595–606. [CrossRef]
     [PubMed]
61. Barbosa, D.J.; Capela, J.P.; Feio-Azevedo, R.; Teixeira-Gomes, A.; Bastos, M.L.; Carvalho, F. Mitochondria:
     Key players in the neurotoxic effects of amphetamines. *Arch. Toxicol.* **2015**, *89*, 1695–1725. [CrossRef]
     [PubMed]

7

Isolation and Structural Characterization of Bioactive Molecules on Prostate Cancer from Mayan Traditional Medicinal Plants

Rafael Sebastián Fort [1,†], Juan M. Trinidad Barnech [1,2,†], Juliette Dourron [2], Marcos Colazzo [3], Francisco J. Aguirre-Crespo [4], María Ana Duhagon [1,5,*] and Guzmán Álvarez [2,*] [ID]

[1]   Laboratorio de Interacciones Moleculares, Facultad de Ciencias, Universidad de la República, Montevideo, C.P. 11400, Uruguay; rfort@fcien.edu.uy (R.S.F.); juan.manuel.trinidad13@gmail.com (J.M.T.B.)

[2]   Laboratorio de Moléculas Bioactivas, CENUR Litoral Norte, Universidad de la República, Ruta 3 (km 363), Paysandú, C.P. 60000, Uruguay; juli.dourron@gmail.com

[3]   Departamento de Química del Litoral, CENUR Litoral Norte, Universidad de la República, Paysandú, C.P. 60000, Uruguay; mcolazzo@gmail.com

[4]   Facultad de Ciencias Químico Biológicas, Universidad Autónoma de Campeche, Campeche, C.P. 24039, Mexico; fjaguirr@uacam.mx

[5]   Departamento de Genética, Facultad de Medicina, Universidad de la República, Montevideo, C.P. 11800, Uruguay

*   Correspondence: mduhagon@fmed.edu.uy (M.A.D.); guzmanalvarezlqo@gmail.com (G.Á.);

†   These authors contributed equally to this work.

Abstract: Prostate cancer is the most common cancer in men around the world. It is a complex and heterogeneous disease in which androgens and their receptors play a crucial role in the progression and development. The current treatment for prostate cancer is a combination of surgery, hormone therapy, radiation and chemotherapy. Therapeutic agents commonly used in the clinic include steroidal and non-steroidal anti-androgens, such as cyproterone acetate, bicalutamide and enzalutamide. These few agents have multiple adverse effects and are not 100% effective. Several plant compounds and mixtures, including grape seed polyphenol extracts, lycopene and tomato preparations, soy isoflavones, and green tea extracts, have been shown to be effective against prostate cancer cell growth. In vivo activity of some isolated compounds like capsaicin and curcumin was reported in prostate cancer murine models. We prepared a library of plant extracts from traditional Mayan medicine. These plants were selected for their use in the contemporaneous Mayan communities for the treatment of different diseases. The extracts were assessed in a phenotypic screening using LNCaP prostate cancer androgen sensitive cell line, with a fixed dose of 25 μg/mL. MTT assay identified seven out of ten plants with interesting anti-neoplastic activity. Extracts from these plants were subjected to a bioguided fractionation to study their major components. We identified three compounds with anti-neoplastic effects against LNCaP cells, one of which shows selectivity for neoplastic compared to benign cells.

Keywords: prostate cancer; in vitro; LNCaP; natural product; plants; Mayan medicine

1. Introduction

Currently, there are many millenary cultures such as the Mayans who use plants to treat diverse human diseases. In some areas of Mexico, large communities of people are only treated by their traditional physicians (called "Chamanes") who reach some success using traditional herbal medicine [1]. Although many plants are used for different purposes, scientific support for their application is still required. Due to the frequent consumption of these plants, there are many reports on their good toxicology that warrant their human use [2,3]. The search for natural products for cancer therapy represents an area of great interest in which plants have been the most important source. As an example, different plant extracts and herbal compounds studied in traditional Chinese medicine showed promising anti-prostate cancer activity [4]. Indeed, many clinically successful anti-cancer drugs are either natural products themselves or have been developed from natural occurring lead compounds [5,6]. One example used in the therapy of prostate cancer (PCa) is docetaxel [7]. Despite their different mechanisms of action, most of these compounds exhibit cytotoxic activity which is useful in cancer therapy where the goal is to kill cancerous cells.

Cancer remains one of the major causes of mortality worldwide and PCa is the most common cancer among males in Western countries [8]. PCa is a complex heterogeneous disease which shows a heterogeneous prognosis [9]. The current treatment for PCa is a combination of surgery, radiation, and chemotherapy. The therapeutic agents commonly used in the first line of PCa treatment include steroidal (cyproterone acetate) and nonsteroidal anti-androgens (like bicalutamide and enzalutamide) [10–12]. Steroids have partial agonistic activity and effects that extend to other hormonal systems, leading to many complications, including serious cardiovascular problems, gynecomastia, loss of libido and erectile dysfunction [10,13]. Non-steroidal anti-androgens also show several side effects, but have an improved oral bioavailability which favors their use over steroidal anti-androgens [12,14].

In the present context, there is a need for new more efficient and specific PCa drugs causing less severe side effects. Successful strategies for drug discovery employ the phenotypic screening of neoplastic cells [15]. Seeking for the discovery of anti-neoplastic compounds, the present investigation evaluate the anti-neoplastic activity of extracts from *Cnidoscolus chayamansa* McVaugh (Euphorbiaceae), *Byrsonima crassifolia* L. Kunth (Malpighiaceae), *Leucaena leucocephala* Lam. de Wit (Fabaceae), *Malmea depressa* Baillon R.E. Fries (Annonaceae), *Ipomoea pes-caprae* L. R. Br. (Convolvulaceae), *Capsicum chinense* Jacq. (Solanaceae), *Terminalia catappa* L. (Combretaceae), *Helicteres baruensis* Jacq. (Sterculiaceae), *Cecropia obstusifolia* Bertol. (Moraceae) and *Coccoloba uvifera* L. (Polygonaceae) and identifies active compounds using the PCa cell line LNCaP. The isolated compounds were structurally characterized by GC/MS and NMR analysis.

C. chayamansa, commonly known as "chaya" (Figure 1) is extensively used in Mexican daily diet due to its high nutritional value, but its anti-tumor activity has not been studied so far. However, it is known to display anti-mutagenic activity in the bacterial cell lines TA100 and TA98 [16]. In addition, ischemia-reperfusion tests performed in mice showed its anti-inflammatory and anti-oxidant activity in the ethanolic extract [16–18]. These data suggests its potential prophylactic and therapeutic use in cancer treatment [19].

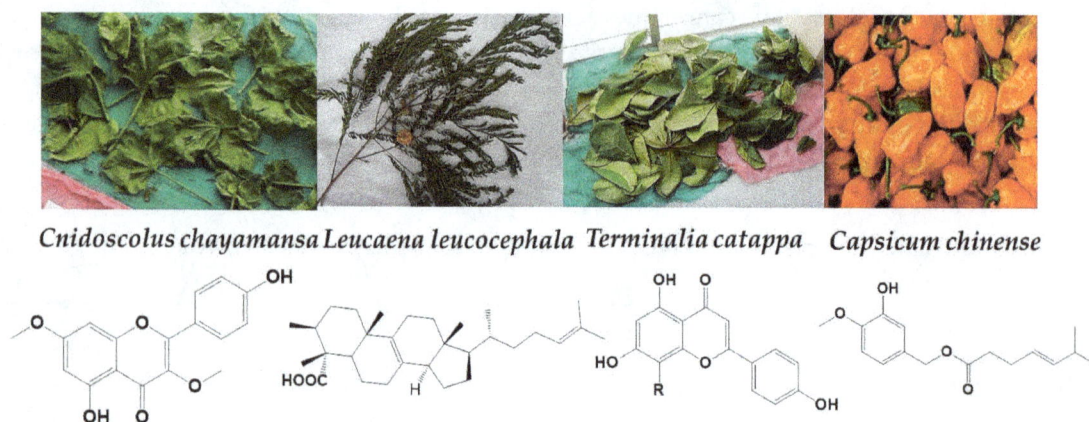

Cnidoscolus chayamansa *Leucaena leucocephala* *Terminalia catappa* *Capsicum chinense*

Figure 1. Pictures of plants assayed in this study and derived compounds previously reported in the literature [18,20–23].

B. crassifolia is a native American orchid species whose leaves produce a drug named birsonimadiol, an anti-inflammatory agent that suppresses the production of nitric oxide (NO) and prostaglandin E_2 (PGE_2), decreasing the gene expression of cyclooxygenase-2 (COX-2), tumor necrosis factor alpha (TNF-alpha) and interleukin 6 (IL-6) in lipopolysaccharide-stimulated macrophages [24]. Since IL-6 is an important determinant of PCa progression [25], the organic extract of *B. crassifolia* constitutes an interesting candidate for PCa treatment.

L. leucocephala, known as "huaje" by the Mayan culture, displays anti-proliferative effects in the cell lines HT-29 (human colon carcinoma), HeLa (human cervical carcinoma), HepG3 (human liver carcinoma) and MCF-7 (human breast adenocarcinoma), being the last one the most affected by the ethanolic extract. These effects are attributed to its promising condensed tannin compounds, which potentially hold health promoting qualities [26]. In addition, *L. leucocephala* extracts showed cytotoxic activity in SCC9 and SAS cells [20], while some of its chemical components have significant chemo-preventive and anti-proliferative properties [27].

M. depressa, also known as "elemuy", was reported to inhibit the growth of HT-29 (human colon carcinoma), MCF-7 (human breast carcinoma) and A-549 (human lung carcinoma) cell lines [28]. Mice trials performed with *I. pes-caprae* in melanoma (B16F10) resulted in a decrease in tumor growth that position it as a complementary treatment to radiotherapy [26].

T. catappa, commonly referred as "almendro", is a tropical and subtropical plant widely used in folk medicine. Since the ethanolic extract obtained from its leaves decreases the invasion of metastatic cells in oral and lung cancer cell lines [22,29], it is an interesting plant to further study. In addition, ethanol extracts of *Terminalia catappa* leaves were shown to exhibit an anti-tumor effect against Ehrlich ascites carcinoma by modulating lipid peroxidation [30].

C. uvifera, known as "niiche" or "Uva de mar", displays anti-oxidant and anti-tyrosinase activities and also inhibits the production of IL-1alpha, TNF-alpha and alpha-MSH in melanocytes subjected to UV radiation [31].

C. chinense, called "chile habanero", is one of the spiciest chilies of the genus, being widely used as a spicy sauce in Mexican food. Some of its compounds have been tested in clinical trials [32–34]. Capsaicin is the major components of *C. chinense* responsible for the burning sensation in the spices of the genus *Capsicum* spp. and is a well-known anti-neoplastic molecule in PCa and others tumors [34–36]; indeed, it has a proven anti-proliferative effect against the LNCaP cell line in a time and concentration dependent manner [37]. Thus, we decided to use *C. chinense* as a positive control for the bioguided fractionation. According to the NIH, there are four molecules derived from this kind of plants in clinical trials linked to cancer (two completed and two in progress) [38,39].

The only plant present in the study that does not present literature associated with cancer is *H. baruensis,* commonly referred as "tsutsup". These families of plants have some toxicological reports and anti-parasitic activity reported, but nothing specific to *H. baruensis* [40,41].

2. Results and Discussion

2.1. Plant Collection and Extract Preparation

Based on prescription frequency, we selected 10 plants from southeastern Mexico (Caribbean region) of more than 300 species used in traditional Mayan medical practice (Table 1). These plants were chosen according to indications of the "chamanes" (the traditional Mayan doctors) and were then classified taxonomically by botanists. Although Mayan doctors recommend the use of these plants to treat human affections, the precision of the diagnosis is hampered by the absence of conventional medical consultation and treatment decisions that largely rely on religious ideas. In this context, to avoid bias in the process, the selection of the plants was independent from the disease in which they are used.

Table 1. Plant collection: general plant information, and extract production yields.

Common Name	Scientific Name	Location	Collection Time	Part of the Plant Used	MeOH Extract (g) *	CH$_2$Cl$_2$ Extract (g) *	Initial Sample (g)	Extraction Yield %
Bejuco de playa	*Ipomoea pes-caprae*	Tulum Beach (20°11′52.00″ N; 87°26′12.38″ O)	may-14	leaves and branches	20.2 (T25)	2.4 (T33)	132	17
Nance	*Byrsonima crassifolia*	Ecological Park Chetumal (18°30′21.25″ N; 88°19′12.79″ O)	sep-13	tree bark	35.5 (T27)	12.6 (T28)	200	24
Uva de mar	*Coccoloba uvifera*	Chetumal bay (18°31′1.79″ N; 88°16′14.46″ O)	may-14	leaves	40.0 (T24)	4 (T23)	214	21
Almendro	*Terminalia catappa*	Chetumal city (18°31′0.55″ N; 88°18′50.27″ O)	may-14	leaves	27.9 (T13)	9 (T6)	250	15
Elemuy	*Malmea depressa*	Santa Rosa town (19°57′51.90″ N; 88°16′17.00″ O)	may-14	leaves and branches	25.6 (T19)	4	164	18
Elemuy	*Malmea depressa*	Santa Rosa town (19°57′51.90″ N; 88°16′17.00″ O)	may-14	root	9.5 (T20)	2.6 (T21)	187	6
Huachi	*Leucaena leucocephala*	Chetumal city (18°31′17.48″ N; 88°18′47.94″ O)	may-14	leaves and branches	26.8 (T2)	9 (T8)	273	13
Chaya	*Cnidoscolus chayamansa*	Chetumal city (18°31′0.55″ N; 88°18′50.27″ O)	may-14	leaves	16.7 (T3)	2 (T4)	100	19
Guarumbo	*Cecropia obstusifolia*	Chetumal city (18°31′26.60″ N; 88°18′49.84″ O)	may-14	leaves	16.7 (T5)	4.5 (T22)	150	14
Tsutsup	*Helicteres baruensis Jacg*	Tulum Beach (20°11′59.42″ N; 87°26′53.68″ O)	may-14	leaves and branches	10.6 (T11)	6 (T14)	113	15
Chile habanero	*Capsicum chinese*	F. Carrillo Puerto town (19°34′50.49″ N; 88° 2′39.57″ O)	may-14	fruit	11.3 (T31)	5 (T38)	55	21

* "T#" is the Nomenclature used to name the extract prepared.

A robust system was used to maximize the extraction of stable molecules. Methanol was used to extract the most hydrosoluble compounds and dichloromethane was used to extract the most lipophilic components. High temperature was used in some steps to enhance solubilization. As shown in Table 1, extraction yield was appropriate to be applied in drug development process considering the good accessibility to the plant material and the simplicity of the instrument and methods used.

2.2. Bioguided Fractionation

The cytotoxic/anti-proliferative activity of the 22 fractions derived from the 10 plants was evaluated in the LNCaP cell line by MTT assays. We obtained the methanolic extract, the dichloromethane extract and some solid material from the filtration of the precipitated material mentioned. Dried plant extracts were dissolved in dimethylsulfoxide (DMSO) and used at a fixed dose of 25 μg/mL in the MTT assay. Putative MTT false positives due to direct reduction of MTT by remnant extract compounds were excluded studying the effect of the extracts on MTT absorbance in the absence of cells [42]. Although, some extracts caused a reduction of MTT, its magnitude is negligible in comparison to the reduction of MTT caused by the cells treated with them (Figure S1). In addition, we carried out a microscopic inspection of the cultures after the treatment to record alterations in cell number and morphology indicative of changes in cell proliferation and cell viability/death respectively. We found that reduction in MTT was always accompanied by changes in either cell number or morphology, which indicates that the reduction of MTT was not caused by a sole change in mitochondrial activity. As shown in Figure 2, we found seven plants whose extracts display in vitro anti-neoplastic activity in LNCaP. *C. obstusifolia*, *I. pes-caprae* and *H. baruensis Jacg* extracts were not cytotoxic/anti-proliferative at the tested concentration. Strikingly, some extracts showed increased activity in the MTT assay compared to the control, which is indicative of a pro-proliferative activity and/or a boosting effect on mitochondrial metabolism (T13, T5 and T11). Among the seven plants with cytotoxic/anti-proliferative activity in LNCaP (Figure 2), *C. chayamansa* (T3F1, T3F2 and T4), *L. leucocephala* (T2 and T8), *T. catappa* (T6), *B. crassifolia* (T28), *C. chinense* (T31), *M. depressa* (T19, T20 and T21) altered MTT absorbance greater than a 50%. Moreover, this threshold is reached by all the fractions from *L. leucocephala* and *M. depressa* showed cytotoxic/anti-proliferative greater than 50% (Figure 2). As expected, *C. chinense* (T31) showed a cytotoxic/anti-proliferative activity that validates this step of the fractionation.

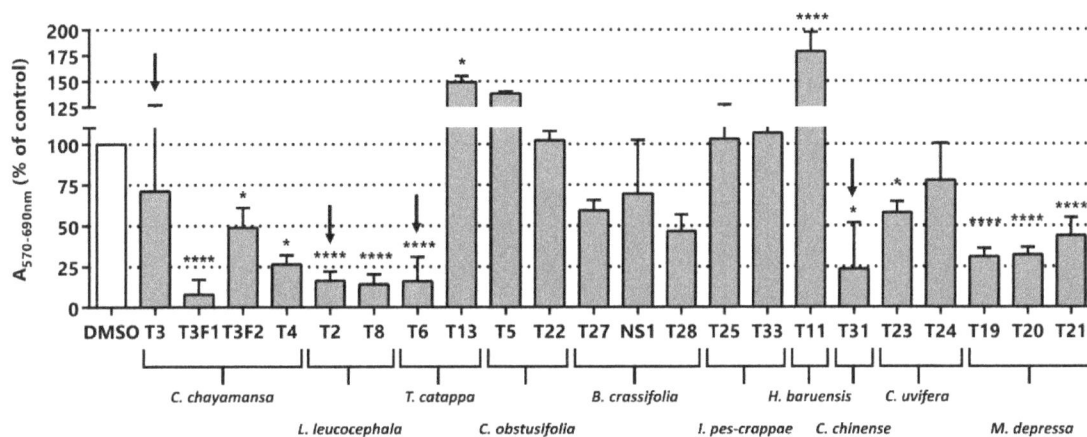

Figure 2. Phenotypic screening. Cytotoxic/anti-proliferative activity of the extracts (25 µg/mL) in LNCaP cells. Black arrows indicate samples selected for the next step of the bioguided fractionation procedure. The nomenclature of the fractions corresponds to a code of the preparation procedure. T3F1 and T3F2 fractions of *C. chayamansa* are derived from the sugar extraction of the methanolic extract with ethyl acetate/water. NS1 it is a solid derived from the T27 fraction isolated by filtration during the evaporation process. Statistical significance is * $p < 0.05$; **** $p < 0.0001$.

Four active extracts were selected to continue the bioguided fractionation (blacks arrows in Figure 2 indicate the selected samples). The selected extracts comprise the methanolic extracts from *L. leucocephala* (T2), *C. chayamansa* (T3), *T. catappa* (T6) and *C. chinense* (T31). The new fractions derived from the fractionation by silica chromatography of the methanolic extract of *L. leucocephala* were again evaluated in LNCaP cells using the MTT assay. However, the MTT activity of these sub-fractions did not improve and even worsened in this purification stage (Figure 3A). The fractions F28, F29 and F34 were the most active fractions of *L. leucocephala*. The yield obtained in the first chromatography was poor and the amount of the material remaining from the next step was even lower. Indeed, there was not enough material to pursue the fractionation of F34. Nevertheless, since the TLC profile of fractions F28 and F29 were similar, they were mixed to continue with a preparative chromatography. As shown in Figure 3B, the cytotoxic/anti-proliferative effect of fraction F10 was similar to the parental fractions (preparative chromatography image available in Figure S2). However, there was not enough material to proceed to further fractionation with this extract. Although there are no reports about the activity of methanolic extracts of *L. leucocephala* in LNCaP cell line, extracts from this plant have been tested in other PCa cells, such as DU145, and some of the compounds responsible for the cytotoxic activity were structurally elucidated [26].

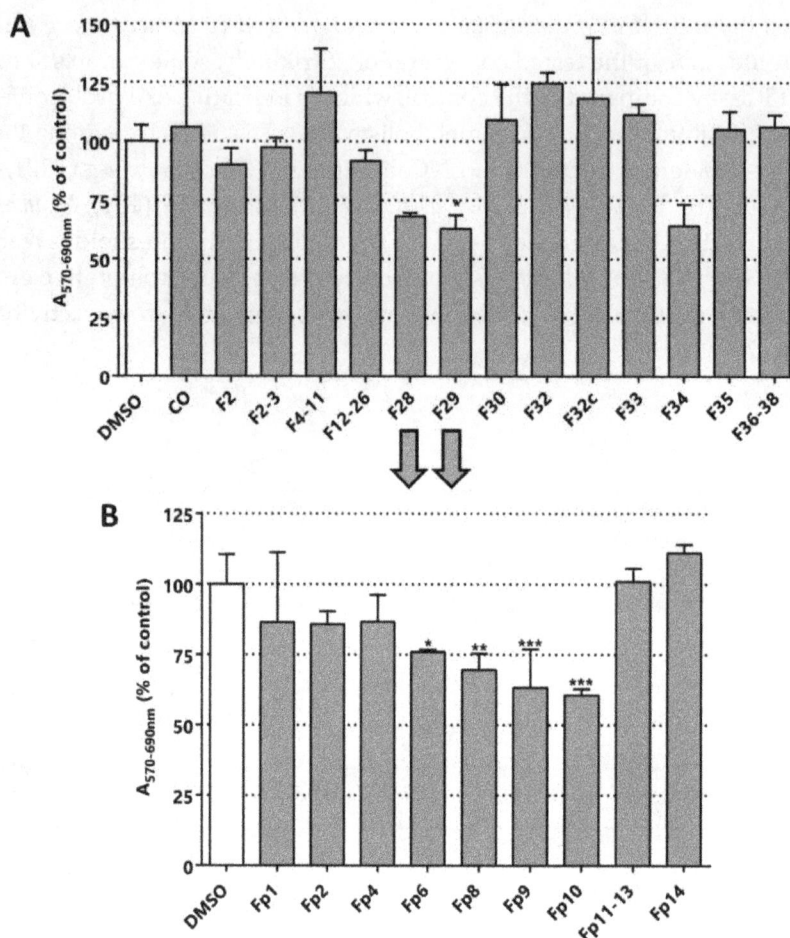

Figure 3. Bioguided fractionation. Cytotoxic/anti-proliferative activity of the *L. leucocephala* extracts (25 µg/mL) in LNCaP cells. (**A**) Evaluation of the fractions obtained from the silica chromatography of the methanolic extract of *L. leucocephala*. CO is the organic phase after the extraction with ethyl acetate/water. (**B**) Evaluation of the fractions obtained by preparative chromatography, particularly fractions F28 and F29. The nomenclature of the fractions corresponds to the chromatographic elution time. Statistical significance is * $p < 0.05$; ** $p < 0.01$; *** $p < 0.001$.

From the purification of T3 fraction (crude fraction from the methanolic extract of *C. chayamansa*) nine sub-fractions were obtained. Contrary to what was observed for *L. leucocephala* T2 extracts, the cytotoxic/anti-proliferative effect of fraction T3 on LNCaP was 31%, whereas the sub-fractions increased the effect to values of 48% in F5-8 and 59% in F31 (Figure 4). These results indicate that in the latter purification there was an enrichment of the active molecule(s).

The fraction F5-8 was submitted to preparative chromatography yielding nine different fractions (chromatography image available in Figure S3). Only Fp9 was active in the MTT assay. Optical microscopy images of the cultures after the treatment with this fraction and its previous fraction confirmed the cytotoxic/anti-proliferative activity determined by MTT (Figure S4). The major compound present in Fp9 fraction was then structurally characterized by NMR and MS (results available in Figures S5 and S6) and the structure is depicted in Figure 4C. The single major molecule corresponds to the methyl ester of the fatty acid 8-methyl-6-nonanoic acid (Figure 4C). Surprisingly, a relatively simple fatty acid was isolated in the form of ester, which surely derives from the successive manipulations with methanol and high temperature. The action of simple fatty acids has been reported in different types of cancer previously [43–46]. The closest related structure found in the literature was 13-methyltetradecanoic acid, which showed in vitro and in vivo anti-neoplastic activity (IC_{50} in prostate cancer cell in vitro DU145 was 62 µM) [47]. This strongly validates our bioguided fractionation procedure and opens a new class of molecules for use in a nature inspired design of new bioactive molecules for PCa. Simple fatty acids are versatile compounds that can be used in different types of reaction, as in the preparation of hybrid molecules. These molecules could be part of a new multi-target drug for PCa.

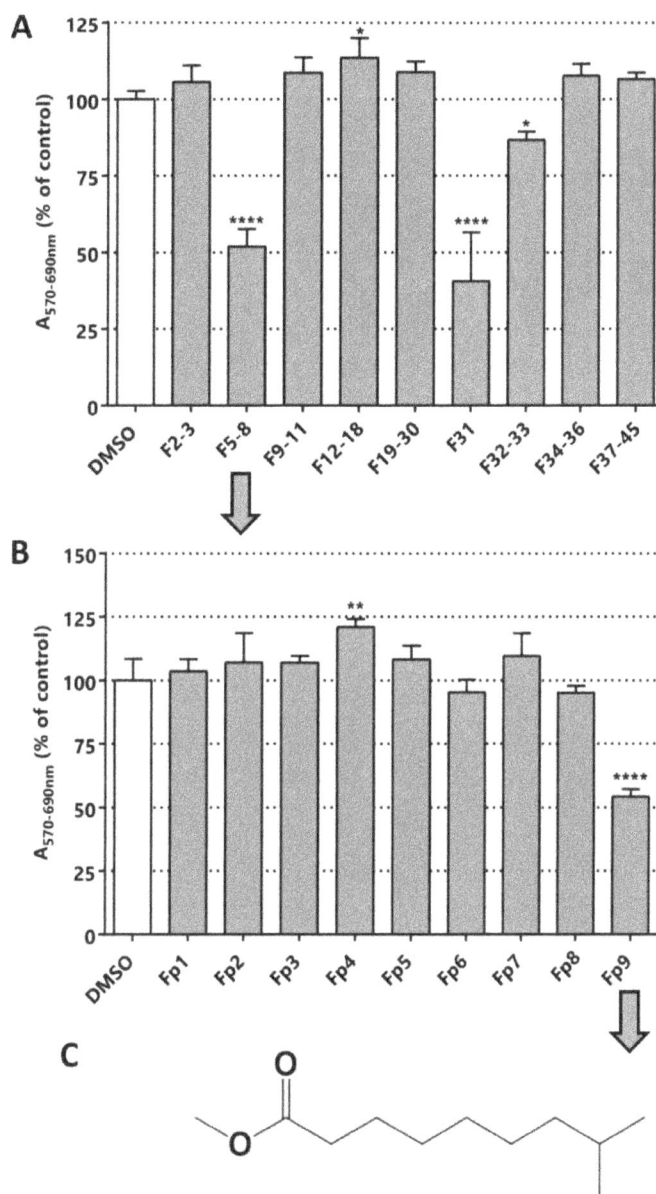

Figure 4. Bioguided fractionation. Cytotoxic/anti-proliferative activity of the *C. chayamansa* extracts (25 μg/mL) in LNCaP cells. (**A**) Evaluation of the fractions obtained from the silica chromatography of the methanolic extract of *C. chayamansa*. (**B**) Evaluation of the fractionations obtained by preparative chromatography of F5-8. (**C**) The structure of the compound identified in fraction Fp9: methyl ester of the fatty acid 8-methyl-6-nonanoic acid. Statistical significance is * $p < 0.05$; ** $p < 0.01$; **** $p < 0.0001$.

The sub-fractionation of *C. chinense* yield seven sub-fractions, three of which were cytotoxic/anti-proliferative against the LNCaP cell line: F0, F11 and F16 (Figure 5). F11 and F16 could be similar molecules due to their elution in neighboring fractions; however, F0 is probably a different molecule. The F0 and F11 fractions were selected for further fractionation and structural elucidation, since they were the most active fractions, decreasing the MTT activity to 35% and 55% respectively (Figure 5). Optical microscopy images of the cultures after the treatment with these fractions confirmed a decrease in cell viability suggested by MTT assay (Figure S7). F0 and F11 underwent silica preparative chromatography. For F0, five different subfractions were isolated (Figure S8), among which F5p was the subfraction with the highest cytotoxic/anti-proliferative effect, reducing MTT activity to 76% (Figure S8). Despite having evidenced cytotoxic effect in LNCaP, the subsequent step of fractionation decreased the MTT effect of the subfractions.

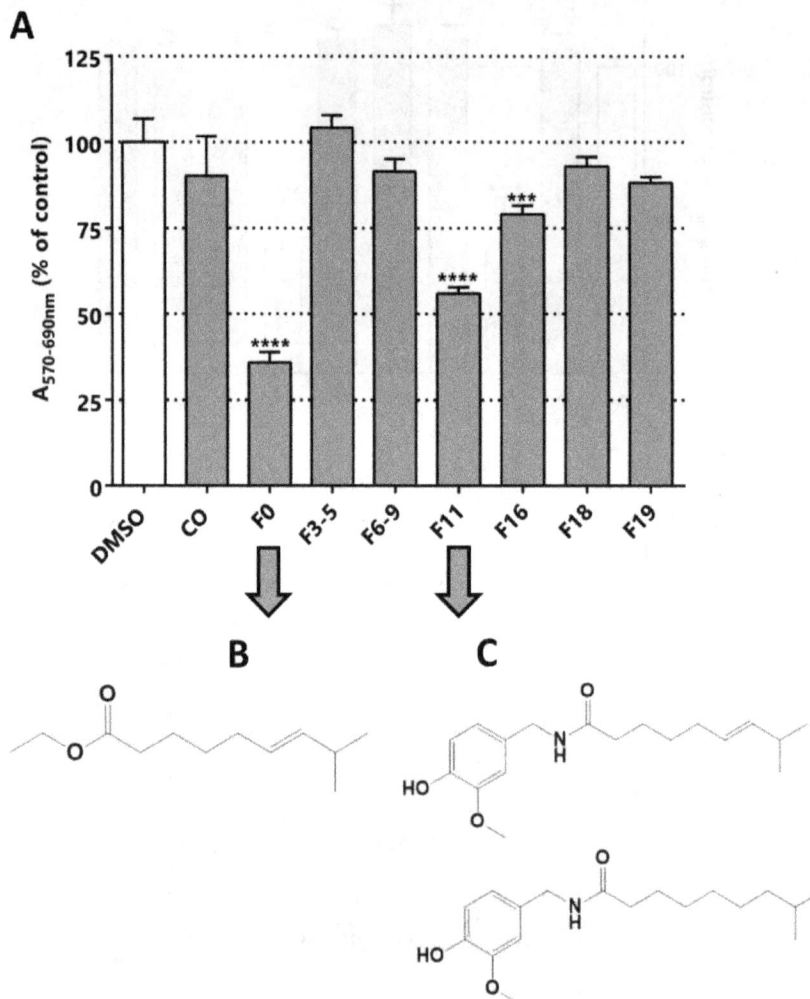

Figure 5. Bioguided fractionation. Cytotoxic/anti-proliferative activity of the *C. chinense* extracts (25 µg/mL) in LNCaP cells. (**A**) Evaluation of all the fractions obtained from the silica chromatography of the methanolic extract of *C. chinense*. The structure of the compounds isolated from the preparative chromatography of (**B**) F0 ((*E*)-ethyl 8-methylnon-6-enoate) and (**C**) F11 (capsaicin and dihydrocapsaicin, respectively) is shown. Statistical significance is *** $p < 0.001$; **** $p < 0.0001$.

From the sub-fractionation of F0, we isolated the active compound (*E*)-ethyl 8-methylnon-6-enoate (Figures 5B and S9). This molecule is a precursor in the biosynthesis of capsaicin, and has not been described as an inhibitor of PCa cells [32,48]. In addition, it is structurally correlated to the compound isolated from *C. chayamansa*, since it is a fatty acid with one unsaturation. Finally, we isolated a mixture of capsaicin and dihydrocapsaicin from F11 (Figures 5C and S1), in a 60/40 proportion. This mixture was reported in the isolation from others types of chili [34,49]. These results confirm our bioguided procedure, because we finally purified the same product from the fruit of the *C. chinense* plant and evidenced the same range of cytotoxic/anti-proliferative effect reported previously for the LNCaP cell line [36,50].

2.3. Selectivity

To explore the selectivity of the isolated compounds we performed a MTT assay using different types of prostate cells lines: benign prostatic hyperplasia (BPH-1) [42], a prostate cancer cell line derived from a brain metastatic site (DU145), a prostate cancer cell line derived from bone metastasis (PC3), and a prostate cancer cell line derived from a lymph node metastasis (LNCaP). (E)-ethyl 8-methylnon-6-enoate was evaluated in a fixed dose of 100 μM for the 4 lines (Figure 6A). As can be seen in Figure 6, the malignant cell lines were affected in their activity, while the benign cell line was not. Remarkably, the MTT activity values for the LNCaP, DU145 and PC3 lines were 76%, 41% and 62%, respectively. This is correlated with the good toxicology profiles showed by these kind of fatty acids in other type of cells and also with their low in vivo toxicity [47]. Additionally, we tested vanillin to evaluate the possible contribution of the polyphenol motif in the anti-neoplastic activity, and curcumin, which has activity against PCa cells, as a positive control (Figure 6B). As can be observed in Figure 6C, vanillin did not affect the tested cell lines, suggesting that this pharmacophore itself is not sufficient for the cytotoxic/anti-proliferative effect observed for capsaicin. As expected, curcumin showed activity in the cell lines studied and selectivity for the neoplastic cells, but it greatly affected the benign cell line.

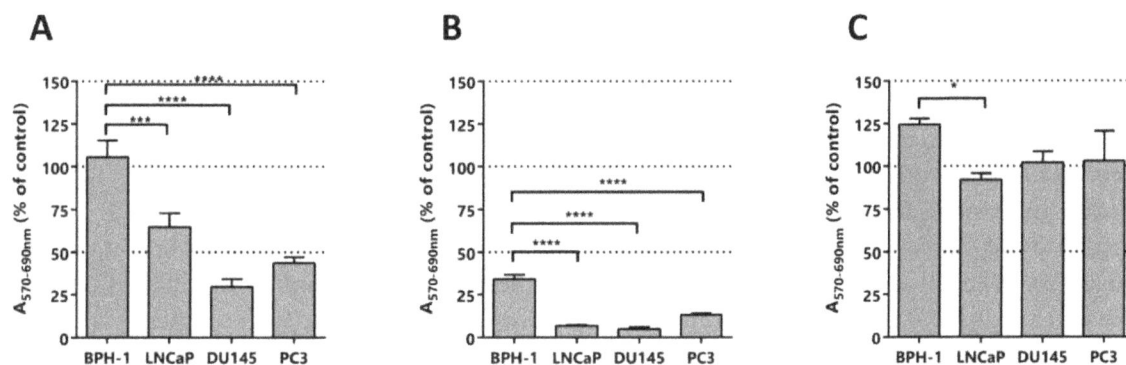

Figure 6. Selectivity assay. Cytotoxic/anti-proliferative activity after treatment of prostate cell lines with the indicated compounds. (**A**) (E)-ethyl 8-methylnon-6-enoate assayed at 100 μM, (**B**) Curcumin assayed at 50 μM and (**C**) vanillin assayed at 50 μM. The percentages of MTT activity of the compounds was calculated relative to control cultures incubated only with DMSO. Prostate cell lines: BPH-1 derived from a benign prostatic hyperplasia (control) and LNCaP, DU145 and PC3 derived from metastatic PCa. Statistical significance is * $p < 0.05$; *** $p < 0.001$; **** $p < 0.0001$.

Finally, the structure-activity relationship was explored to understand the relation between the vinyl and vanillin motif in the cytotoxic activity observed. We used curcumin as a known anti-neoplastic drug hit, a molecule isolated from *Curcuma longa* which is used as a food spice worldwide and has strong structural relations with the capsicum family (Figure 7).

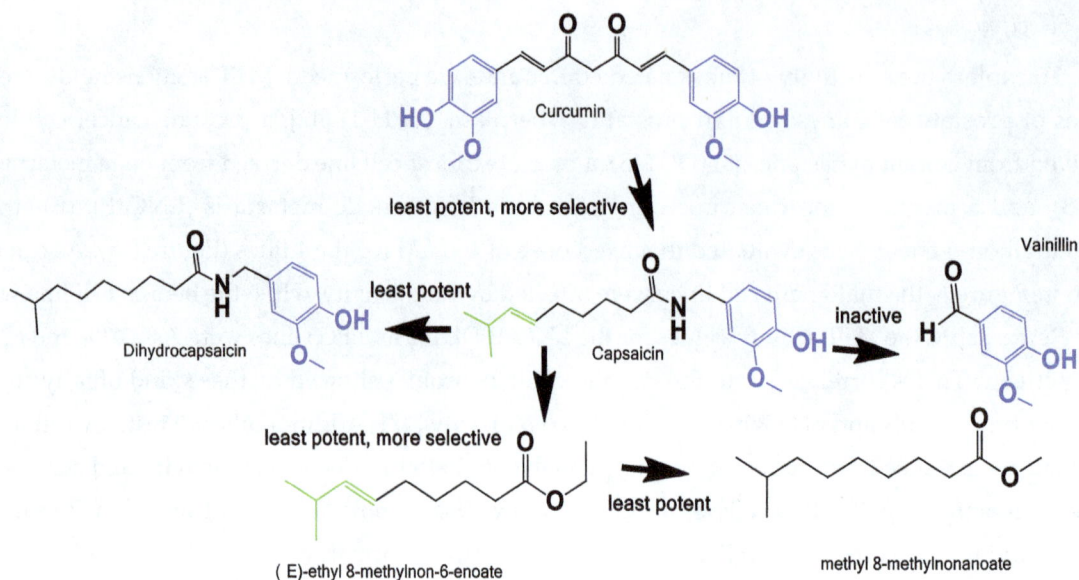

Figure 7. Structure activity relationship. Exploration of the possible pharmacophore responsible for the cytotoxic/anti-proliferative activities against LNCaP. Color codes indicate the vanillin motif (blue), and vinyl motif (green). The "potency" refers to the activity of the compound in LNCaP and the selectivity towards malignant vs benign cells.

The curcumin was reported to be active in different cancer cell line models, infection and diseases [51–54]. Although it is labeled as a pan assay interference (PAINS) compound [55], there is a lot of toxicological information supporting its safety. Indeed, it is actually widely consumed in many diets around the world [56]. In this work, we evidenced that curcumin has similar activity in all the prostate cell models assessed (Figure 6B and Table 2). In addition, vanillin has been used as proof of the activity of the vanillin motif, and was innocuous at 100 µM (Figure 6C). Our observations and the review of the literature, allow us to propose that the region of the vanillin ring linked with the carbonyl amide bond could be an important motif involved in the cytotoxic/anti-proliferative activity. This region could be the area of the molecule that potentially interacts with the vanillin transitory receptor type 1 (TRPV1), a non-selective calcium channel involved in the burning sensation that has been proposed as one of the anti-neoplastic mechanisms of capsaicin [35,57].

Table 2. IC$_{50}$ for curcumin and (*E*)-ethyl 8-methylnon-6-enoate.

	BPH-1	DU145	PC3	LNCaP
Curcumin IC$_{50}$ (µM)	11 ± 2	12 ± 3	8 ± 1	2 ± 1
(E)-Ethyl 8-methylnon-6-enoate at 100 µM (%) *	0	76	62	41

* % of inhibition of the cell growth at 100 µM.

The conjecture mentioned above is based on the fact that the molecules known to interact with TRPV1 are the capsaicinoids called "capsiate", i.e., capsaicin and resiniferatoxin (RTX) [58]. They have only one common motif: the vanillin ring with the amide bond on carbon 1, where the bond can be amide (capsaicin and RTX) or ester (capsiate). TRPV1 mRNA and protein levels show a positive correlation with the level of malignancy of the tumors in PCa samples from patients, placing TRPV1 as a candidate biomarker and also a target for drugs [59]. In the LNCaP and PC-3 cell lines, this receptor is present and active, as in benign prostatic hyperplastic tissue samples, so the cell lines can be used to assays of TRPV1 activity [38]. The fatty acid motif in capsaicin seems to influence the selectivity between benign and neoplastic cells; it also has an intrinsic anti-neoplastic activity independent of the vanillin motif. Curcumin has higher activity than capsaicin, but there is not selectivity in the assayed cells. Curcumin has two vanillin motif without the fatty acid motifs, and also a Michael acceptor region, which together could explain its reduced selectivity (Figure 6). Therefore, the fatty acid is a promising motif to use in a drug design program inspired by nature. Finally, it could be useful in the design of new hybrid molecules with recognized anti-neoplastic compounds.

3. Experimental Section

3.1. Plant Material Collection

The most popular "chamanes" in the area of Quintana Roo, where the mayor community of Mayan descendants lives, where identified. Then, these traditional doctors were interviewed to find ethnobotanic information about the plant used for disease treatment. Ten plants were selected based on the prescription frequency. The "chamanes" shared their collection spaces and helped to identify the plants. The different species of plants were classified after a botanical verification using voucher samples. The information related to the time and location of the plants collected is indicated in Table 1. An identified voucher sample has been deposited in the herbarium of the Autonomous University of Campeche.

3.2. Extract Preparation

The collected samples were first separated according to the part of the plant, for example, leaves, flowers fruits, etc. With this first separation we had more than one sample for each species of plant. The extracts were prepared in a classical format. After the collection, the plant material was dried in an oven at 50–60 °C for approximately twelve hours. Then the dry material was ground to powder grade in a mill (MF 10.2 Impact Grinding Head), weighed and extracted. Preferably 150 and 250 g of the plant powder were dissolved with 600–800 mL of solvent. Two types of extraction were carried out, one with methanol and the other with dichloromethane. The methanolic extract was obtained from the macerate of the plant material incubated with methanol for 4 h (600–800 mL), then the solvent was collected by filtration and a new amount of solvent was added for 4 more hours. This process was repeated four times. The same method was used to prepare the dichloromethane extract, using dichloromethane in the same way as methanol. Finally, the total methanolic and dichloromethane extract was evaporated to dryness in vacuum and the crude was stored at room temperature in hermetic bottles for later use. When two phases were observed during the evaporation process in the crude extract, an extraction was performed using ethyl acetate/water.

3.3. Chromatographic Studies and Isolation of Active Constituents

The extract was adsorbed on silica gel and chromatographed on a silica gel column eluted with mixtures of petroleum ether-EtOAc-CH_2Cl_2 at increasing polarities. The eluted fractions were evaluated by TLC in the same condition. Elution with methanol at 10% yielded the polar material retained on the top of the column. The fractions were biological evaluated to identify the active fraction and a sub-sequent chromatography separation was made from them. The end point in some cases was an isolated compound.

3.4. Determination of the Chemical Structures

Structures of isolated fractions and purified compounds were analyzed by extensive spectroscopic methods including GS-MS, UV, IR, ^{1}H-NMR, ^{13}C-NMR, COSY, HSQC, HMBC, DEPT, NOE-diff and NOESY experiments, using deuterated chloroform and the instrument default parameters. ^{1}H- and ^{13}C-NMR spectra, and the rest of the experiments (COSY, NOE-diff, HSQC, HMBC, DEPT, and NOESY) were obtained on an AVANCE DPX-400 spectrometer (Bruker Rheinstetten, Germany) at 22.16 °C. UV and IR spectra were recorded at room temperature using ACTGene-Nanodrop (Piscataway, NJ, USA) and Shimadzu (Kyoto, Japan) IR PRESTIGE-21 spectrophotometers, respectively. GC–MS analyses were performed on a HP 5890 chromatograph Series II Gas Chromatograph (Hewlett-Packard,

Avondale, PA, USA) coupled to a VG Trio 2 mass spectrometer (VG Instruments, Danvers, MA, USA) using a DB-5 fused silica capillary column, 30 m × 0.25 mm i.d., 0.25 μm film thickness (J&W Scientific, Folsom, CA, USA). Injections were made in the splitless mode with a helium head pressure of 0.85 MPa (velocity: 0.35 ms^{-1}). The injector, the transfer line and the source temperatures were set to 315, 300 and 220 °C respectively. The temperature program was: 80 °C for 1 min followed by a gradient at 4 °C min^{-1} to 300 °C, final temperature held for 30 min. Scan rate was adjusted to 1s per scan from 50 to 700 amu. The "non-aromatic hydrocarbon" fraction was dissolved in 50 μl of hexane before injection of a 1 μL aliquot. Automated Mass Spectral Deconvolution and Identification System software (AMDIS), version 2.1, provided by the National Institute of Standards and Technology (NIST, Gaithersburg, MD USA, web address: http://chemdata.nist.gov/massspc/amdis/index.html) has been used for post-processing the MS data files [60].

3.5. MTT Assay

BPH-1, LNCaP, PC-3 and DU145 human cell lines were obtained from the ATCC (Manassas, VA, USA). All the cell lines were maintained in RPMI 1640 (R7755) supplemented with 10% FBS (PAA™) and penicillin/streptomycin. To perform the cytotoxicity assay 1×10^4 cells per well were seeded in a 96 well plate in a final volume of 200 μL of medium. The extracts or fractions were incubated for 24 h to evaluate the anti-neoplastic effect in the cell lines [61]. For selectivity assay compounds we incubated during 48 h. To proceed with the MTT assay, 20 μL of 3-(4,5-dimethylthiazol-2-yl)-2,5-diphenyl-2H-tetrazolium bromide (MTT) 5 mg/mL solution dissolved in 1× PBS was added to the wells and incubated for 4 h at 37 °C in a 5% CO_2 controlled atmosphere. Next, the medium was aspirated,100 μL of DMSO was added to each well and the plate was incubated at room temperature for 15 min in the dark with moderate orbital shaking. Before the addition of MTT to the culture medium, all the plates were observed under the optical microscope and a semi-quantitative evaluation of changes in cell number and morphology was performed. Optical density (OD) was read on a plate spectrophotometer (Varioskan® Flash Multimode, Thermo Scientific, Waltham, MA, USA) at 570 nm (for formazan absorbance measurement) and 690 nm (for background measurement) wavelengths. The methanolic and dichloromethane extracts, as well as the fractions of the chromatographies, were tested in cell lines at a fixed concentration of 25 μg/mL (on 0.3% v/v of DMSO) and, based on their activity, they were subjected to other subfractionation methods (bioguided fractionation). All the fractions were centrifuged to eliminate insoluble particles. All the analyses were done at least in triplicates. For the statistical analyses the Dunnett's multiple comparison tests, one-way ANOVA and Student's t test on GraphPad Prism 6 [62] were used.

4. Conclusions

In this work, the in vitro anti-neoplastic activity of ten plants used in traditional Maya medicine were evaluated in the LNCaP cell line as a PCa biological model. *C. chayamansa, C. chinense, C. uvifera, L. leucocephala, M. depressa* and *T. catappa* showed the best cytotoxic/anti-proliferative activity. In addition, the process of bioguided fractionation of the plant extracts was standardized using the LNCaP cell line. The procedure was validated by the isolation of capsaicin from the extract of the fruit of *C. chinense*. Additionally, two novel simple fatty acids with in vitro anti-neoplastic activity were identified: 8-methyl 6-nonenoic acid ethyl ester from *C. chinense* and 8-methyl-6-nonanoic acid methyl ester from *C. chayamansa*. Finally, the selectivity for these molecules was evaluated, observing that the 8-methyl 6-nonenoic acid ethyl ester affected the malignant cells considerably more than the benign one.

Author Contributions: J.M.T.B., R.S.F. and G.Á. (made the experiment, analyzed the data and wrote the paper), J.D. (collaborated in some experiments), F.J.A.-C (made the primary extract and collection of the plants), G.Á. and

M.A.D. (designed and coordinated the research and experiments and analyzed the data), G.Á., J.M.T.B. and R.S.F. wrote the draft manuscript and M.A.D. revised it. All authors read and approved the final manuscript.

Funding: This research was funded by Secretaría de Relaciones Exteriores (SRE) Mexico for a travel grant of GA and PRODEP Incorporación Nuevos Profesores for financial support to carry out this research (FJA). The APC was funded by Universidad de la República full time professor grant. PEDECIBA-Biología, Duhagon MA. ANII-PhD fellowships, Fort RS.

Acknowledgments: To the Chamanes from Carrillo Puerto (Mexico) for sharing their knowledge. To Secretaría de Relaciones Exteriores (SRE) Mexico for a travel grant of GA and PRODEP Incorporación Nuevos Profesores for financial support to carry out this research. To PEDECIBA Uruguay for the financial support.

References

1. Bautista-Cruz, A.; Arnaud-Viñas, M.R.; Martínez-Gutiérrez, G.A.; Soledad Sánchez-Medina, P.; Pacheco, R.P. The traditional medicinal and food uses of four plants in Oaxaca, Mexico. *J. Med. Plants Res.* **2011**, *5*, 3404–3411.

2. Kumar, S.; Jawaid, T.; Dubey, S. Therapeutic Plants of Ayurveda; A Review on Anticancer. *Pharmacogn. J.* **2011**, *3*, 1–11. [CrossRef]

3. Déciga-Campos, M.; Rivero-Cruz, I.; Arriaga-Alba, M.; Castañeda-Corral, G.; Angeles-López, G.E.; Navarrete, A.; Mata, R. Acute toxicity and mutagenic activity of Mexican plants used in traditional medicine. *J. Ethnopharmacol.* **2007**, *110*, 334–342. [CrossRef] [PubMed]

4. Wang, X.; Fang, G.; Pang, Y. Chinese medicines in the treatment of prostate cancer: From formulas to extracts and compounds. *Nutrients* **2018**, *10*, 283. [CrossRef] [PubMed]

5. De Petrocellis, L.; Arroyo, F.J.; Orlando, P.; Schiano Moriello, A.; Vitale, R.M.; Amodeo, P.; Sánchez, A.; Roncero, C.; Bianchini, G.; Martín, M.A.; et al. Tetrahydroisoquinoline-Derived Urea and 2,5-Diketopiperazine Derivatives as Selective Antagonists of the Transient Receptor Potential Melastatin 8 (TRPM8) Channel Receptor and Antiprostate Cancer Agents. *J. Med. Chem.* **2016**, *59*, 5661–5683. [CrossRef] [PubMed]

6. Hosseini, A.G. Cancer therapy with phytochemicals: Evidence from clinical studies. *Avicenna J. Phytomedicine* **2015**, *5*, 84–97.

7. Henry, J.Y.; Lu, L.; Adams, M.; Meyer, B.; Bartlett, J.B.; Dalgleish, A.G.; Galustian, C. Lenalidomide enhances the anti-prostate cancer activity of docetaxel in vitro and in vivo. *Prostate* **2012**, *72*, 856–867. [CrossRef] [PubMed]

8. Hu, Y.; Fu, L. Targeting cancer stem cells: A new therapy to cure cancer patients. *Am. J. Cancer Res.* **2012**, *2*, 340–356. [PubMed]

9. Klarmann, G.J.; Hurt, E.M.; Mathews, L.A.; Zhang, X.; Maria, A.; Mistree, T.; Thomas, S.B.; Farrar, W.L. Invasive Prostate Cancer Cells Are Tumor Initiating Cells That Have A Stem Cell-Like Genomic Signature. *Clin Exp Metastasis* **2009**, *26*, 433–446. [CrossRef] [PubMed]

10. Handratta, V.D.; Vasaitis, T.S.; Njar, V.C.O.; Gediya, L.K.; Kataria, R.; Chopra, P.; Newman, D.; Farquhar, R.; Guo, Z.; Qiu, Y.; et al. Novel C-17-heteroaryl steroidal CYP17 inhibitors/antiandrogens: Synthesis, in vitro biological activity, pharmacokinetics, and antitumor activity in the LAPC4 human prostate cancer xenograft model. *J. Med. Chem.* **2005**, *48*, 2972–2984. [CrossRef] [PubMed]

11. Vicentini, C.; Festuccia, C.; Angelucci, A.; Gravina, G.L.; Muzi, P.; Eleuterio, E.; Miano, R.; Marronaro, A.; Tubaro, A.; Bologna, M. Bicalutamide dose-dependently inhibits proliferation in human prostatic carcinoma cell lines and primary cultures. *Anticancer Res.* **2002**, *22*, 2917–2922. [PubMed]

12. Furr, B.J.A.; Tucker, H. The preclinical development of bicalutamide: Pharmacodynamics and mechanism of action. *Urology* **1995**, *47*, 13–25. [CrossRef]

13. Bobach, C.; Tennstedt, S.; Palberg, K.; Denkert, A.; Brandt, W.; De Meijere, A.; Seliger, B.; Wessjohann, L.A. Screening of synthetic and natural product databases: Identification of novel androgens and antiandrogens. *Eur. J. Med. Chem.* **2015**, *90*, 267–279. [CrossRef] [PubMed]

14. Liedtke, A.J.; Adeniji, A.O.; Chen, M.; Byrns, M.C.; Jin, Y.; Christianson, D.W.; Marnett, L.J.; Penning, T.M. Development of Potent and Selective Indomethacin Analogs for the Inhibition of AKR1C3 (Type 5 17 β-Hydroxysteroid Dehydrogenase/Prostaglandin F Synthase) in Castrate-Resistant Prostate Cancer. *J. Med. Chem.* **2013**, *56*, 2429–2446. [CrossRef] [PubMed]

15. Hamid, R.; Rotshteyn, Y.; Rabadi, L.; Parikh, R.; Bullock, P. Comparison of alamar blue and MTT assays for high through-put screening. *Toxicol. In Vitro* **2004**, *18*, 703–710. [CrossRef] [PubMed]

16. Loarca-Piña, G.; Mendoza, S.; Ramos-Gómez, M.; Reynoso, R. Antioxidant, antimutagenic, and antidiabetic activities of edible leaves from *Cnidoscolus chayamansa* Mc. Vaugh. *J. Food Sci.* **2010**, *75*, H68–H72. [CrossRef] [PubMed]

17. García-Rodríguez, R.V.; Gutiérrez-Rebolledo, G.A.; Méndez-Bolaina, E.; Sánchez-Medina, A.; Maldonado-Saavedra, O.; Domínguez-Ortiz, M.Á.; Vázquez-Hernández, M.; Muñoz-Muñiz, O.D.; Cruz-Sánchez, J.S. *Cnidoscolus chayamansa* Mc Vaugh, an important antioxidant, anti-inflammatory and cardioprotective plant used in Mexico. *J. Ethnopharmacol.* **2014**, *151*, 937–943. [CrossRef] [PubMed]

18. Pérez-González, M.Z.; Gutiérrez-Rebolledo, G.A.; Yépez-Mulia, L.; Rojas-Tomé, I.S.; Luna-Herrera, J.; Jiménez-Arellanes, M.A. Antiprotozoal, antimycobacterial, and anti-inflammatory evaluation of *Cnidoscolus chayamansa* (Mc Vaugh) extract and the isolated compounds. *Biomed. Pharmacother.* **2017**, *89*, 89–97. [CrossRef] [PubMed]

19. Gorrini, C.; Harris, I.S.; Mak, T.W. Modulation of oxidative stress as an anticancer strategy. *Nat. Rev. Drug Discov.* **2013**, *12*, 931–947. [CrossRef] [PubMed]

20. Chung, H.-H.; Chen, M.-K.; Chang, Y.-C.; Yang, S.-F.; Lin, C.-C.; Lin, C.-W. Inhibitory effects of *Leucaena leucocephala* on the metastasis and invasion of human oral cancer cells. *Environ. Toxicol.* **2017**, *32*, 1765–1774. [CrossRef] [PubMed]

21. Abu Zarin, M.; Wan, H.Y.; Isha, A.; Armania, N. Antioxidant, antimicrobial and cytotoxic potential of condensed tannins from Leucaena leucocephala hybrid-Rendang. *Food Sci. Hum. Wellness* **2016**, *5*, 65–75. [CrossRef]

22. Chu, S.C.; Yang, S.F.; Liu, S.J.; Kuo, W.H.; Chang, Y.Z.; Hsieh, Y.S. In vitro and in vivo antimetastatic effects of Terminalia catappa L. leaves on lung cancer cells. *Food Chem. Toxicol.* **2007**, *45*, 1194–1201. [CrossRef] [PubMed]

23. Pino, J.; Sauri-Duch, E.; Marbot, R. Changes in volatile compounds of Habanero chile pepper (*Capsicum chinense* Jack. cv. Habanero) at two ripening stages. *Food Chem.* **2006**, *94*, 394–398. [CrossRef]

24. Pérez Gutiérrez, R.M. Anti-inflammatory effect of birsonimadiol from seeds of *Byrsonima crassifolia*. *Food Sci. Biotechnol.* **2016**, *25*, 561–566. [CrossRef]

25. Nguyen, D.P.; Li, J.; Tewari, A.K. Inflammation and prostate cancer: The role of interleukin 6 (IL-6). *BJU Int.* **2014**, *113*, 986–992. [CrossRef] [PubMed]

26. Manigauha, A.; Kharya, M.D.; Ganesh, N. In vivo antitumor potential of Ipomoea pes-caprae on melanoma cancer. *Pharmacogn. Mag.* **2015**, *11*, 426–433. [CrossRef] [PubMed]

27. She, L.; Liu, C.; Chen, C.; Li, H.; Li, W.; Chen, C. The anti-cancer and anti-metastasis effects of phytochemical constituents from *Leucaena leucocephala*. *Biomed. Res.* **2017**, *28*, 2893–2897.

28. Gutierrez-Lugo, M.T.; Barrientos-Benítez, T.; Luna, B.; Ramirez-Gama, R.M.; Bye, R.; Linares, E.; Mata, R. Antimicrobial and cytotoxic activities of some crude drug extracts from Mexican medicinal plants. *Phytomedicine* **1996**, *2*, 341–347. [CrossRef]

29. Yang, S.F.; Chen, M.K.; Hsieh, Y.S.; Yang, J.S.; Zavras, A.I.; Hsieh, Y.H.; Su, S.C.; Kao, T.Y.; Chen, P.N.; Chu, S.C. Antimetastatic effects of *Terminalia catappa* L. on oral cancer via a down-regulation of metastasis-associated proteases. *Food Chem. Toxicol.* **2010**, *48*, 1052–1058. [CrossRef] [PubMed]

30. Tigari, P.; Dupadahalli, K.; Kamurthy, H.; Nadendla, R.; Pandya, N. Antitumor and antioxidant status of *Terminalia catappa* against Ehrlich ascites carcinoma in Swiss albino mice. *Indian J. Pharmacol.* **2013**, *45*, 464. [CrossRef] [PubMed]

31. Silveira, J.E.P.S.; Pereda, M.d.C.V.; Eberlin, S.; Dieamant, G.C.; Di Stasi, L.C. Effects of *Coccoloba uvifera* L. on UV-stimulated melanocytes. *Photodermatol. Photoimmunol. Photomed.* **2008**, *24*, 308–313. [CrossRef] [PubMed]

32. Aza-González, C.; Núñez-Palenius, H.G.; Ochoa-Alejo, N. Molecular biology of capsaicinoid biosynthesis in chili pepper (*Capsicum* spp.). *Plant Cell Rep.* **2011**, *30*, 695–706. [CrossRef] [PubMed]

33. Amruthraj, N.J.; Raj, P.; Saravanan, S.; Lebel, L.A. In vitro studies on anticancer activity of capsaicinoids from *Capsicum chinense* against human hepatocellular carcinoma cells. *Int. J. Pharm. Pharm. Sci.* **2014**, *6*, 254–558.

34. Mori, A.; Lehmann, S.; O'Kelly, J.; Kumagai, T.; Desmond, J.C.; Pervan, M.; McBride, W.H.; Kizaki, M.; Koeffler, H.P. Capsaicin, a component of red peppers, inhibits the growth of androgen-independent, p53 mutant prostate cancer cells. *Cancer Res.* **2006**, *66*, 3222–3229. [CrossRef] [PubMed]

35. Ziglioli, F.; Frattini, A.; Maestroni, U.; Dinale, F.; Ciuffreda, M.; Cortellini, P. Vanilloid-mediated apoptosis in prostate cancer cells through a TRPV-1 dependent and a TRPV-1-independent mechanism. *Acta Biomed. l'Ateneo Parm.* **2009**, *80*, 13–20.

36. Bode, A.M.; Dong, Z. The two faces of capsaicin. *Cancer Res.* **2011**, *71*, 2809–2814. [CrossRef] [PubMed]

37. Ramos-Torres, Á.; Bort, A.; Morell, C.; Rodríguez-Henche, N.; Díaz-Laviada, I. The pepper's natural ingredient capsaicin induces autophagy blockage in prostate cancer cells. *Oncotarget* **2016**, *7*, 1569–1583. [CrossRef] [PubMed]

38. O'Neill, J.; Brock, C.; Olesen, A.E.; Andresen, T.; Nilsson, M.; Dickenson, A.H. Unravelling the mystery of capsaicin: A tool to understand and treat pain. *Pharmacol. Rev.* **2012**, *64*, 939–971. [CrossRef] [PubMed]

39. Rollyson, W.D.; Stover, C.A.; Brown, K.C.; Perry, H.E.; Cathryn, D.; Stevenson, C.A.M.; Ball, J.G.; Valentovic, M.A.; Dasgupta, P. Bioavailability of capsaicin and its implications for drug delivery William. *J. Control. Release* **2010**, *196*, 96–105. [CrossRef] [PubMed]

40. Balogun, S.O.; Da Silva, I.F.; Colodel, E.M.; De Oliveira, R.G.; Ascêncio, S.D.; De Oliveira Martins, D.T. Toxicological evaluation of hydroethanolic extract of Helicteres sacarolha A. St.- Hil. et al. *J. Ethnopharmacol.* **2014**, *157*, 285–291. [CrossRef] [PubMed]

41. Mukul-Yerves, J.M.; Del Rosario Zapata-Escobedo, M.; Montes-Pérez, R.C.; Rodríguez-Vivas, R.I.; Torres-Acosta, J.F. Parásitos gastrointestinales y ectoparásitos de ungulados silvestres en condiciones de vida libre y cautiverio en el trópico mexicano. *Rev. Mex. Ciencias Pecu.* **2014**, *5*, 459–469. [CrossRef]

42. Abel, S.D.A.; Baird, S.K. Honey is cytotoxic towards prostate cancer cells but interacts with the MTT reagent: Considerations for the choice of cell viability assay. *Food Chem.* **2018**, *241*, 70–78. [CrossRef] [PubMed]

43. Kuhajda, F.P.; Jennert, K.; Wood, F.D.; Hennigart, R.A.; Jacobs, L.B.; Dick, J.D.; Pasternack, G.R. Fatty acid synthesis: A potential selective target for antineoplastic therapy. *Proc. Nati. Acad. Sci.* **1994**, *91*, 6379–6383. [CrossRef]

44. Swinnen, J.V.; Roskams, T.; Joniau, S.; Van Poppel, H.; Oyen, R.; Baert, L.; Heyns, W.; Verhoeven, G. Overexpression of fatty acid synthase is an early and common event in the development of prostate cancer. *Int. J. Cancer* **2002**, *98*, 19–22. [CrossRef] [PubMed]

45. Bégin, M.E.; Ells, G.; Das, U.N.; Horrobin, D.F. Differential killing of human carcinoma cells supplemented with n-3 and n-6 polyunsaturated fatty acids. *J. Natl. Cancer Inst.* **1986**, *77*, 1053–1062. [PubMed]

46. De Schrijver, E.; Brusselmans, K.; Heyns, W.; Cells, C. RNA Interference-mediated Silencing of the Fatty Acid Synthase Gene Attenuates Growth and Induces Morphological Changes and Apoptosis of LNCaP Prostate Cancer Cells. *Cancer Res.* **2003**, *63*, 3799–3804. [PubMed]

47. Yang, Z.; Liu, S.; Chen, X.; Chen, H.; Huang, M.; Zheng, J. Induction of Apoptotic Cell Death and in Vivo Growth Inhibition of Human Cancer Cells by a Saturated Branched-Chain Fatty Acid, 13-Methyltetradecanoic Acid. *Cancer Res.* **2000**, *60*, 505–509. [PubMed]

48. Gahungu, A.; Ruganintwali, E.; Karangwa, E.; Zhang, X.; Mukunzi, D. Volatile compounds and capsaicinoid content of fresh hot peppers (*Capsicum chinense*) scotch bonnet variety at red stage. *Adv. J. Food Sci. Technol.* **2011**, *3*, 211–218.

49. Musfiroh, I.D.A.; Mutakin, M.; Angelina, T.; Muchtaridi, M. Capsaicin level of various Capsicum fruits. *Int. J. Pharm. Pharm. Sci.* **2013**, *5*, 248–251.

50. Laratta, B.; De Masi, L.; Sarli, G.; Pignone, D. Hot peppers for happiness and wellness: A rich source of healthy and biologically active compounds. *XV EUCARPIA Meet. Genet. Breed. Capsicum Eggplant* **2011**, *1*, 233–240.

51. Anderson, T.M.D. Anticancer Potential of Curcumin Preclinical and Clinical Studies. *Anticancer Res.* **2003**, *23*, 363–398.

52. Gafner, S.; Lee, S.K.; Cuendet, M.; Barthélémy, S.; Vergnes, L.; Labidalle, S.; Mehta, R.G.; Boone, C.W.; Pezzuto, J.M. Biologic evaluation of curcumin and structural derivatives in cancer chemoprevention model systems. *Phytochemistry* **2004**, *65*, 2849–2859. [CrossRef] [PubMed]

53. Lin, L.; Shi, Q.; Nyarko, A.K.; Bastow, K.F.; Wu, C.-C.; Su, C.-Y.; Shih, C.C.-Y.; Lee, K.-H. Antitumor agents. 250. Design and synthesis of new curcumin analogues as potential anti-prostate cancer agents. *J. Med. Chem.* **2006**, *49*, 3963–3972. [CrossRef] [PubMed]

54. Padmanaban, G. Curcumin as an Adjunct Drug for Infectious Diseases. *Trends Pharmacol. Sci.* **2016**, *37*, 3–5. [CrossRef] [PubMed]

55. Wang, R.; Chen, C.; Zhang, X.; Zhang, C.; Zhong, Q.; Chen, G.; Zhang, Q.; Zheng, S.; Wang, G.; Chen, Q.H. Structure-Activity Relationship and Pharmacokinetic Studies of 1,5-Diheteroarylpenta-1,4-dien-3-ones: A Class of Promising Curcumin-Based Anticancer Agents. *J. Med. Chem.* **2015**, *58*, 4713–4726. [CrossRef] [PubMed]

56. Adapala, N.; Chan, M.M. Long-term use of an antiinflammatory, curcumin, suppressed type 1 immunity and exacerbated visceral leishmaniasis in a chronic experimental model. *Lab. Invest.* **2008**, *88*, 1329–1339. [CrossRef] [PubMed]

57. Kobata, K.; Kawaguchi, M.; Watanabe, T. Enzymatic Synthesis of a Capsinoid by the Acylation of Vanillyl Alcohol with Fatty Acid Derivatives Catalyzed by Lipases. *Biosci. Biotechnol. Biochem.* **2002**, *66*, 319–327. [CrossRef] [PubMed]

58. Kobata, K.; Tate, H.; Iwasaki, Y.; Tanaka, Y.; Ohtsu, K.; Yazawa, S.; Watanabe, T. Isolation of coniferyl esters from Capsicum baccatum L., and their enzymatic preparation and agonist activity for TRPV1. *Phytochemistry* **2008**, *69*, 1179–1184. [CrossRef] [PubMed]

59. Czifra, G.; Varga, A.; Nyeste, K.; Marincsák, R.; Tóth, B.I.; Kovács, I.; Kovács, L.; Bíró, T. Increased expressions of cannabinoid receptor-1 and transient receptor potential vanilloid-1 in human prostate carcinoma. *J. Cancer Res. Clin. Oncol.* **2009**, *135*, 507–514. [CrossRef] [PubMed]

60. Finck, Y.; Aydin, N.; Pellaton, C.; Gorin, G.; Gülaçar, F. Combination of gas chromatography-mass spectrometry and mass spectral deconvolution for structural elucidation of an unusual C29-steroid detected in a complex sedimentary matrix. *J. Chromatogr. A* **2004**, *1049*, 227–231. [CrossRef]

61. Kawasaki, B.T.; Hurt, E.M.; Kalathur, M.; Duhagon, M.A.; John, A.; Kim, Y.S.; Farrar, W.L. Effects of the sesquiterpene lactone parthenolide on prostate tumor-initiating cells: An integrated molecular profiling approach. *Prostate* **2009**, *69*, 827–837. [CrossRef] [PubMed]

62. Fort, R.S.; Mathó, C.; Geraldo, M.V.; Ottati, M.C.; Yamashita, A.S.; Saito, K.C.; Leite, K.R.M.; Méndez, M.; Maedo, N.; Méndez, L.; et al. Nc886 is epigenetically repressed in prostate cancer and acts as a tumor suppressor through the inhibition of cell growth. *BMC Cancer* **2018**, *18*, 1–13. [CrossRef] [PubMed]

8

An Antioxidant Potential, Quantum-Chemical and Molecular Docking Study of the Major Chemical Constituents Present in the Leaves of *Curatella americana* Linn

Mayara Amoras Teles Fujishima [1,2,3], Nayara dos Santos Raulino da Silva [2],
Ryan da Silva Ramos [2], Elenilze Figueiredo Batista Ferreira [1,2], Kelton Luís Belém dos Santos [2],
Carlos Henrique Tomich de Paula da Silva [4], Jocivania Oliveira da Silva [1,3],
Joaquín Maria Campos Rosa [5] and Cleydson Breno Rodrigues dos Santos [1,2,5,*]

[1]   Posgraduate Program of Pharmaceutical Innovation, Federal University of Amapá, 68902-280 Macapá, AP, Brazil; mayarafuji@hotmail.com (M.A.T.F.); elenilze@yahoo.com.br (E.F.B.F.); jocivania@unifap.br (J.O.d.S.)
[2]   Laboratory of Modeling and Computational Chemistry, Department of Biological and Health Sciences, Federal University of Amapá, 68902-280 Macapá, AP, Brazil; nsraulino@gmail.com (N.d.S.R.d.S.); ryanquimico@hotmail.com (R.d.S.R.); keltonbelem@hotmail.com (K.L.B.d.S.)
[3]   Laboratory of Toxicology, Department of Biological and Health Sciences, Federal University of Amapá, 68902-280 Macapá, AP, Brazil
[4]   Computational Laboratory of Pharmaceutical Chemistry, Faculty of Pharmaceutical Sciences of Ribeirão Preto, 14040-903 São Paulo, Brazil; tomich@fcfrp.usp.br
[5]   Department of Pharmaceutical Organic Chemistry, University of Granada, 18071 Granada, Spain; jmcampos@ugr.es
*   Correspondence: breno@unifap.br

Abstract: Reactive oxygen species (ROS) are continuously generated in the normal biological systems, primarily by enzymes as xanthine oxidase (XO). The inappropriate scavenging or inhibition of ROS has been considered to be linked with aging, inflammatory disorders, and chronic diseases. Therefore, many plants and their products have been investigated as natural antioxidants for their potential use in preventive medicine. The leaves and bark extracts of *Curatella americana* Linn. were described in scientific research as anti-inflammatory, vasodilator, anti-ulcerogenic, and hypolipidemic effects. So, the aim of this study was to evaluate the antioxidant potentials of leaf hydroalcoholic extract from *C. americana* (HECA) through the scavenging DPPH assay and their main chemical constituents, evaluated by the following quantum chemical approaches (DFT B3LYP/6-31G**): Maps of Molecular Electrostatic Potential (MEP), Frontier Orbital's (HOMO and LUMO) followed by multivariate analysis and molecular docking simulations with the xanthine oxidase enzyme. The hydroalcoholic extract showed significant antioxidant activity by free radical scavenging probably due to the great presence of flavonoids, which were grouped in the PCA and HCA analysis with the standard gallic acid. In the molecular docking study, the compounds studied presented the binding free energy (ΔG) values close each other, due to the similar interactions with amino acids residues at the activity site. The descriptors Gap and softness were important to characterize the molecules with antioxidant potential by capturing oxygen radicals.

Keywords: *Curatella americana* L.; natural antioxidant; quantum chemical; xanthine oxidase

1. Introduction

Free radicals or reactive oxygen species (ROS), including superoxide anions, hydroxyl radicals, and hydrogen peroxide are continuously generated in normal biological systems. Especially under stress, our body produces more ROS resulting in oxidative stress [1].

The intracellular production of ROS is associated with many cellular events including activation of enzymes such as xanthine oxidase (XO). This is a form of xanthine oxidoreductase, which is molybdenum-containing and uses O_2 as the terminal electron acceptor during the purine metabolism; it is also implicated in human disease due to its capacity to generate uric acid and ROS such as hydrogen peroxide (H_2O_2) and superoxide (O_2-) [2]. The XO has been involved in the pathogenesis of chronic heart failure, cardiomyopathy in diabetes and chronic wounds [3–7].

The inappropriate scavenging of these ROS or xanthine oxidase inhibition generally result in degradation of protein, lipid peroxidation, and DNA oxidation, which have been linked to aging, skin inflammatory disorders, many chronic diseases such as cancer, atherosclerosis besides contributing with the development of degenerative diseases as Alzheimer's disease [1,8–10].

Several studies demonstrated that the intake of natural antioxidants has been associated with the promotion of health and prevention of diseases [11–13]. Natural antioxidants, including phenolic compounds, have diverse biological effects, such as anti-inflammatory, anti-carcinogenic and antiatherosclerotic effects, because of their antioxidant activity [14–16], many plants and their products have been investigated as natural antioxidants for their potential use in the preventive medicine.

Curatella americana L. is a member of the *Dileniaceae* family, popularly known in Brazil as "lixeira" or "cajueiro-bravo." This species is an evergreen woody shrub that is characteristic of Neotropical Savanna, occurring from southern Mexico to Bolivia and in almost all savanna region of Brazil, [17–19]. Into Amazonian savanna *C. americana* it is one of the most frequent species found in Amapa, Amazonas, Para and Roraima states [20,21]. In the Brazilian folk medicine, it is used for inflammation, arthritis, bronchitis, high blood pressure [22]; the leaf decoction is used as an antiseptic and astringent [23]; the bark infusion is used for the treatment of cold, wounds healing and ulcers [24].

The extracts of the leaves and bark of *C. americana* are described in the literature for its anti-inflammatory, analgesic, antihypertensive, vasodilator, anti-ulcerogenic, antimicrobial, and hypolipidemic effects [25–29]. The computational investigation of natural compounds using molecular modeling by the DFT method allowed to evaluate chemical reactivity, molecular stability and molecular electrostatic potential maps (MEPs) to investigate the probable constituents with biological activity [30].

The aim of this study was to evaluate the antioxidant potentials of the hydroalcoholic extract of leaves of *C. americana* (HECA) through the scavenging DPPH assay, followed by the evaluation of the major chemical constituents by quantum chemical studies (DFT B3LYP/6-31G**), such as Maps of Molecular Electrostatic Potential (MEP), Frontier Orbital's (HOMO and LUMO), multivariate analysis (PCA and HCA) and transference of electron compared with gallic acid to identify chemical descriptors that may characterize molecules with antioxidant potential. The molecular docking simulations with the xanthine oxidase enzyme (PDB codes 3 NRZ) was used to evaluate another possible action mechanism of the antioxidant potential in preventing ROS formation and relate the most promising molecules to their chemical characteristics.

2. Results and Discussion

2.1. Chemical Constituents and Molecular Modeling of Curatella americana L.

Phytochemical analyses of the leaves of *C. americana* L. already published, revealed the presence of phenolic compounds, flavonoids, terpenes, saponins and steroids according to studies performed by El-Azizi et al. and Gurni and Kubitzki [31,32], that identified the following compounds: (**1**) Avicularin; (**2**) Quercetin; (**3**) Quercetin-3-*O*-galactopyranoside; (**4**) Quercetin galactoarabinoside; (**5**) Quercetin-3-glucoside; (**6**) Quercetin-3-*O*-Alpha-L-rhamnoside; (**7**) Procyanidin; (**8**) β-Amyrin;

(**9**) Betulinic acid; (**10**) Lupeol; (**11**) gallic acid; (**12**) Foeniculin (see Figure 1). The identified molecules were used in the molecular modeling study.

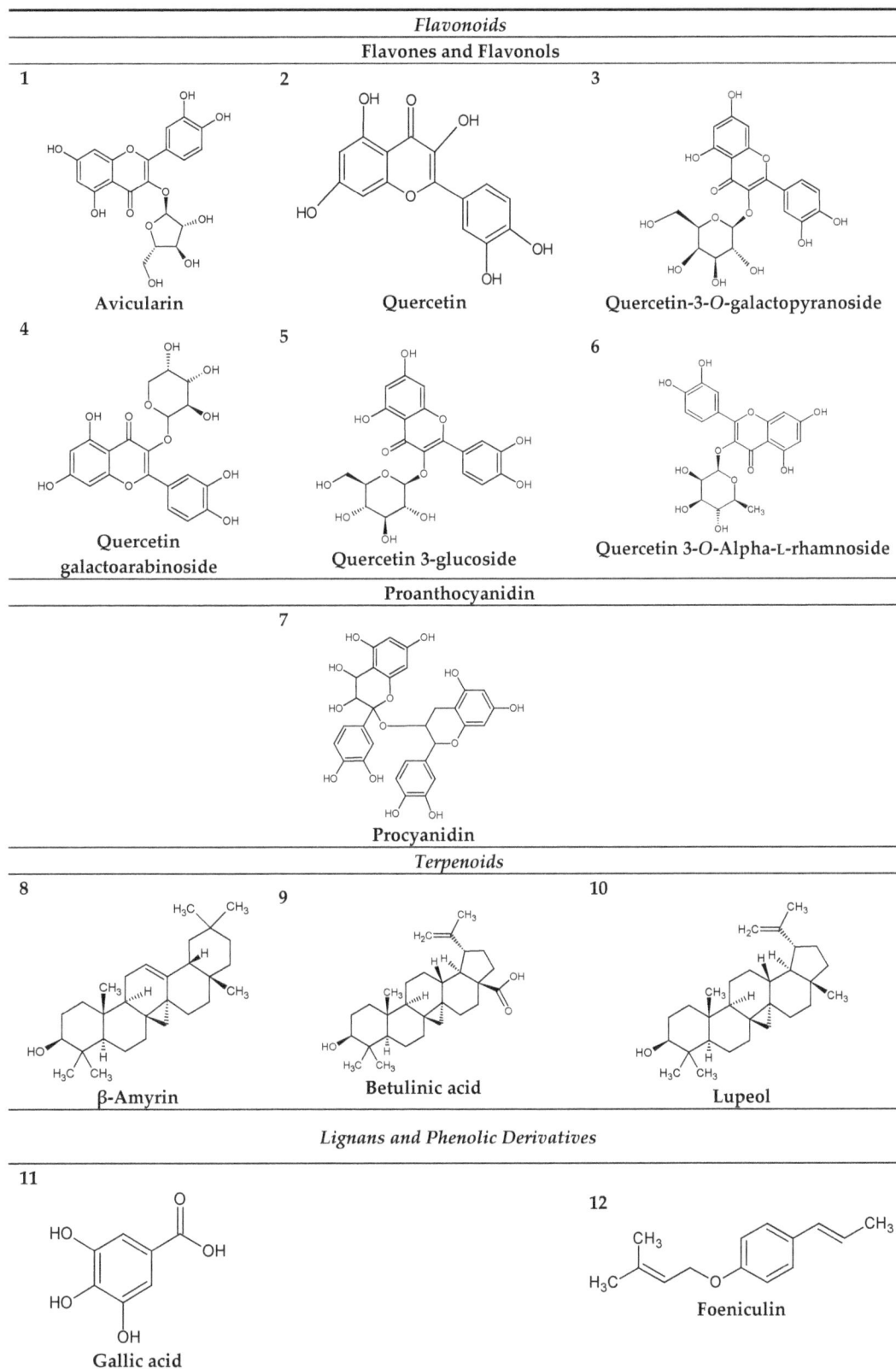

Figure 1. Chemical constituents of the leaves the *C. americana* L.

2.2. DPPH Scavenging Assay

The hydroalcoholic extract of the leaves of *C. americana* (HECA) is rich in phenolic compounds, mainly flavonoids, which have been proposed to exert beneficial effects in multiple disease states due to their antioxidant properties [11,13]. Flavonoids can scavenge a wide range of reactive oxygen species (ROS) by their classical hydrogen-donating antioxidant activity, as well as inhibition of ROS formation [33,34]. The DPPH scavenging potential of HECA and standard reference compound (positive control), Gallic acid, is presented in Figure 2.

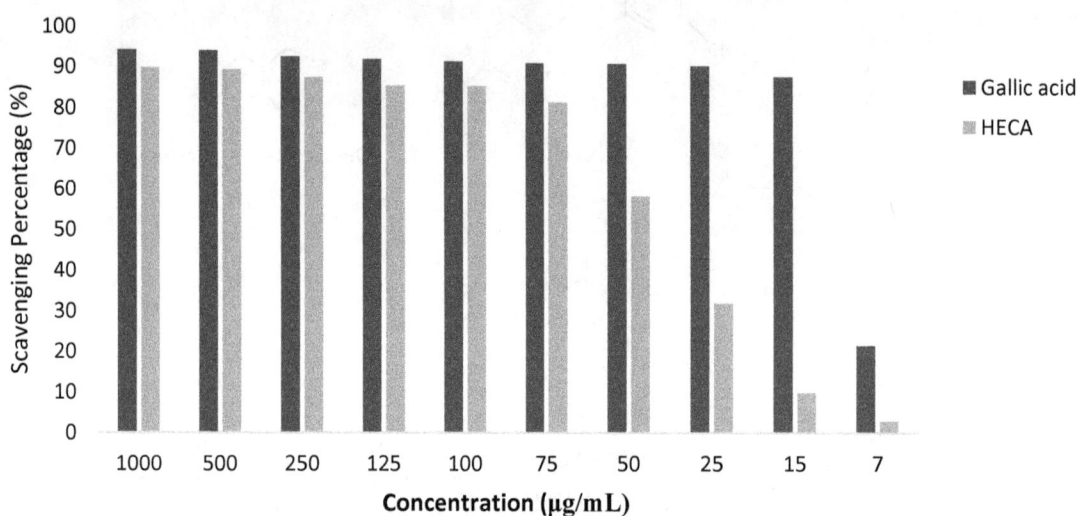

Figure 2. DPPH radical scavenging potential of gallic acid as the reference compound and hydroalcoholic extract of *Curatella americana* (HECA). The mean of scavenging percentage was significative different in all concentrations at $p < 0.01$.

With an estimative based in an exponential model, the 50% concentration inhibitory (IC_{50}) was calculated, $R^2 = 0.8$. Although there are a lot of antioxidant constituents in HECA, even in gallic acid, the activity was moderate, showing an IC_{50} of 45 $\mu g \cdot mL^{-1}$, lower than that previously identified by Lopes et al. [29], the differences in the methodology to obtain the hydroalcoholic extract must be considered. Besides that, it is important to emphasize that the control is an isolated substance and, therefore, would be indispensable to perform the quantum chemical studies to evaluate the most promising molecules with the antioxidant potential of HECA. Most of the compounds identified in the HECA were flavonoids admittedly as potent antioxidants, such as gallic acid (compound **11**) and quercetin (compound **2**); this fact can explain the great potential pharmacological of HECA mainly for the important hypolipidemic and anti-inflammatory activity of this species.

2.3. Molecular Modelling

2.3.1. Maps of Molecular Electrostatic Potential (MEP) and Frontier Orbitals (HOMO and LUMO)

The maps of molecular electrostatic potential (MEP) show the regions featured by colors that vary depending on the potential/charges. The positive regions (blue/green) indicate the portion of the molecule with the higher probability to suffer a nucleophilic attack, while the negative regions (green/red) indicate the regions that will perform nucleophilic attacks [35]; see Figure S1 in the supplementary material.

The analyses of the *C. americana* L. constituents showed that the positive regions presented a uniformity or pattern, mainly due to the hydrogens (H) directly bonded to the oxygens atom (hydroxyls –OH). The positive electrostatic potentials maximum of the compounds varied from 0.02926 a.u (compound **12**) to 0.08821 a.u (compound **2**). The compounds **8**, **9**, **10** and **12** presented the less positive regions, evidencing that in this portion there is a higher probability of occurring nucleophilic attacks than the other molecules.

There is a pattern in the distribution of the negative regions in the molecules, being located mainly in the hydroxyls (–OH) and oxygen atoms (O) bonded to other elements is explained by the higher oxygen electronegativity. Therefore, the minimum electrostatic potential for the molecules varied from −0.09952 a.u (compound **1**) to −0.04836 a.u. (compound **12**), confirming the qualitative analysis of the regions, wherein compound **1** presented less electrostatic potential (negative region); probably this region will perform more nucleophilic attacks than compound **12**. In addition, the variation of electrostatic potentials, the **2–6** and **7–12** compounds deserve some feature in the qualitative analysis by showing close values to compounds **1** and **11** (gallic acid), respectively.

The frontier orbitals are capable of providing information about the Highest Occupied Molecular Orbital (HOMO) energies and the Lowest Unoccupied Molecular Orbital (LUMO) energies, besides acting as electron-donors and electron-acceptors, respectively [36]. Thus, the higher the HOMO energy, the higher the capacity to realize nucleophilic attacks, that is, donating electrons; it is an important electronic parameter for describing the antioxidant ability because it can be related to electron transfer reactions [37,38].

Gallic acid (compound **11**) has demonstrated significant antioxidant effects and has been used as the standard in antioxidant assays [39]. Thereby, it is important to provide quantum chemical information about this compound to improve the search of others with similar antioxidant activity. The HOMO value for gallic acid was −1.2327 eV and the LUMO energy was 0.2414 eV; both were lower than others compounds values. In the HOMO, the regions are distributed in the entire molecule, while in the LUMO, these regions are concentrates in its aromatic ring (Figure S2). The analysis of the orbital HOMO showed that the regions are located predominantly over the aromatics rings (over the double bond) and isolated over the carbon atoms of this aromatic ring. Compound **9** presented the lowest value of HOMO = −6.4722 eV while **7** showed the highest value of HOMO = −0.0435 eV followed by the compounds **2** and **12**. It is important to emphasize that compounds **2** (Quercetin) is one of the most studied and potent antioxidant flavonoids that can scavenge ROS (metal- and nonmetal-induced), probably due to its free 3–OH, which to increase the stability of the radical flavonoid [40]. Therefore, compound **9** presents the lowest probability to perform nucleophilic attacks regarding the other compounds studied. Besides, compounds **8** (HOMO = −6.0213 eV) and **10** (HOMO = −6.3092 eV) presented values close to compound **9**, which may have the same capacity, confirming the qualitative analyses in MEP.

Regarding the orbital LUMO analyses, they show the regions more susceptible to suffer nucleophilic attacks because of it character electron-acceptor, thus, the lower the energy of LUMO, the lower the resistance to accept electrons [41]. Even the LUMO does not show similarities or patterns when compared; it was possible to observe that the regions are close to the aromatic rings, over the hydrogen atoms (H) that stabilize the valence of carbons atoms (C) in these rings and mainly over the carbons that perform double bond in the aromatic rings.

The minimum values (−0.1570 eV, 0.0065 eV) and maximum (0.7959 eV) were represented by compounds **12**, **2** and **8**, respectively. Thus, between the orbitals LUMO, compounds **8** and **10** (LUMO = 0.7619 eV) have the higher resistance to suffer nucleophilic attacks or accept electrons than the other ones.

2.3.2. Multivariate Analysis PCA and HCA

After the determination of all molecular descriptors, the quantum chemical and QSAR variable values were auto-scored or standardized to give each variable an equal weight in mathematical terms to develop a multivariate analysis step. PCA was used to reduce the number of variables and select the most relevant ones, i.e., those responsible for classification of the compounds into two groups (more reactive and less reactive) based on the quantum chemical analysis of gap properties of the gallic acid, because the gap value indicates the chemical reactivity and molecular stability [42]. Good separation was obtained using five variables, see Table 1.

Table 1. Descriptors most relevant for the principal component analysis.

Compounds	HE (kcal/mol)	LogP	DMT (Debye)	GAP (eV)	1/η (eV)
1	−40.230	−5.100	2.1057	0.462	4.3285
2	−31.530	−4.010	6.6104	0.447	4.4653
3	−42.990	−5.480	5.7241	0.194	10.2795
4	−39.770	−5.100	6.6674	0.469	4.2559
5	−42.959	−5.480	5.6174	0.568	3.5167
6	−37.220	−4.690	6.3514	0.186	10.6985
7	−49.340	−5.910	4.8393	0.064	30.8818
8	0.250	8.090	1.5464	6.817	0.2934
9	−3.510	7.260	2.3235	6.643	0.3010
10	−0.640	8.030	1.5438	7.071	0.2828
11	−25.049	−2.090	3.7109	1.474	1.3568
12	−1.060	2.530	1.7570	0.185	10.7611

HE: Hydration energy; LogP: lipophilicity coefficient; DMT: Dipole moment total; 1/η: molecular softness; GAP: stability measure.

The model was constructed with the three principal components (PC1, PC2, and PC3) which describes 96.2259% of the overall variance as follows: PC1 = 74.6975%, PC2 = 15.1881% and PC3 = 6.3403%, losing just 3.7741% of the original information. PC1 contains 74.6975% of the original data, and the combination of the first two components (PC1 + PC2) contains 89.8856% of the total information. The principal components can be written as a linear combination of the selected descriptors. The mathematical expression for PC1 and PC2 are shown below:

$$PC1 = 0.4901HE + 0.5064LogP - 0.4281DMT + 0.4719GAP - 0.3121 (1/\eta), \tag{1}$$

$$PC2 = 0.0978HE + 0.1308LogP - 0.4199DMT - 0.0329GAP + 0.8922 (1/\eta), \tag{2}$$

The multivariate analysis (PCA and HCA) permitted to distinguish the compounds as the most reactive and less reactive through the stability measure, the GAP. This descriptor results from the difference between the LUMO-HOMO, compounds with low GAP values are generally reactive while molecules with high GAP values have higher molecular stability and lower reactivity [43]. A large gap implies good thermodynamic stability of the compound, whereas a small gap suggests an easy electronic transition, so we hypothesize is that the molecules with antioxidant potential are less stable and, therefore, more reactive.

The compounds with lowest GAP values varied between 1.47 eV (compound **11**—gallic acid) to 0.06 eV (compound **7**—procyanidin), see Table 1. These constituents are less stable and more reactive being grouped in the left (Figure 3). These compounds had higher contributions for the descriptors 1/η and DMT (Figure 4).

As a matter of fact, these compounds are flavones, flavonols and phenolic derivatives that through their ringed structures, conjugated double bonds and the presence of functional groups in the ring, can prevent the formation and scavenging of reactive oxygens species [40].

The phenolic compounds have been considered promising natural photoprotectors due to their potent antioxidant activity. Studies with cells and extracts of plants rich in polyphenols, including gallic acid, procyanidin and a mixture of flavonoids, demonstrated the protective action against the UV-induced damage in DNA through direct antioxidant action [44,45].

The values show that compounds **8**, **9** and **10** are the lowest reactive in the leaves of *Curatella americana*, due to the highest values of GAP (6.81 eV, 6.64 eV, and 7.07 eV, respectively), being grouped in the PCA at the right portion of the graph (Figure 3). These compounds had contributions from the descriptors LogP and HE; it is interesting to note that they had the lowest capacity to donate electrons due to their HOMO.

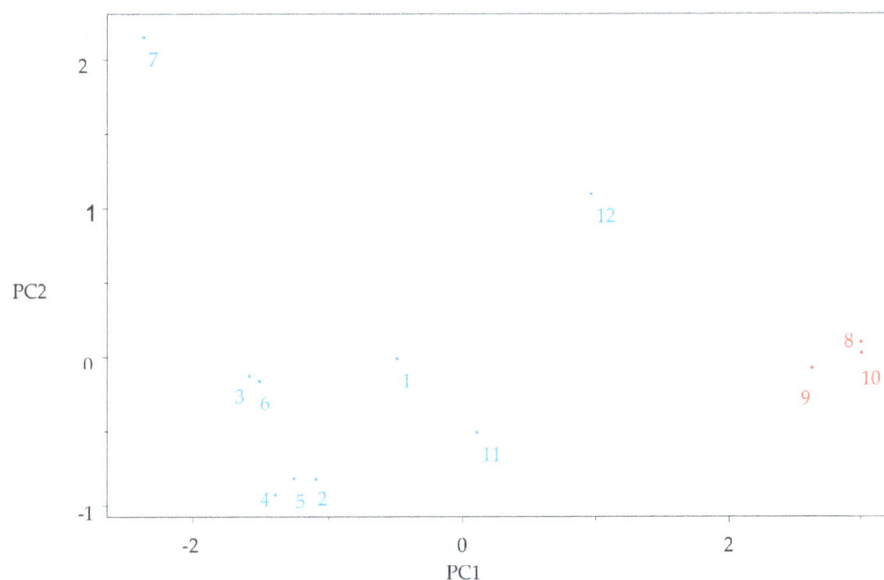

Figure 3. The plot of PC1–PC2 scores for *Curatella americana* chemical constituents. Red color indicates less reactive compounds and blue color indicate more reactive compounds.

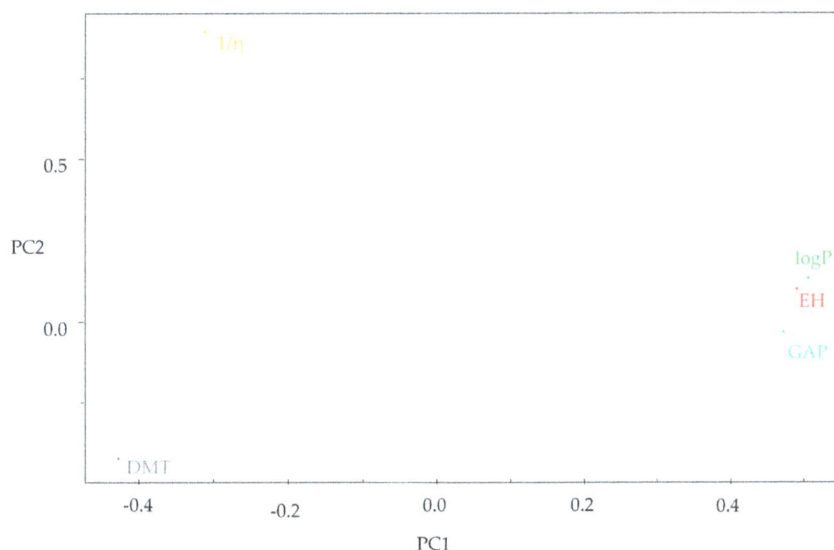

Figure 4. The plot of the PC1–PC2 loadings with the five descriptors selected.

The hydration energy (HE) is related to the drug capacity to absorb or release energy when in contact with an aqueous solvent. It is important to infer the transport and distribution for the different plasmatic biophases, as well as attraction and interaction of the drug with its receptor. Negative values indicate an exothermic reaction while positive values indicate an endothermic reaction; in other words, the more negative the values for HE, the more water soluble the molecule. The HE negatives values of the compounds vary from −49.340 kcal/mol (compound **7**) to −0.640 kcal/mol (compound **10**), thus, the procyanidin (compound **7**), showed the best solubility. Besides, this compound showed a higher softness ($1/\eta$) value (30.8818 eV) and this descriptor was important for the grouping in the PCA. The molecular softness represents the facility a molecule to deform [40]. Therefore, the higher the softness, the lower the energy necessary for the transition electron from HOMO to LUMO probably generating more stable radicals after the donation of electrons in function of the possibility of the unpaired electrons be able to transit to the LUMO region with less energy.

Procyanidin has been considered an important antioxidant, presenting important effects in protecting human neutrophil and erythrocytes hemolysis caused by ROS [46,47]. In a double-blinded with two treatments, placebo and a control treatment study, the consumption of capsules rich in this compound for four weeks reduced bloody ambulatory pressure probably due to its antioxidant effects [48].

The lipophilicity coefficient (LogP) is a property that quantitatively measures the lipophilia of the compounds, one of the most important molecular properties for drug absorption [49]. It is possible to observe that there is a relation between HE and LogP, because of negative values of HE being related to the compounds' hydrophilicity, while the positive values are related to lipophilicity and this characteristic is exposed by the LogP, i.e., when higher is the HE values, higher will be the LogP value.

Therefore, the terpenoid compounds **8** (β-Amyrin) showed higher values for HE (0.250 kcal/mol) and consequently higher values for LogP (8.090) and hence, it is the most lipophilic molecule. The other two terpenoids, compounds **9**, **10** and compound **12** (foeniculum), although presenting negative values for HE, close to zero, showed positives values for LogP, having important lipophilicity too, see Table 1. These characteristics of the terpenoids added to the low HOMO values, small softness and the high GAP value, showing less reactivity and consequently higher stability, suggest that this class does not show important antioxidant activity by scavenging ROS, although studies performed with plants rich in these compounds have demonstrated a potent antioxidant activity [16], maybe the other compounds in the studied extracts contribute to this activity.

In the HCA technique, the distances between a pair of samples are computed and compared. Small distances imply that the compounds are similar, while non-similar samples will be separated by relatively large distances. The scale of similarity ranges from 0 for samples with no similarity to 1 for samples with great similarity. The dendrogram in Figure 5 shows that the HCA results confirmed the PCA analysis.

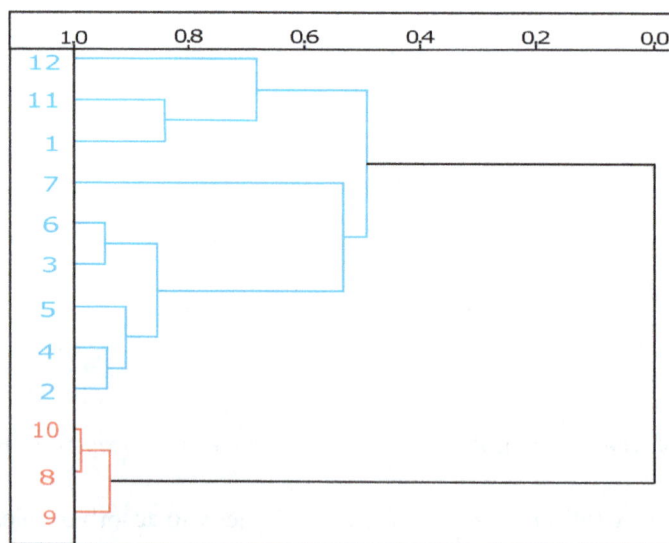

Figure 5. HCA dendrogram for *Curatella americana* constituents showing them separated into two main classes (red color indicates less reactive and blue color indicate more reactive compounds).

2.3.3. Theoretical Mechanism to Antioxidant Activity via Electron Abstraction

Antioxidant activity is highly related to the electron donation capacity. The hydrogen transfer step has been highlighted, but the antioxidant activity does not only depend on the energy strength of the O–H bond. The stabilization of the cation-radical and radical species formed should also be considered [50–52]. Therefore, we evaluated via ionization potential value (IP) and spin density compounds **7** (procyanidin), **11** (gallic acid) and **12** (foeniculin). Glycosylated flavonoids were disregarded because they had lower antioxidant activity than their free aglycones [53,54] and terpenoids because they had lower HOMO values and in the PCA analysis were grouped separately from the known antioxidant compounds. Procyanidin and foeniculin presented high HOMO values besides low Gap values, showing low molecular stability and high chemical reactivity.

The ionization potential (IP) represents the facility of an electron donation, and abstraction of electron; the molecules with the lowest IP values are more active. The ionization energies for a radical can be also used as a measure of stability of the corresponding cation, when the ionization energy is lower, the radical should be more stable [55,56]. The calculated values for the selected molecules are shown in Table 2.

Table 2. Theoretical Properties obtained for the compounds studied.

Molecules	HOMO (eV)	E_{Neutro} (Kcal/mol)	E_{Cation} (Kcal/mol)	IP (Kcal/mol)
7	−0.0435	−1340,833.36	−1340,680.69	152.67
11	−1.2327	−405,680.81	−405,505.18	175.62
12	−0.3429	−388,768.73	−388,611.82	156.90

$E_{Neutron}$: neutro energy; E_{Cation}: Cation energy.

According to the calculated IP values, molecule **7** (procyanidin) shows higher antioxidant activity than molecules **12** (foeniculin) and **11** (gallic acid), confirming the qualitative analyses of the multivariate analyses (PCA and HCA). Besides that, its radical is probably more stable.

An efficient antioxidant is one that donates the electron with ease and then in this process becomes more stable. The stabilization studied here is in function of the resonance process, after the donation, the molecule rearranges the electrons so that they do not to remain in the reactive radical form. The density spin shows the contribution of the atoms in the stabilization of the molecule, since we will have unpaired electrons. The resonance structures of cation free-radicals by electron abstraction can be observed by spin density distributions for the compounds selected, see Figure 6.

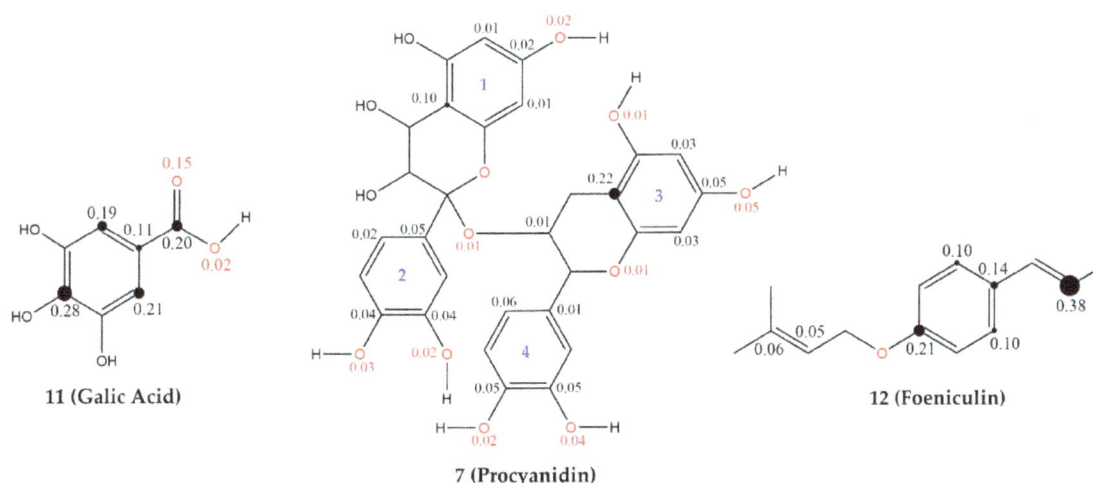

Figure 6. Spin densities in the cation free-radical of selected compounds.

Gallic acid (**11**) presented higher spin distribution, ranging from 0.02 to 0.28 in the structure with global contribution in the benzene ring of 0.79, despite the presence of hydroxyls bound in the aromatic ring, they do not participate in the stabilization, only acetyl bound to the aromatic ring. However, gallic acid has the highest IP value (175.62 Kcal/mol) among the studied compounds.

Procyanidin had the lowest IP value (152.67 Kcal/mol) and, therefore, it was the molecule with greater ease for electron donation. Its radical cation presented a more uniform distribution of spin in the structure, with global contribution of the rings 1, 2, 3 and 4 from 0.14, 0.15, 0.33 and 0.17, respectively. Despite the low contribution of ring 2, it is possible to observe the stabilization and greater probability of electron output in this ring by HOMO (supplementary material Figure S2). It is important to note that the cation radical formed from this molecule presents lower energy indicating greater stability, it is possible that the more uniform distribution of the electrons in the molecule after the exit of one electron contributes to radical stability, this behavior can be related to the high softness of this molecule that could allow better electronic transition.

In relation to the structure of Foeniculin (**12**), there was a greater contribution of propenyl among the analyzed structures (value of 0.38). The resonance occurs with the hyperconjugation of the carbon of the radical, thus sacrificing an electron for the donation, after the presence the aromatic ring leaves the molecule stable due to resonance.

2.3.4. Molecular Docking Study

To evaluate the action mechanism of potential antioxidants in preventing ROS formation, we performed a molecular docking study of the compounds with the xanthine oxidase enzyme. According to the studies of Cao et al. [2], hypoxanthine is first hydroxylated by XO at C-2 to form xanthine and then converted it to uric acid, in a reductive half-reaction in which the substrate is oxidatively hydroxylated at the molybdenum (Mo) center, hence, also generating ROS. The inhibition of xanthine oxidase would be a strategy to treat and prevent diseases that result in the accumulation of uric acid and consequently the ROS [57,58].

Although the most known inhibitor drug of XO has been allopurinol, we chose using febuxostat as the reference, because the allopurinol behaves as an analog of hypoxanthine, which is self-oxidation to form oxypurinol (the active inhibitory metabolite) resulting in the reduction of O_2-, so remaining the production of ROS [58]. Instead, febuxostat is reported to be significantly more potent, probably because it fills the pocket of XO obstructing substrate binding. Thus, febuxostat should not be affected by enzyme redox state and interaction with XO and does not induce ROS formation [59].

The structure derived from X-ray of hypoxanthine complex with xanthine oxidase PDB codes 3 NRZ (*Bos taurus*) was selected for molecular docking studies of the HECA chemical constituents due to good parameters for experimental resolution (1.8 Å). The control ligands used in the molecular docking study were Hypoxanthine (HPX) and Febuxostat (FBX), Figure 7, downloaded at PDB server in sdf format ensuring the bioactive conformation. For validation of the docking method, the hypoxanthine structure with crystallographic information was submitted to docking until the best-docked ligand conformation that had a root mean square deviation (RMSD) of 1.64 Å. According to Hevener et al. [60], Santos et al. [61] and Cruz et al. [62] the binding prediction mode using the docking, affirm that when the RMSD is less than 2.0 Å on the crystallographic pose of the ligand can be considered satisfactory. Therefore, our results with the methodological proposal using these parameters are optimal and satisfactory.

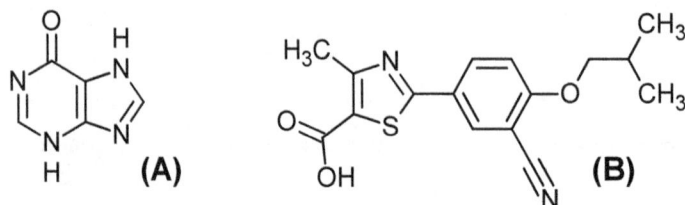

Figure 7. Control Ligands 2D structure: (**A**) hypoxanthine (HPX) and (**B**) Febuxostat (FBX).

The molecular docking method identified a conformation that allows the ligand also to interact with the active sites for hypoxanthine (PDB 3 NRZ) that around the α-helix between the amino acids residues 878–882, 1012–1014 and for β-sheet between the amino acids residues 801–805, 912–915, 1007–1011, 1076–1079. For the ligand, it is possible to see common hydrogen bonds with residues Arg880 and Glu802. There is also a hydrophobic interaction with residues Phe914, Phe1009, Ala1078 and Ala1079 as observed by Cao et al. [2].

The evaluation of affinity showed that foeniculin (compound 12) has a higher binding affinity (−6.9 Kcal/mol) in relation to the studied compounds and that it had a variation ±0.7 Kcal/mol in comparison to the HPX, and the other structure with better affinity, gallic acid (compound 11), had a variation of ±0.4 Kcal/mol, see Figure 8.

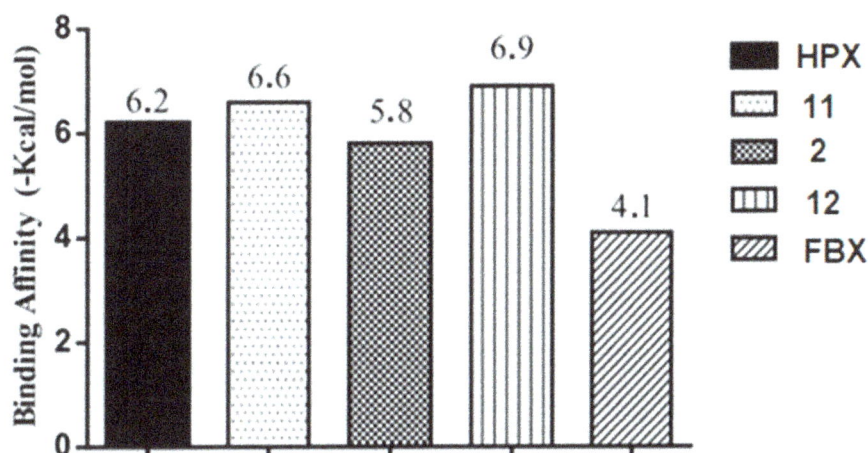

Figure 8. Binding affinity provided by AutoDock/Vina software of the compounds **11** (Gallic acid), **2** (Quercetin) and **12** (Foeniculin) and control ligand febuxostat (FBX). Ligand complexed hypoxanthine (HPX) for XO (organism *Bos taurus*).

However, gallic acid interacts with Glu1261 in the active site which is responsible for the deprotonation of the prosthetic group Mo-OH in the enzyme; this residue is universally conserved in the families of the enzymes containing molybdenum. After deprotonation, the nucleophilic attack occurs on the substrate promoting the oxidation reaction, generating ROS. In this way, gallic acid could behave as a competitive inhibitor of XO. Although foeniculin has high affinity, the presence of the highly reactive chemical group (the isoprene) and delocalization of π-type electrons (resonance), which would be rapidly oxidized by the enzyme generating ROS. The low gap (0.185 eV) of this molecule and the lowest positive electrostatic potentials, confirms its high chemical reactivity and it smaller capacity to suffer a nucleophilic attack.

We can also observe higher interaction numbers of febuxostat, which is a potent inhibitor of the enzyme xanthine oxidase. We found similar interactions with those published by Okamoto et al. [59], except for the interaction with the Ser876, Ala1078, and Ala1079. The interaction Ala1079 was found in all compounds selected, but the Ser876 only was found in the febuxostat and quercetin (compound **2**). Figure 9 shows the interactions for the docked structures that had the best affinities. Amino acids residues, quantitative data of distances and binding free energies (ΔG) between the compounds and XO receptor are shown in Table 3.

By analyzing the interaction sites for quercetin (compound **2**, see Figure 9) and comparing with the interaction sites of the febuxostat, we observed that the results were similar with the active sites (XO) having amino acid residues which are around the α-helix in the Ser876, Leu1014; and for β-sheet in the amino acids residues Leu873, Phe914, Val1011 and Ala1079, that with exception of Thr1010 presented just with the quercetin (compound **2**) agree with the literature [2]. In fact, the quercetin has been demonstrated to be an important inhibitor of XO in vitro, probably behaving as the febuxostat preventing the access of the substrate in the active site of the enzyme [63,64].

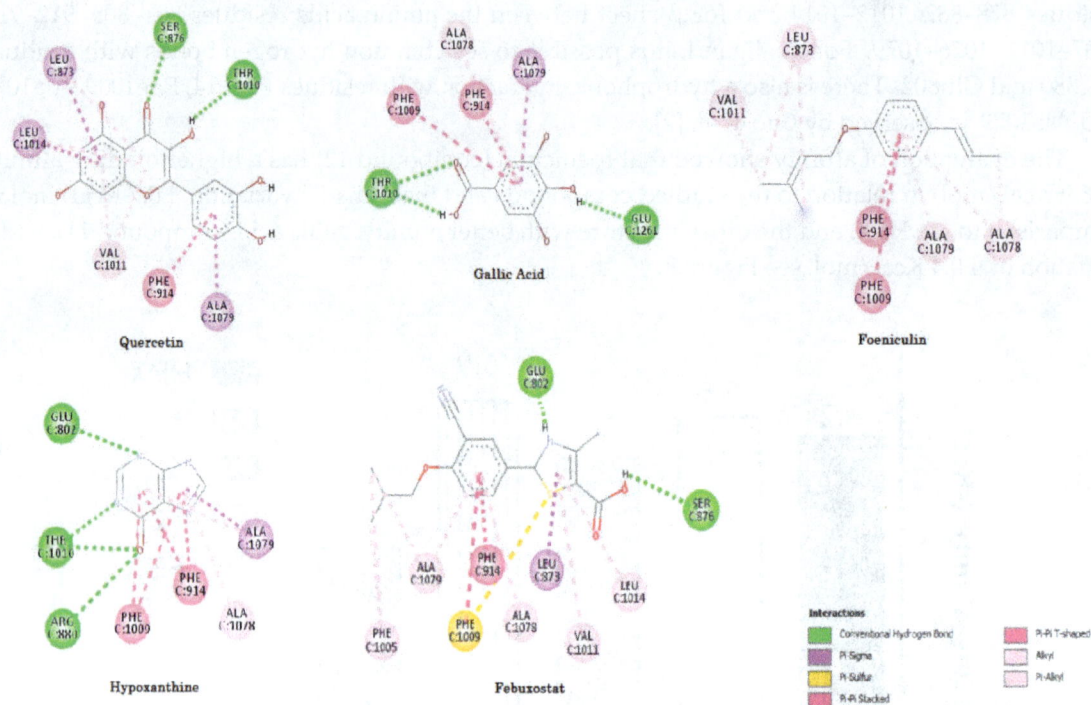

Figure 9. Interactions of the compounds with XO enzyme. Nominal interactions, aminoacids, and distances can be seen in Table 3.

Table 3. Interactions between ligands with therapeutic target XO (organism *Boss taurus*).

	Amino Acid	Distance (Å)	Type	Binding Free Energy (kcal/mol)
	Leu873	3.5408	Pi-Sigma	
		4.8720	Pi-Alkyl	
	Ser876	2.3000	Conventional Hydrogen Bond	
	Phe914	3.7825	Pi-Pi Stacked	
2 vs. XO	Thr1010	2.0916	Conventional Hydrogen Bond	−6.76
	Val1011	5.2238	Pi-Alkyl	
		5.4506	Pi-Alkyl	
	Leu1014	5.0207	Pi-Alkyl	
		2.8423	Pi-Sigma	
	Phe914	3.6159	Pi-Pi Stacked	
	Phe1009	5.4325	Pi-Pi T-shaped	
	Thr1010	2.0504	Conventional Hydrogen Bond	
		2.8382	Conventional Hydrogen Bond	
11 vs. XO	Ala1078	4.9487	Pi-Alkyl	−4.4
	Ala1079	3.6445	Pi-Sigma	
	Glu1261	1.9196	Conventional Hydrogen Bond	
	Leu873	4.4308	Alkyl	
		4.9122	Alkyl	
	Phe914	3.5349	Pi-Pi Stacked	
	Phe1009	4.8397	Pi-Pi Stacked	
	Val1011	4.4798	Alkyl	
12 vs. XO	Ala1078	4.9457	Pi-Alkyl	−7.13
		4.1350	Alkyl	
	Ala1079	4.1423	Pi-Alkyl	
	Glu802	3.2579	Conventional Hydrogen Bond	
	Arg880	3.0805	Conventional Hydrogen Bond	
	Phe914	3.4234	Pi-Pi Stacked	
		3.8092	Pi-Pi Stacked	
	Phe1009	4.7907	Pi-Pi T-shaped	
HPX vs. XO		5.2023	Pi-Pi T-shaped	−5.65
	Thr1010	3.1183	Conventional Hydrogen Bond	
		2.8251	Conventional Hydrogen Bond	
	Ala1078	4.6549	Pi-Alkyl	
	Ala1079	3.9407	Pi-Sigma	
		4.8965	Pi-Alkyl	

Table 3. *Cont.*

	Amino Acid	Distance (Å)	Type	Binding Free Energy (kcal/mol)
	Glu802	1.9544	Conventional Hydrogen Bond	
	Leu873	3.7514	Pi-Sigma	
	Ser876	2.8449	Conventional Hydrogen Bond	
	Phe914	3.8848	Pi-Pi Stacked	
	Phe1005	3.8139	Pi-Alkyl	
		4.6647	Pi-Alkyl	
FBX vs. XO	Phe1009	4.4818	Pi-Pi T-shaped	−6.1
		5.5513	Pi-Sulfur	
	Val1011	4.8667	Pi-Alkyl	
	Leu1014	4.2479	Pi-Alkyl	
	Ala1078	4.4684	Pi-Alkyl	
	Ala1079	4.7224	Pi-Alkyl	
		3.7013	Alkyl	

It is possible to verify that, among the standard and control compounds (ligands HPX and FBX), the increase in the number of interactions would result in the lowering of binding free energy, which indicates a higher degree of the spontaneity of the interactions [65]. On the other hand, we observed that the FBX interacted with Leu873, Ser876, Val1011 and Leu1014 as the quercetin (compound **2**) which had the binding free energy lower than FBX while the foeniculin (compound **12**) that had a lowest binding free energy ($\Delta G = -7.13$ kcal/mol), showed only Leu873 and Val1011 residues in common with FBX and quercetin, suggesting that these residues are the most important than the amount of interactions. It is important to emphasize that these four residues are in the solvent-accessible channel leading to the molybdenum center, explaining the potential inhibitor of quercetin [66].

It is interesting to note that the compounds do not have significant structural similarity; however, the compounds studied had binding free energy values approximate to each other, due to the similarity of the interactions with the amino acids residues.

3. Materials and Methods

3.1. Plant Material

Curatella americana leaves were collected from Macapa in Amapa State, Brazil, in the month of february 2015. A sampling location ($00°9'75.251'$ S, $51'8'57.6733''$ W) was marked by a global position measuring (GPS Garmin nüvi 40). The scientific identification of the vegetable material was held in the Herbarium of the Federal University of Amapá under the registration number 010266 for future reference.

Preparation of Plant Extract

Dry and pulverized leaves were extracted with 70% ethanol, in the proportion of 1:3 (*w/v*). The crude extract was filtered in vacuum using Whattman® filter. The hydroalcoholic extract was evaporated under vacuum rotatory evaporator (IKA® RV 05 basic), lyophilized and kept at −20 °C in a freezer until further use.

3.2. DPPH Scavenging Assay

The 1,1-diphenyl-2-picrylhydrazine (DPPH) is a stable free radical that react with compounds that can donate a hydrogen atom that decolorizes the DPPH solution. Therefore, it can be utilized for the evaluation of the free scavenging activity. The assay was performed according to the methodology previously published [67–69].

Briefly, the reaction mixture solution consisted of 2.7 mL of DPPH solutions (40 µg/mL) in methanol and 300 µL of HECA (10^3 to 7.0 µg/mL) that was mixed thoroughly and incubating in darkness. After 30 min, the decline of radical concentration was measured by spectrophotometry visible at 517 nm using Biospectro SP-22. The experiment was performed in triplicate, and the mean absorption was analyzed for each concentration. Methanol was taken as the control, and the gallic acid

(Sigma-Aldrich®, Missouri EUA, MO, USA) in the same concentrations of the extract was taken as the reference standard compound. The percentage of antioxidant activity was calculated according to Cefali et al. [67].

$$\text{Scavenging percentage (\%)} = 1 - (Abs_{(treatment)}/Abs_{(control)}) \times 100 \qquad (3)$$

where $Abs_{(control)}$ and $Abs_{(treatment)}$ is the absorbance of the control and the treatment respectively. To establish the half-maximal inhibitory concentration (IC_{50}) of DPPH free scavenging, the samples were tested in serial dilutions (7, 15, 25, 50, 75, 100, 125, 250, 500 and 1000 µg/mL) and analyzed by linear regression models with exponential specification, the results were evaluated by one way of variance (ANOVA) followed by Tuckey test at $p < 0.05$.

3.3. Molecular Modeling

3.3.1. Maps of Molecular Electrostatic Potential (MEP) and Frontier Orbital's (HOMO and LUMO)

Molecular modeling started with the construction of the 12 identified compounds using GaussView 3.0 [70], and all computational calculations were performed using the Gaussian 09 program [71]. The 12 compounds identified in the leaves of C. americana were optimized in the density functional theory method (DFT) in theory level B3LYP/6-31G** and the frequencies were also calculated in the same method, there were no negative frequencies, thereby ensuring the minimum energy structure. After, the MEP's generated from the atomic charge. The constructions of the MEPs and the frontier orbitals (HOMO and LUMO) were visualized with the aid of Molekel program [72].

The atomic charges used in this study were obtained with the keyword POP = CHELPG using the electrostatic potential [73]. With this strategy, it was possible to obtain the best potential quantum molecular series of points defined around the molecule, and atomic charges offer the general advantage of being physically more satisfactory than Mulliken charges [74]. The descriptors represent different sources of chemical information (features) regarding molecules that are important for the quantitative description of the molecular structure and to finding appropriate predictive models [75].

3.3.2. Multivariate Analysis PCA and HCA

The analysis of inters sample and intervariable relationships were performed via Principal Component Analysis (PCA) and Hierarchical Cluster Analysis (HCA). PCA was used to reduce the number of variables and select the most relevant properties to the classification of the compounds into two groups (more stable and less stable) based in the quantum chemical analysis of the gap properties of the gallic acid compound, because the gap value indicates chemical reactivity and molecular stability [76].

After that, the structures were determined in three dimensions (3D), twelve quantum chemical and seven QSAR descriptors were selected to construct a data matrix. The QSAR descriptors included, i.e., total surface area (TSA), molecular volume (MV), molar refractivity (MR), molar polarizability (MP), coefficient of lipophilicity (LogP), molecular mass (MM) and hydration energy (HE) according to the HyperChem 6.02 [77]. The molecular descriptors were selected to provide valuable information about the influence of electronic, steric, hydrophilic and hydrophobic features, according to studies realized by Santos et al. [42].

The quantum chemical descriptors were: energy (TE), energy of the highest occupied molecular orbital (HOMO), a level below the energy of the highest occupied molecular orbital (HOMO-1), two level below the energy of the highest occupied molecular orbital (HOMO-2), lowest unoccupied molecular orbital energy (LUMO), a level above the energy of the lowest unoccupied molecular orbital (LUMO + 1), two level above the energy of the lowest unoccupied molecular orbital (LUMO + 2), difference in energy between HOMO and LUMO (GAP = HOMO − LUMO), Mulliken electronegativity (χ), molecular hardness (η), molecular softness ($1/\eta$) and Dipolo moment total (DMT).

The descriptors selected by PCA were used to perform the HCA, which was used in processing in an autoscale with the Euclidean distance metric and Incremental Linkage method. The objective of HCA was to show the compounds distributed in groups more and less stables for confirming of the PCA results. The multivariate data analysis was performed by employing the Pirouette 3.01 [78].

3.3.3. Theoretical Mechanism to the Antioxidant Activity

In this work, the geometry optimization of the flavonoid derivatives has been carried out using density functional theory (DFT). The calculations were performed with the Gaussian 09 molecular package [71] and prior to any DFT calculations; all structures were submitted to PM3 [79] geometry conformational search. After the PM3 initial optimizations, the structures were reoptimized using the B3LYP/6-31G** level of theory [80]. We calculated for compounds **7** (procyanidin), **11** (galic acid) and **12** (foeniculin), the following properties: (i) ionization potential (IP) and (ii) spin density, as described by Mendes et al. [53] and Borges et al. [81]. The IP was calculated as the energy difference between a neutral molecule and the respective cation free radical as showed below:

$$IP = EX^{\bullet+} - EX \tag{4}$$

3.3.4. Molecular Docking Study

Molecular docking simulation between xanthine oxidase enzyme, chemical constituents from *C. americana*, and control ligands were undertaken via AutoDock 4.2/Vina 1.1.2 by PyRx 0.8 software with default parameters by the genetic algorithm, following the protocol described by Pereira et al. and Padilha et al. [82,83]. The population size was 100, selection-pressure 1.1, the number of operations was 10,000, the number of islands was 1, the niche size was 2, operator weights for migrating was 0, mutate was 100, and crossover was 100. The coordinates $X = 44.0000$, $Y = 34.0000$ and $Z = 24.000$ (grid box) from the pocket of interest was chosen based on interactions between the amino acids and a 10 Å radius sphere were defined. Ten solutions were calculated for each chemical constituent, and minimum binding energy conformations were analyzed to evaluate the best binding free energy (ΔG), binding affinity and the selectivity of the chemical constituents in therapeutic targets.

4. Conclusions

In the present study, the DPPH assay was used to evaluate the antioxidant activity of *Curatella americana* L., then the study of quantum chemicals was performed to obtain a relation between electronic properties and antioxidant capacity of the chemical constituents. It was possible to characterize the compounds as well as their characteristics of electro donor/electro accepter compared to the gallic acid standard. Multivariate analysis (PCA and HCA) allowed us to identify chemical descriptors that may be related to the antioxidant activity by grouping the most reactive compounds with gallic acid. The Gap and softness descriptors were shown to be important in the grouping of known antioxidant compounds such as procyanidin and quercetin and its derivatives, demonstrating that less stable molecules, that is, lower Gap values, are more antioxidant because they are more reactive. In addition, these compounds presented higher softness, especially procyanidin, indicating ease for the transition electron, confirmed by the calculations of IP and spin density. Therefore, descriptors such as Gap and softness allied to the electronic characteristics of the molecule can be used as criteria for the selection of potentially antioxidant compounds quickly and efficiently even for those compounds with recognized antioxidant activity via hydrogen abstraction as the phenolics.

The evaluation of the species regarding the possibility of prevention of the formation of ROS investigated by molecular docking simulations with XO confirmed the data from the literature showing the potential inhibitory activity of XO by the quercetin. However, we did not relate quantum chemical characteristics to this inhibitory potential.

The presence of important antioxidant compounds in the *C. americana* L. species can explain the pharmacological actions described in scientific research and in folk medicine. Therefore, it would be imperative to investigate the potential of this species and the main compounds as a natural antioxidant for the use in the pharmaceutical industry.

Author Contributions: M.A.T.F. performed the in vitro experiment, PCA and HCA analysis, aided in the molecular docking study and wrote the paper; N.d.S.R.d.S. and K.L.B.d.S. designed the structures and developed the MEP and Frontier Orbital's; E.F.B.F. helped in the methodology of DPPH; R.d.S.R. developed the molecular docking; C.H.T.d.P.d.S. developed the quantum chemical calculations; J.M.C.R.: revised the paper; J.O.d.S. conceived the in vitro experiment; C.B.R.S. conceived and designed the experiments and revised the paper.

Funding: This research received no external funding.

Acknowledgments: Wegliane Campelo da Silva Aparício, a taxonomist at the Department of Biology, Federal University of Amapá, Macapa, AP, Brazil for specimen plant identification.

References

1. Roy, J.; Galano, J.; Durand, T.; Guennec, J.; Lee, J.C.Y. Physiological role of reactive oxygen species as promoters of natural defenses. *FASEB J.* **2017**, *31*, 3729–3745. [CrossRef] [PubMed]

2. Cao, H.; Pauff, J.M.; Hille, R. Substrate orientation and catalytic specificity in the action of xanthine oxidase the sequential hydroxylation of hypoxanthine to uric acid. *J. Biol. Chem.* **2010**, *285*. [CrossRef] [PubMed]

3. Fernandez, M.L.; Upton, Z.; Shooter, G.K. Uric acid and xanthine oxidoreductase in wound healing. *Curr. Rheumatol. Rep.* **2014**, *16*, 396–403. [CrossRef] [PubMed]

4. Landmesser, U.; Spiekermann, S.; Dikalov, S.; Tatge, H.; Wilke, R.; Kohler, C.; Harrison, D.G.; Drexler, H. Vascular oxidative stress and endothelial dysfunction in patients with chronic heart failure role of xanthine-oxidase and extracellular superoxide dismutase. *Circulation* **2002**, *106*, 3073–3078. [CrossRef] [PubMed]

5. Phan, T.T.; Wang, L.; See, P.; Grayer, R.J.; Chan, S.Y.; Lee, S.T. Phenolic compounds of chromolaena odorata protect cultured skin cells from oxidative damage: Implication for cutaneous wound healing. *Biol. Pharm. Bull.* **2001**, *24*, 1373–1379. [CrossRef] [PubMed]

6. Thang, P.T.; Teik, L.S.; Yung, C.S. Anti-oxidant effects of the extracts from the leaves of Chromolaena odorata on human dermal fibroblasts and epidermal keratinocytes against hydrogen peroxide and hypoxanthine–xanthine oxidase induced damage. *Burns* **2001**, *27*, 319–327. [CrossRef]

7. Wilson, A.J.; Gill, E.K.; Abudalo, R.A.; Edgar, K.S.; Watson, C.J.; Grieve, D.J. Reactive oxygen species signalling in the diabetic heart: Emerging prospect for therapeutic targeting. *Heart* **2018**, *104*, 293–299. [CrossRef] [PubMed]

8. Działo, M.; Mierziak, J.; Korzun, U.; Preisner, M.; Szopa, J.; Kulma, A. The potential of plant phenolics in prevention and therapy of skin disorders. *Int. J. Mol. Sci.* **2016**, *17*, 160. [CrossRef] [PubMed]

9. Rahman, K. Studies on free radicals, antioxidants, and co-factors. *Clin. Interv. Aging* **2007**, *2*, 219–236. [PubMed]

10. Reinisalo, M.; Kårlund, A.; Koskela, A.; Kaarniranta, K.; Karjalainen, R.O. Polyphenol stilbenes: Molecular mechanisms of defence against oxidative stress and aging-related diseases. *Oxid Med. Cell. Longev.* **2015**, *2015*, 340–520. [CrossRef] [PubMed]

11. Ganesan, K.; Xu, B. A critical review on polyphenols and health benefits of black soybeans. *Nutrients* **2017**, *9*, 455. [CrossRef] [PubMed]

12. Gulcin, I. Antioxidant activity of food constituents: An overview. *Arch. Toxicol.* **2012**, *86*, 345–391. [CrossRef] [PubMed]

13. Liu, K.; Zhou, R.; Wang, B.; Mi, M.T. Effect of resveratrol on glucose control and insulin sensitivity: A meta-analysis of 11 randomized controlled trials1–3. *Am. J. Clin. Nutr.* **2014**, *99*, 1510–1519. [CrossRef] [PubMed]

14. Jayathilake, C.; Rizliya, V.; Liyanage, R. Antioxidant and free radical scavenging capacity of extensively used medicinal plants in Sri Lanka. *Procedia Food Sci.* **2016**, *6*, 123–126. [CrossRef]

15. Elisha, I.L.; Dzoyem, J.P.; McGaw, L.J.; Botha, F.S.; Eloff, J.N. The anti-arthritic, anti-inflammatory, antioxidant activity and relationships with total phenolics and total flavonoids of nine South African plants used traditionally to treat arthritis. *BMC Complement. Altern. Med.* **2016**, *16*, 307–317. [CrossRef] [PubMed]

16. Krishnaiah, D.; Sarbatly, R.; Nithyanandam, R. A review of the antioxidant potential of medicinal plant species. *FBP* **2011**, *89*, 217–233. [CrossRef]

17. Lima, C.C.; Lemos, R.P.L.; Conserva, L.M. Dilleniaceae family: An overview of its ethnomedicinal uses, biological and phytochemical profile. *J. Pharmacogn. Phytochem.* **2014**, *3*, 181–204.

18. Ratter, J.A.; Bridgewater, S.; Ribeiro, J.F. Analysis of the floristic composition of the Brazilian cerrado vegetation III: Comparison of the woody vegetation of 376 areas. *Edinb. J. Bot.* **2003**, *60*, 57–109. [CrossRef]

19. Villarroel, D.; Catari, J.C.; Calderon, D.; Mendez, R.; Feldpausch, T. Structure, composition and tree diversity of two areas in the Cerrado sensu stricto in the Chiquitanía (Santa Cruz, Bolivia). *Ecol. Boliv.* **2010**, *45*, 116–130.

20. Amaral, D.D.; Costa-Neto, S.V.; Jardim, M.A.G.; Santos, J.U.M.; Bastos, M.D.N.C. *Curatella americana* L. (Dilleniaceae): Primeira ocorrência nas restingas do litoral da Amazônia. *Rev. Bras. Biocienc.* **2016**, *14*, 257–262.

21. Barbosa, R.I.; Nascimento, S.P.; Amorim, P.A.F.; Silva, R.F. Notas sobre a composição arbóreo-arbustiva de uma fisionomia das savanas de Roraima, Amazônia Brasileira. *Acta Bot. Bras.* **2005**, 19. [CrossRef]

22. De Medeiros, P.M.; Ladio, H.A.; Albuquerque, P.U. Patterns of medicinal plant use by inhabitants ofBrazilian urban and ruralareas:A macroscale investigation based on available literature. *J. Ethnopharmacol.* **2012**, *150*, 729–746. [CrossRef] [PubMed]

23. Vila Verde, G.M.; Paula, J.R.; Caneiro, D.M. Levantamento etnobotânico das plantas medicinais do cerrado utilizadas pela população de Mossâmedes (GO). *Rev. Bras. Farmacogn.* **2003**, *13*, 64–66. [CrossRef]

24. Souza, C.D.; Felfili, J.M. Uso de plantas medicinais na região de Alto Paraíso de Goiás, GO, Brasil. *Acta Bot. Bras.* **2006**, *20*, 135–142. [CrossRef]

25. Alexandre-Moreira, M.; Piuvezam, M.; Araújo, C.; Thomas, G. Studies on the anti-inflammatory and analgesic activity of *Curatella americana* L. *J. Ethnopharmacol.* **1999**, *67*, 171–177. [CrossRef]

26. Toledo, C.E.; Britta, E.A.; Ceole, L.F.; Silva, E.R.; de Mello, J.C.; Dias Filho, B.P.; Nakamura, C.V.; Ueda-Nakamura, T. Antimicrobial and cytotoxic activities of medicinal plants of the Brazilian cerrado, using Brazilian cachaca as extractor liquid. *J. Ethnopharmacol.* **2011**, *133*, 420–425. [CrossRef] [PubMed]

27. Guerrero, M.F.; Puebla, P.; Carron, R.; Martin, M.L.; Arteaga, L.; Roman, L.S. Assessment of the antihypertensive and vasodilator effects of ethanolic extracts of some Colombian medicinal plants. *J. Ethnopharmacol.* **2002**, *80*, 37–42. [CrossRef]

28. Hiruma-Lima, C.A.; Rodrigues, C.M.; Kushima, H.; Moraes, T.M.; Lolis, S.F.; Feitosa, S.B.; Magri, L.P.; Vilegas, W. The anti-ulcerogenic effects of *Curatella americana* L. *J. Ethnopharmacol.* **2009**, *121*, 425–432. [CrossRef] [PubMed]

29. Lopes, R.H.O.; Macorini, L.F.B.; Antunes, K.A.; de Toledo Espindola, P.P.; Alfredo, T.M.; da Rocha, P.d.S.; Pereira, Z.F.; dos Santos, E.L.; de Picoli Souza, K. Antioxidant and hypolipidemic activity of the hydroethanolic extract of *Curatella americana* L. leaves. *Oxid Med. Cell. Longev.* **2016**, *2016*, 6. [CrossRef] [PubMed]

30. Cunha, E.L.; Santos, C.F.; Braga, F.S.; Costa, J.S.; Silva, R.C.; Favacho, H.A.S.; Hage-Melim, L.I.S.; Carvalho, J.C.T.; da Silva, C.H.T.P.; Santos, C.B.R. Computational investigation of antifungal compounds using molecular modeling and prediction of ADME/Tox properties. *J. Comput. Theor. Nanosci.* **2015**, *12*, 3682–3691. [CrossRef]

31. El-Azizi, M.M.; Ateya, A.M.; Svoboda, G.H.; Schiff, P.L.; Slatkin, D.J., Jr.; Knapp, J.E. Chemical constituents of *Curatella americana* (Dilleniaceae). *J. Pharm. Sci.* **1980**, *69*, 360–361. [CrossRef] [PubMed]

32. Gurni, A.A.; Kubitzki, K. Flavonoid chemistry and systematics of the dilleniaceae. *Biochem. Syst. Ecol.* **1981**, *9*, 109–114. [CrossRef]

33. Khlebnikov, A.I.; Schepetkin, I.A.; Domina, N.G.; Kirpotinab, L.N.; Quin, M.T. Improved quantitative structure-activity relationship models to predict antioxidant activity of flavonoids in chemical, enzymatic, and cellular systems. *Bioorg. Med. Chem.* **2007**, *15*, 1749–1770. [CrossRef] [PubMed]

34. Williams, R.J.; Spencer, J.P.E.; Rice-Evans, C. Flavonoids: Antioxidants or signalling molecules? *Free Radic. Biol. Med.* **2004**, *36*, 838–849. [CrossRef] [PubMed]

35. Silva, N.S.R.; Santos, C.F.; Gonçalves, L.K.S.; Braga, F.S.; Almeida, J.R.; Lima, C.S.; Brasil, D.S.B.; Silva, C.H.T.P.; Hage-Melim, L.I.S.; Santos, C.B.R. Molecular modeling of the major compounds of sesquiterpenes class in copaiba oil-resin. *Br. J. Pharm. Res.* **2015**, *7*, 247–263. [CrossRef]

36. Santos, C.B.R.; Lobato, C.C.; Sousa, M.A.C.; Macêdo, W.J.C.; Carvalho, J.C.T. Molecular modeling: Origin, fundamental concepts and applications using structure-activity relationship and quantitative structure-activity relationship. *RITS* **2014**, *2*, 91–115. [CrossRef]

37. Contreras, R.; Domingo, L.R.; Andrés, J.; Pérez, P.; Tapia, O. Nonlocal (Pair site) reactivity from second-order static density response function: Gas- and solution-phase reactivity of the acetaldehyde enolate as a test case. *J. Phys. Chem. A* **1999**, *103*, 1367–1375. [CrossRef]

38. Heaton, C.A.; Miller, A.K.; Powell, R.L. Predicting the reactivity of fluorinated compounds with copper using semi-empirical calculations. *J. Fluorine Chem.* **2001**, *107*, 1–3. [CrossRef]

39. Thring, T.S.A.; Hili, P.; Naughton, D.P. Anti-collagenase, anti-elastase and anti-oxidant activities of extracts from 21 plants. *BMC Complement. Altern. Med.* **2009**, *9*, 27. [CrossRef] [PubMed]

40. Heim, K.E.; Tagliaferro, A.R.; Bobilya, D.J. Flavonoid antioxidants: Chemistry, metabolism and structure-activity relationships. *J. Nutr. Biochem.* **2002**, *13*, 572–584. [CrossRef]

41. Arroio, A.; Honório, K.M.; Silva, A.B.F. Propriedades químico-quânticas empregadas em estudos das relações estrutura atividade. *Quim. Nova* **2010**, *33*, 694–699. [CrossRef]

42. Santos, C.B.R.; Vieira, J.B.; Lobato, C.C.; Hage-Melim, L.I.S.; Souto, R.N.P.; Lima, C.S.; Costa, E.V.M.; Brasil, D.S.B.; Macêdo, W.J.C.; Carvalho, J.C.T. A SAR and QSAR study of new artemisinin compounds with antimalarial activity. *Molecules* **2014**, *19*, 367–399. [CrossRef] [PubMed]

43. Zhang, G.; Musgrave, C.B. Comparison of DFT methods for molecular orbital eigenvalue calculations. *J. Phys. Chem. A* **2007**, *111*, 1554–1561. [CrossRef] [PubMed]

44. Almeida, L.; Pinto, A.; Monteiro, C.; Monteiro, H.; Belo, L.; Fernandes, J.; Bento, A.; Duarte, T.; Garrido, J.; Bahia, M. Protective effect of *C. sativa* leaf extract against UV mediated-DNA damage in a human keratinocyte cell line. *J. Photochem. Photobiol. B Biol.* **2015**, *144*, 28–34. [CrossRef] [PubMed]

45. Calvo-Castro, L.; Syed, D.N.; Chamcheu, J.C.; Vilela, F.M.P.; Pérez, A.M.; Vaillant, F.; Miguel, R.; Mukhtar, H. Protective effect of tropical highland blackberry juice (*Rubus adenotrichos* Schltdl.) against UVB-mediated damage in human epidermal keratinocytes and in a reconstituted skin equivalent model. *Photochem. Photobiol.* **2013**, *89*, 1199–1207. [CrossRef] [PubMed]

46. Arwa, P.S.; Zeraik, M.L.; Ximenes, V.F.; Fonseca, L.M.; Bolzani, V.S.; Silva, D.H.S. Redox-active biflavonoids from *Garcinia brasiliensis* as inhibitors of neutrophil oxidative burst and human erythrocyte membrane damage. *J. Ethnopharmacol.* **2015**, *174*, 410–418. [CrossRef] [PubMed]

47. Zhu, Q.Y.; Schramm, D.D.; Gross, H.B.; Holt, R.R.; Kim, S.H.; Yamaguchi, T.; Kwik-Uribe, C.L.; Keen, C.L. Influence of cocoa flavanols and procyanidins on free radical-induced human erythrocyte hemolysis. *Clin. Dev. Immunol.* **2005**, *12*, 27–34. [CrossRef] [PubMed]

48. Draijer, R.; Graaf, Y.; Slettenaar, M.; Groot, E.; Wright, C.I. Consumption of a polyphenol-rich grape-wine extract lowers ambulatory blood pressure in mildly hypertensive subjects. *Nutrients* **2015**, *7*, 3138–3153. [CrossRef] [PubMed]

49. Lipinski, C.A.; Lombardo, F.; Dominy, B.W.; Feeney, P.J. Experimental and computational approaches to estimate solubility and permeability in drug discovery and development settings. *Adv. Drug Deliv. Rev.* **1997**, *23*, 3–25. [CrossRef]

50. Cao, H.; Cheng, W.X.; Li, C.; Pan, X.-L.; Xie, X.G.; Li, T.H. DFT study on the antioxidant activity of rosmarinic acid. *J. Mol. Struct. THEOCHEM* **2005**, *719*, 177–183. [CrossRef]

51. Wright, J.S.; Johnson, E.R.; Dilabio, G.A. Predicting the activity of phenolic antioxidants: Theoretical method, analysis of substituent effects, and application to major families of antioxidants. *J. Am. Chem. Soc.* **2001**, *123*, 1173–1183. [CrossRef] [PubMed]

52. Scotti, L.; Scotti, M.T.; Cardoso, C.; Pauletti, P.; Castro-Gamboa, I.; Bolzani, V.S.; Velasco, M.V.R.; Menezes, C.M.S.; Ferreira, E.I. Modelagem molecular aplicada ao desenvolvimento de moléculas com atividade antioxidante visando ao uso cosmético. *Braz. J. Pharm. Cienc.* **2007**, *43*, 153–166. [CrossRef]

53. Mendes, A.P.S.; Borges, R.S.; Neto, A.M.J.C.; Macedo, L.G.M.; Silva, A.B.F. The basic antioxidant structure for flavonoid derivatives. *J. Mol. Model.* **2012**, *18*, 4073–4080. [CrossRef] [PubMed]

54. Amic, D.; Lucic, B. Reliability of bond dissociation enthalpy calculated by the PM6 method and experimental TEAC values in antiradical QSAR of flavonoids. *Biorg. Med. Chem.* **2010**, *18*, 28–35. [CrossRef] [PubMed]

55. Zhan, C.G.; Nichols, J.A.; Dixon, D.A. Ionization potential, electron affinity, electronegativity, hardness, and electron excitation energy: Molecular properties from density functional theory orbital energies. *J. Phys. Chem. A* **2003**, *107*, 4184–4195. [CrossRef]

56. Jursic, B.S. Determining the stability of three-carbon carbocations and carbanions through computing ionization energies, electron affinities and frontier molecular orbital energy gaps for corresponding radicals, cations and anions. *J. Mol. Struct. THEOCHEM* **2000**, *505*, 233–240. [CrossRef]

57. Higgins, P.; Dawson, J.; Lees, K.R.; McArthur, K.; Quinn, T.J.; Walters, M.R. Xanthine oxidase inhibition for the treatment of cardiovascular disease: A systematic review and meta-analysis. *Cardiovasc. Ther.* **2012**, *30*, 217–226. [CrossRef] [PubMed]

58. Malik, U.Z.; Hundley, N.J.; Romero, G.; Radi, R.; Freeman, B.A.; Tarpey, M.M.; Kelley, E.E. Febuxostat inhibition of endothelial-bound XO: Implications for targeting vascular ROS production. *Free Radic. Biol. Med.* **2011**, *51*, 179–184. [CrossRef] [PubMed]

59. Okamoto, K.; Eger, B.T.; Nishino, T.; Kondo, S.; Pai, E.F.; Nishino, T. An extremely potent inhibitor of xanthine oxidoreductase crystal structure of the enzyme-inhibitor complex and mechanism of inhibition. *J. Biol. Chem.* **2003**, *278*, 1848–1855. [CrossRef] [PubMed]

60. Hevener, K.E.; Zhao, W.; Ball, D.M.; Babaoglu, K.; Qi, J.; White, S.W.; Lee, R.E. Validation molecular docking programs for virtual screening against dihydropteroate synthase. *J. Chem. Inform. Model.* **2009**, *49*, 444–460. [CrossRef] [PubMed]

61. Santos, C.B.R.; Ramos, R.S.; Ortiza, B.L.S.; Silva, G.M.; Giuliatti, S.; Navarrete, J.L.A.; Carvalho, J.C.T. Oil from the fruits of *Pterodon emarginatus* Vog.: A traditional anti-inflammatory. Study combining in vivo and in silico. *J. Ethnopharmacol.* **2018**, *222*, 107–120. [CrossRef] [PubMed]

62. Cruz, J.V.; Neto, M.F.A.; Silva, L.B.; Ramos, R.d.S.; Costa, J.d.S.; Brasil, D.S.B.; Lobato, C.C.; da Costa, G.V.; Bittencourt, J.D.A.H.M.; da Silva, C.H.T.P.; et al. Identification of novel protein kinase receptor type 2 inhibitors using pharmacophore and structure-based virtual screening. *Molecules* **2018**, *23*, 453. [CrossRef] [PubMed]

63. Li, Y.; Frenz, C.M.; Li, Z.; Chen, M.; Wang, Y.; Li, F.; Cheng, L.; Sun, J.; Bohlin, L.; Li, Z.; et al. Virtual and in vitro bioassay screening of phytochemical inhibitors from flavonoids and isoflavones against xanthine oxidase and cyclooxygenase-2 for gout treatment. *Chem. Biol. Drug. Des.* **2013**, *81*, 537–544. [CrossRef] [PubMed]

64. Pauff, J.M.; Hille, R. Inhibition studies of bovine xanthine oxidase by luteolin, silibinin, quercetin, and curcumin. *J. Nat. Prod.* **2009**, *72*, 725–731. [CrossRef] [PubMed]

65. Costa, J.S.; Costa, K.S.L.; Cruzb, J.V.; Ramos, R.S.; Silva, L.B.; Brasil, D.S.B.; Tomich, C.S.; Rodrigues, C.B.; Macêdo, W.J.C. Virtual screening and statistical analysis in the design of new caffeine analogues molecules with potential epithelial anticancer activity. *Curr. Pharm. Des.* **2017**, *23*, 576–594. [CrossRef]

66. Cao, H.; Pauff, J.M.; Hille, R. Xray crystal structure of a xanthine oxidase complex with the flavonoid inhibitor quercetin. *J. Nat. Prod.* **2014**, *77*, 1693–1699. [CrossRef] [PubMed]

67. Cefali, L.C.; Cazedey, E.C.L.; Souza-Moreira, T.M.; Correa, M.A.; Salgado, H.R.N.; Isaac, V.L.B. Antioxidant activity and validation of quantification method for lycopene extracted from tomato. *J. AOAC Int.* **2015**, *98*, 1340–1345. [CrossRef] [PubMed]

68. Lopes-Lutz, D.; Alviano, D.S.; Alviano, C.S.; Kolodziejczyk, P.P. Screening of chemical composition, antimicrobial and antioxidant activities of Artemisia essential oils. *Phytochemistry* **2008**, *69*, 1732–1738. [CrossRef] [PubMed]

69. Pitaro, S.P.; Fiorani, L.V.; Jorge, N. Potencial antioxidante dos extratos de manjericão (*Ocimum basilicum* Lamiaceae) e orégano (*Origanum vulgare* Lamiaceae) em óleo de soja. *Rev. Bras. Plantas Med.* **2012**, *14*, 686–691. [CrossRef]

70. Frisch, M.J.; Trucks, G.W.; Schlegel, H.B.; Scuseria, G.E.; Robb, M.A.; Cheeseman, J.R. *GAUSSVIEW 3.07*; Gaussian Inc.: Pittsburgh, PA, USA, 1992.

71. Frisch, M.J.; Trucks, G.W.; Schlegel, H.B.; Scuseria, G.E.; Robb, M.A.; Cheeseman, J.R.; Scalmani, G.; Barone, V.; Petersson, G.A.; Nakatsuji, H.; et al. *GAUSSIAN 09, Revision A.02*; Gaussian Inc.: Wallingford, CT, USA, 2009.

72. Varetto, U. *MOLEKEL 4.1*; Swiss National Supercomputing Centre: Manno, Switzerland, 2009.

73. Breneman, C.M.; Wiberg, K.B. Determining atom-centered monopoles from molecular electrostatic potentials. The need for high sampling density in formamide conformational analysis. *J. Comput. Chem.* **1990**, *11*, 361–373. [CrossRef]

74. Singh, U.C.; Kollman, P.A. An approach to computing electrostatic charges for molecules. *J. Comput. Chem.* **1984**, *5*, 129–145. [CrossRef]

75. Estrada, E.; Molina, E. Novel local (fragment-based) topological molecular descriptors for QSPR/QSAR and molecular design. *J. Mol. Graph. Mod.* **2001**, *20*, 54–64. [CrossRef]

76. Santos, C.B.R.; Lobato, C.C.; Braga, F.S.; Costa, J.S.; Favacho, H.A.S.; Carvalho, J.C.T.; Macêdo, W.J.C.; Brasil, D.S.B.; Tomich, C.S.; Hage-Melim, L.I.S. Rational design of antimalarial drugs using molecular modeling and statistical analysis. *Curr. Pharm. Des.* **2015**, *21*, 4112–4127. [CrossRef] [PubMed]

77. *CHEMPLUS, Modular Extensions to HyperChem*; Version Release 6.02; HuperClub Inc.: Gainesville, FL, USA, 2000.

78. *PIROUETTE*, Version 3.01; Infometrix Inc.: Seattle, WA, USA, 2001.

79. Stewart, J.J.P. Optimization of parameters for semi-empirical methods J-method. *J. Comput. Chem.* **1989**, *10*, 209–220. [CrossRef]

80. Lee, C.; Yang, W.; Parr, R.G. Development of the colle-salvetti correlatrion-energy formula into a functional of the eletron density. *Phys. Rev.* **1988**, *37*, 785–789. [CrossRef]

81. Borges, R.S.; Batista, J., Jr.; Viana, R.B.; Baetas, A.C.; Orestes, E.; Andrade, M.A.; Honório, K.M.; Silva, A.B.F. Understanding the molecular aspects of tetrahydrocannabinol and canabidiol as antioxidants. *Molecules* **2013**, *18*, 12663–12674. [CrossRef] [PubMed]

82. Pereira, A.L.; Santos, G.B.; Franco, M.S.; Federico, L.B.; Silva, C.H.; Santos, C.B. Molecular modeling and statistical analysis in the design of derivatives of human dipeptidyl peptidase IV. *J. Biomol. Struct. Dyn.* **2017**, *36*, 318–334. [CrossRef] [PubMed]

83. Padilha, E.C.; Serafim, R.B.; Sarmiento, D.Y.R.; Santos, C.F.; Santos, C.B.; Silva, C.H. New PPARα/γ/δ optimal activator rationally designed by computational methods. *Braz. Chem. Soc.* **2016**, *27*, 1636–1647. [CrossRef]

9

A Novel Protocol using Small-Scale Spray-Drying for the Efficient Screening of Solid Dispersions in Early Drug Development and Formulation, as a Straight Pathway from Screening to Manufacturing Stages

Aymeric Ousset [1] ⓘ, Rosanna Chirico [2], Florent Robin [2], Martin Alexander Schubert [2], Pascal Somville [2] and Kalliopi Dodou [1,*] ⓘ

[1]   School of Pharmacy and Pharmaceutical Sciences, Faculty of Health Sciences and Wellbeing, University of Sunderland, Sunderland SR13SD, UK; aymeric.ousset@gmail.com

[2]   UCB Pharma S.A., Product Development, B-1420 Braine l'Alleud, Belgium; Rosana.Chirico@ucb.com (R.C.); Florent.Robin@ucb.com (F.R.); Martin-Alexander.Schubert@gmx.net (M.A.S.); Pascal.Somville@ucb.com (P.S.)

*   Correspondence: kalliopi.dodou@sunderland.ac.uk

Abstract: This work describes a novel screening strategy that implements small-scale spray-drying in early development of binary amorphous solid dispersions (ASDs). The proposed methodology consists of a three-stage decision protocol in which small batches (20–100 mg) of spray-dried solid dispersions (SDSDs) are evaluated in terms of drug–polymer miscibility, physical stability and dissolution performance in bio-predictive conditions. The objectives are to select the adequate carrier and drug-loading (DL) for the manufacturing of robust SDSD; and the appropriate stabilizer dissolved in the liquid vehicle of SDSD suspensions, which constitutes the common dosage form used during non-clinical studies. This methodology was verified with CDP146, a poorly water soluble (<2 μg/mL) API combined with four enteric polymers and four stabilizers. CDP146/HPMCAS-LF 40:60 (w/w) and 10% (w/v) PVPVA were identified as the lead SDSD and the best performing stabilizer, respectively. Lead SDSD suspensions (1–50 mg/mL) were found to preserve complete amorphous state during 8 h and maintain supersaturation in simulated rat intestinal fluids during the absorption window. Therefore, the implementation of spray-drying as a small-scale screening approach allowed maximizing screening effectiveness with respect to very limited API amounts (735 mg) and time resources (9 days), while removing transfer steps between screening and manufacturing phases.

Keywords: amorphous solid dispersions; screening; spray-dryer; downscaling; polymers; miscibility; dissolution; supersaturation; stability

---

1. Introduction

Non-clinical testing is a mandatory step of drug development that aims to evaluate the pharmacodynamics, pharmacokinetics and toxicity profiles of new chemical entities (NCEs) so that safe initial dose level can be identified for the first human exposure [1]. In general, liquid suspension formulations represent the most common dosage form used during non-clinical studies because of their ease of preparation and applicability to the vast majority of non-clinical species [2,3]. Suspension formulations consist of the dispersion of drug solid particles throughout an aqueous medium containing additional excipients, typically emulsifying, suspending or ionizing agents as well as surfactants and solvents [4]. This standard non-clinical formulation is generally administrated to animals via oral gavage. Therefore, oral non-clinical formulations such as liquid suspensions differ from conventional oral dosage forms used during clinical trials since tablets or capsules are not adapted for the dosing of most non-clinical species [5].

However, as the number of NCEs with poorly water soluble properties is continuously increasing during drug discovery phase, the conduction of non-clinical studies becomes challenging [3,6]. In this regard, the use of amorphous solid dispersions (ASD) has become a common strategy to tackle low solubility and improve absorption of the active pharmaceutical ingredient (API) in early drug development and formulation [7]. One of the major benefits of using ASD dosed as suspension formulation in comparison to the crystalline drug is the capability of producing adequate exposure of the API during non-clinical studies [8]. The strategy of solid dispersions consists of the drug amorphization and its dispersion into a polymeric carrier [9]. Spray-drying is considered as the solvent based process of reference for the manufacturing of solid dispersions in the pharmaceutical industry [10]. The key expectations regarding the development of a solid dispersion are the successful manufacturing of the amorphous form of the drug, its stability during the shelf life of the product and its capacity to maintain supersaturation during dissolution test [11].

Because, the selection of the appropriate polymer and drug-loading (DL) prior to the manufacturing of spray-dried solid dispersions (SDSDs) should be addressed in the first stage of the product's development, the use of miniaturized screening methodologies have gained a large interest in the pharmaceutical industry. More specifically, solvent casting screening has been particularly used in the industrial sector due to its capacity to operate in an automated mode allowing the testing of a maximum number of carriers while using a minimum amount of drug product [12,13].

However, the effect of the preparation method on the properties of screened ASDs and, more generally, on the outcome of the screening is often underestimated [14]. The fact that standard screening methodologies e.g., solvent casting and quench cooling are not representative of the operating mode and process conditions of regular spray-dryer, increases the risk to generate 'false negative and positive' results [15,16]. These samples are known to display different properties in terms of drug–polymer miscibility, glass transition temperature (T_g), physical stability, inter-components interactions and dissolution kinetics between screening and manufacturing scale [15,17–19]. This limits the prediction accuracy of conventional screening approaches because API-polymer systems can be abandoned prematurely during screening phases or can present limited potential when manufactured. The frequency of conventional screening methods to generate 'false negatives/positives' is not evaluated in a systematic way and increases the risk of inappropriate carrier selection. Finally, transfer from screening phases to laboratory scale production generally requires time and resources as a set of new experiments need to be carried out in order to finetune optimal DL and determine appropriate processing conditions [8].

Considering the increasing number of poorly soluble NCEs requiring formulation to ASDs, and the drawbacks of the current screening processes, there is a need for the development of a more reliable screening method that would also be time-efficient and simple enough to be used on a routine basis by the industry. In this regard, this work aims to propose a novel screening strategy at preclinical scale that integrates laboratory spray-drying throughout all phases of API development from the screening phases to the first SDSD batch production to support GLP non-clinical studies. The novelty of this work is to overcome preconceived ideas about the use of laboratory spray-drying at small-scale and demonstrates its suitability to operate in the case of resource limited compounds as a practical solution for pharmaceutical scientists

The present paper describes a new step-wise strategy for the (i) the screening of binary SDSD in early drug and formulation, and (ii) the development of SDSD dosed as non-clinical suspension formulation for oral administration. This novel screening approach was applied for CDP146: a poorly water soluble API from the UCB pipeline that is a candidate for the treatment of epilepsy. Firstly, the screening of appropriate polymer and optimal DL for the manufacturing of the lead SDSD that combines the best performance in terms of physical stability and solubility improvement was conducted during the first two stages of the proposed protocol. To do that the performance of

API-polymer combinations made of four polymeric carriers (HPMCP HP50, HPMCAS-LF, Eudragit L100 and Eudragit L100-55) was examined. In the present study, the selection of enteric polymers is explained by their particular interest during non-clinical studies due to their ability to protect drug from recrystallization in gastric fluid and delay supersaturation until the drug reaches the upper small intestine so that absorption is maximized [20,21]. Furthermore, typical DL used during non-clinical studies is usually in the range 25–40% (w/w) [8,18]. Thus, a DL of 40% (w/w) was initially tested as it would allow reaching high doses (of up to 1 g/kg of drug administrated per day) in toxicology dose escalation studies while limiting the amount of excipients administrated to the animals with regard to toxicity and tolerability. From experience, DL higher than 40% (w/w) can negatively impact the dissolution performance of ASDs by acting as a driving force for recrystallization. Secondly, the previously identified lead SDSD was prepared as liquid oral suspension formulation. The term 'oral formulation' refers to the preparation of SDSD suspended in the vehicle made of an aqueous medium containing HPC-SSL as standard suspending agent and one additional stabilizer. Although, the role of the carrier in ASD blend is to prevent drug from recrystallization in the solid state and during dissolution, the high doses usually tested during non-clinical studies generally require the use of an additional stabilizer dissolved in the liquid vehicle to ensure no physical change of the drug in the suspension that can negatively impact exposure. Accordingly, four conventional crystallization inhibitor agents including SDS, HPMC, Vitamin ETPGS and PVPVA have been screened. The choice of the above stabilizers and their concentration in the oral formulation vehicle have been carefully selected to minimize potential adverse effects and toxicity to the tested animals [4].

2. Material and Methods

2.1. Materials

Crystalline CDP146 was obtained from UCB Pharma, Product Development department (Braine l'Alleud, Belgium). The chemical structure of CDP146 is depicted in Figure 1. This compound has a molecular weight of 375.45 g/mol, a T_g of 95 °C, a melting temperature (T_m) of 198.1 °C. The API solubility in water was determined at 37 °C after 24 h under stirring (250 rpm) with drug content in excess within the aqueous medium. Following this procedure, the drug solubility was found to be below 2 µg/mL from pH 1.2 to pH 10.0.

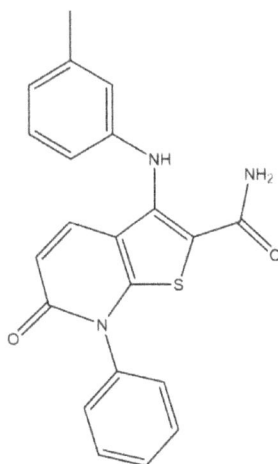

Figure 1. Chemical structure of CDP146.

Four enteric polymers were evaluated as potential carriers for ASD: hydroxypropylmethylcellulose phthalate (HPMCP HP50) and hydroxypropylmethylcellulose acetate succinate fine grade (HPMCAS-LF) obtained from Shin-Etsu (Tokyo, Japan), copolymer of methacrylic acid and methyl methacrylate 1:1 (Eudragit L100) and copolymer of methacrylic acid and ethyl acrylate copolymer 1:1

(Eudragit L100-55) purchased from Evonik (Essen, Germany). Table 1 summarizes the physico-chemical and thermal properties of the selected carriers.

Table 1. Physico-chemical properties of screened polymers for CDP146 ASD development.

Polymer	M_w (g/mol) [a]	Dissolution pH [a]	T_g (°C) [b]	T Degradation (°C) [c]
HPMCP-HP50	78,000	>5.0	140	160
HPMCAS-LF	18,167	>5.5	122	170
Eudragit L100	125,000	>6.0	192	165
Eudragit L100-55	320,000	>5.5	122	165

[a] data obtained from available literature [22]; [b] data experimentally obtained by modulated differential scanning calorimetry (mDSC); [c] data experimentally obtained by thermogravimetric analysis (TGA).

Four stabilizers were tested with regard to the stabilization of suspension formulation: copolymer of N-vinyl-2-pyrrolidone and vinyl acetate (PVPVA) from Ashland (Covington, KY, USA), sodium dodecyl sulfate (SDS) from Merck (Darmstadt, Germany), hydroxypropylmethylcellulose (HPMC) and vitamin ETPGS from Sigma Aldrich (Saint-Louis, MO, USA). Hydroxypropylcellulose (HPC-SSL) from Nisso (Düsseldorf, Germany) was used for oral formulation preparation. Simulated intestinal fluids (SIF) powder was obtained from Biorelevant.com (London, UK) and used to simulate rat intestinal fluid. All other materials and solvents used were of reagent and analytical grade, respectively.

2.2. Methods

2.2.1. Screening Strategy

General Considerations

Figures 2 and 3 describe the experimental protocol summary and the flow chart representation of the proposed screening strategy, respectively. As seen in Figure 3, the proposed screening protocol uses a three-stage decision tree including "Feasibility evaluation of SDSD manufacturing", "Screening of polymer and stabilizer" and "Oral formulation development". API and time consumption have been estimated while considering the screening of four polymers at two DLs (e.g., 30 and 40% (w/w)) for the manufacturing of binary SDSD, and four stabilizers dissolved in the liquid vehicle of the oral non-clinical formulation.

- As a preliminary step of screening protocol, a common solvent or binary solvent mixture of interest that allows dissolving both drug and polymer, needs to be identified. A solute concentration higher than 2% (w/v) is defined as acceptance criteria for spray-drying development to achieve a reasonable yield, process time and solvent consumption to comply with HSE considerations [8,23].
- In the first Stage (S1), the potential of screened carriers was evaluated based on their ability to generate glass solutions by spray-drying. The evaluation of drug–polymer miscibility in the early stage of drug development is known to offer a reliable assessment of the ASD potential [24–26]. Specifically, the formation of glass solution system where amorphous drug is molecularly dispersed in the carrier, combines the best performance in terms of physical stability and solubility improvement [27]. On the contrary, semi-crystalline and phase-separated ASDs are known to provide limited potential of solubility enhancement and higher tendency for drug recrystallization during both dissolution and upon storage [28,29]. Commonly used excipients for the preparation of solid dispersions include cellulose, polyvinlylpyrrolidone, poloxamer, polyethylene glycol or polymethacrylate derivatives [30]. These polymers are recognized as "generally regarded as safe" (GRAS) excipients. Additional criteria such as T_g, hygroscopicity, solubility in organic solvents, viscosifying properties, pH of hydration in water and solid solution capacity need to be considered regarding the carrier selection for the manufacturing of solid dispersions by spray-drying [31].

- In the second Stage (S2), the physical stability of API-polymer systems identified as glass solutions was assessed up to one week. In parallel, the dissolution properties of these ASDs was examined with and without stabilizers dissolved in aqueous medium. Therefore, the influence of the stabilizer in the dosing vehicle of the oral formulation and its ability to maintain drug supersaturation and parachute effect during dissolution tests were investigated. The use of stabilizer in the dosing vehicle of suspensions allows converting the API into suitable dosage form for administration to non-clinical species. The wide variety of stabilizers commonly used during non-clinical studies allows overcoming the diversity of molecule specific exposure limitations so that the formulation maintains stability, homogeneity and dosability within the range of doses tested [5].

- In the last Stage (S3), the long-term stability of the lead SDSD identified during Stage 2 was investigated for up to 3 months. Moreover, the lead SDSD was prepared as non-clinical suspension formulation in the vehicle containing the stabilizer of interest. Then, the oral formulation was prepared at various doses generally tested during non-clinical studies. Its stability prior to administration and dissolution performance in bio-predictive conditions were assessed.

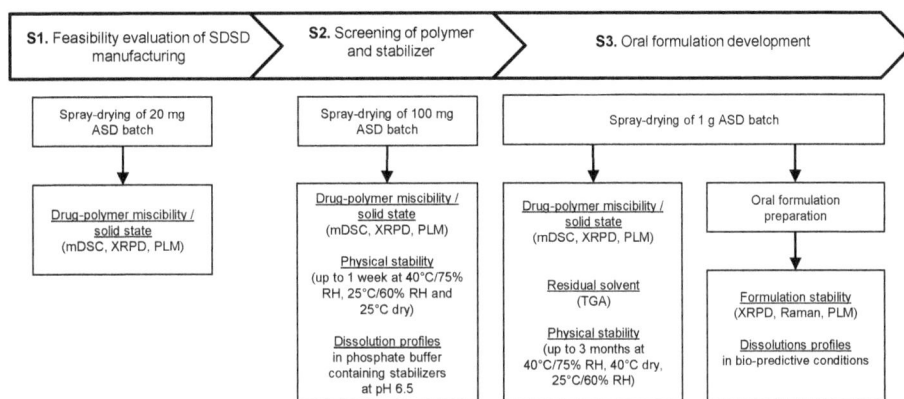

Figure 2. Summary of the experimental protocol applied in the proposed screening strategy.

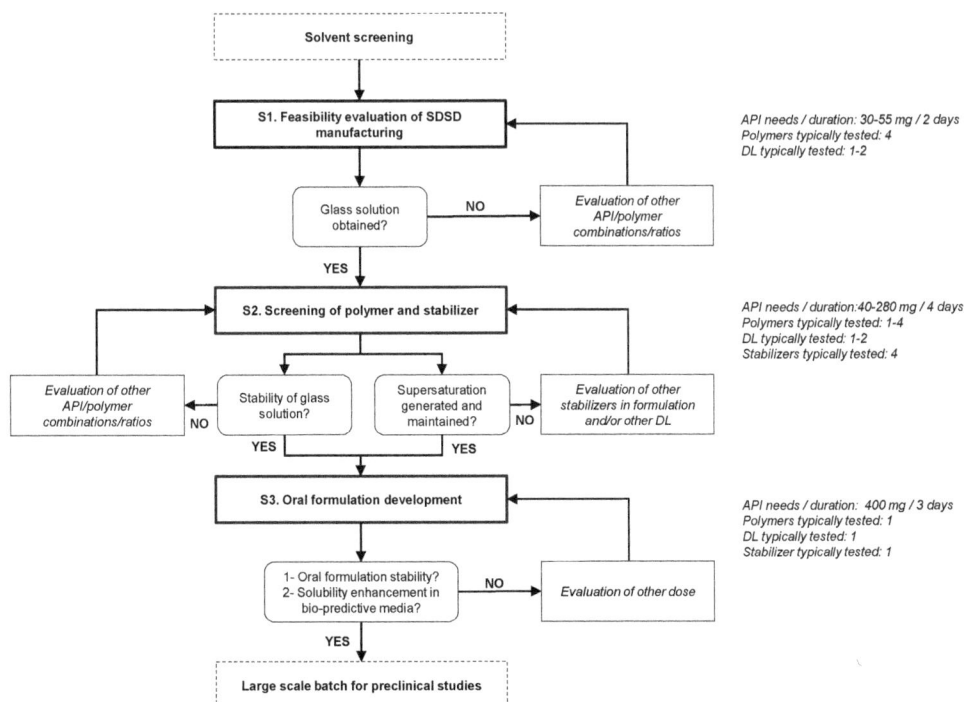

Figure 3. Flow chart representation of the three-stages' decisional screening strategy.

Application to CDP146 ASD Screening

- Feasibility evaluation of SDSD manufacturing (Stage 1)

Productions of 20 mg batches of 40:60 (w/w) CDP146 ASDs with HPMCP HP50, HPMCAS-LF, Eudragit L100 and Eudragit L100-55 were performed using the laboratory scale ProCept 4M8-TriX spray-dryer (Zelzate, Belgium). This equipment was selected due to its capability to operate with feed solution volume as low as 0.5 mL and up to 24 L/8 h [32,33]. API-polymer solutions were prepared in Dichloromethane (DCM)/Ethanol (EtOH) 2:1 (v/v) at 50 mg/mL. The feed solution was pumped to the nozzle via a peristaltic pump Watson Marlow 530S (Falmouth, Cornwall, UK) and adjusted at 1 g/min. Atomization of the feed solution into fine droplets was achieved using a bifluid nozzle with a diameter of 1.2 mm and an atomizing air pressure of 1.50 bars. Solvent evaporation was performed by using a drying gas airflow of 0.30 m^3/min at an inlet temperature of 60 °C. A lateral cooling airflow of 100 L/min was applied to transfer powder from the bottom of the drying chamber to the small cyclone (height/diameter of 210 mm/40 mm) where particle separation occurs. The present manufacturing conditions have been specifically optimized to maximize the yield of small-scale batches of solid dispersions. In addition, a customized 3D printed funnel has been particularly developed to allow powder collection into a standard aluminum pan (TA Instruments, Leatherhead, UK) used for modulated differential scanning calorimetry (mDSC) analysis. This powder collection system allows reducing material loss during powder handling and eases the transfer for subsequent analytical characterization. After processing, the collected powders were stored in a vacuum oven for 48 h before analysis. Duplicate SDSD productions were conducted per API-polymer combination to assess reproducibility: one batch was analyzed by mDSC while the repeated sample was analyzed by X-ray powder diffraction (XRPD).

- Screening of polymer and stabilizer (Stage 2)

100 mg batches of 40:60 (w/w) CDP146 solid dispersions identified as 'glass solutions' during Stage 1 were produced by spray-drying. The same process and formulation conditions used for the 20 mg batch productions were maintained. In this particular case, spray-dried material was collected in a 2 mL glass vial (Waters, Saint-Quentin-en-Yvelines, France) connected to the 3D printed system. SDSDs were analyzed by mDSC and XRPD, respectively, to confirm up-scaling robustness and comparability between Stage 1 and Stage 2 with regard to miscibility and solid state. The physical stability of produced solid dispersions was assessed after one week upon storage under both stress and ambient storage conditions. About 10 mg of spray-dried powder were placed in an incubator at 40 °C/75% Relative humidity (RH), 25 °C/60% RH and 25 °C dry storage conditions. The aforementioned storage conditions were selected in line with the ICHQ1A(R2) guidelines. After one week, SDSDs were analyzed by mDSC, XRPD and polarized light microscopy (PLM) to detect the presence of potential drug crystals formed upon storage.

An accurate weight of 2.5 mg of SDSD (equivalent to 1 mg of API) was dosed into 1 mL of dissolution medium consisting of 50 mM phosphate buffer at pH 6.5 with stabilizers. Five dissolution media with different stabilizer compositions were tested: Vehicle A (no stabilizers), Vehicle B (1% (w/v) HPMC), Vehicle C (0.2% (w/v) SDS), Vehicle D (1% (w/v) vitamin ETPGS) and Vehicle E (10% (w/v) PVPVA). The dissolution profile of pure crystalline CDP146 was obtained in each dissolution medium so that the solubility improvement (%) of screened SDSD can be evaluated. The aforementioned dissolution conditions represent non-sink conditions with respect to the crystalline drug so that the ability of screened ASD to generate and maintain supersaturation can be assessed during the duration of the test [34]. Dissolution tests were carried out manually in 10 mL glass tube (VWR, Heverlee, Belgium). Mixtures were maintained at 37 °C under magnetic stirring at 250 rpm using Thermo Mixer C unit (Eppendorf, Hamburg, Germany). Samples of 100 μL were collected after 5, 30, 60, 120, 180, 240, 360 and 1440 min and transferred into 0.45 μm ultrafree filter units (Merck Millipore, Burlington, MA, USA). Samples were centrifugated at 8000 rpm during 2 min. The filtrate was pipetted, properly diluted in H$_2$O/Acetonitrile (ACN) 1/1 (v/v) and analyzed in High performance liquid chromatography (HPLC).

- Oral formulation development (Stage 3)

1 g of lead ASD of CDP146 was produced by spray-drying using the laboratory scale ProCept 4M8-TriX spray-dryer (Zelzate, Belgium). Drug–polymer solutions were prepared in the binary solvent mixture of interest DCM/EtOH 2:1 (v/v) at 50 mg/mL. The feed solution flow rate was adjusted at 5 g/min. An atomizing air pressure of 0.65 bars was applied to a 1.2 mm bifluid nozzle to create a spray. The drying gas airflow was set at 0.35 m^3/min and maintained at 65 °C. The lateral cooling air was kept constant at 100 L/min and dried particles were separated from the exhaust air within the medium cyclone (height/diameter of 242 mm/60 mm). After processing, the spray-dried material was stored in a vacuum oven for 48 h before analysis to eliminate the last traces of residual solvent.

The solid state and miscibility of spray-dried material was analyzed by XRPD, PLM and mDSC, respectively, to confirm the results obtained during previous screening steps. Residual solvent analysis was carried by Thermogravimetric analysis (TGA). The long term stability of the lead SDSD of CDP146 was investigated up to 3 months at 40 °C/75% RH, 40 °C dry storage conditions and 25 °C/60% RH. Solid state evolution and residual solvent content were determined after 2 weeks, 1, 2 and 3 months. This would help to gain insight into the shelf life of the formulated drug.

In order to obtain ASD suspension, SDSD powder was dispensed in a 100 mM citrate buffer (pH 4) vehicle containing 1% (w/v) HPC-SSL, 0.1% (w/v) antifoam and the stabilizer agent of interest identified during the second step of the screening procedure. Oral liquid formulation was prepared at various API concentrations of 1, 10, 30 and 50 mg/mL. Powder was accurately weighed into 4 mL Nalgene polypropylene vial (Thermo Fischer Scientific, Waltham, MA, USA), and half of the required amount of vehicle was added. The mixture was manually mixed during one minute in order to wet all solid particles. Then, the rest of the vehicle was poured into the mixture and the formulation was magnetically stirred at 350 rpm for at least 30 min to remove the presence of air bubbles in the stirring at 350 rpm.
mixture and homogenize the suspension. The formulation stability and homogeneity was determined by XRPD, PLM and Raman spectroscopy up to 8 h corresponding to a working day, under magnetic

Dissolution profiles of CDP146 suspension formulation were obtained at various doses in bio-predictive conditions representative for the rat species. First, 2 mL of freshly prepared oral formulation was pipetted into a 10 mL glass tube. 2.4 mL of a medium containing HCl and NaCl (6.19 g/L) at pH 3.2, used to simulate the gastric medium of rat was added to the mixture. The dissolution was carried out at 37 °C under magnetic stirring at 250 rpm using Thermo Mixer C unit (Eppendorf, Hamburg, Germany). Temperature and magnetic stirring were maintained constant during the entire dissolution tests. Samplings of 100 µL were taken after 1, 5, 10, 15 and 30 min. After 30 min of dissolution in simulated rat gastric fluid, 1 mL of the mixture was transferred and diluted with 1 mL of 100 mM phosphate buffer at pH 5.0 containing SIF powder (35.6 mM). This vehicle was used to simulate the composition of the first compartment of rat intestinal fluid. This procedure was repeated twice with the second and third compartment of rat intestinal fluids that consist of 100 mM phosphate buffer at pH 5.0 containing SIF powder (14 mM) and 100 mM phosphate buffer at pH 6.0 containing SIF powder (4 mM), respectively. A dilution factor of 2 from the gastric to each intestinal fluid was applied to be representative for physiological conditions. Samplings of 100 µL were taken after 1, 5, 10, 15, 30, 60, 90 and 120 min. All samples were filtered on 0.45 µm ultrafree filter units (Merck Millipore, Burlington, MA, USA) and centrifuged at 8000 rpm during 2 min. Appropriate dilution in H$_2$O/ACN 1/1 (v/v) was performed and API content was determined in HPLC.

2.2.2. Analytical or Characterization Methods

Modulated Differential Scanning Calorimetry

The phase behavior and thermal properties of SDSD were analyzed in mDSC using TA Instruments Q1000 calorimeter (TA Instruments, Leatherhead, UK). The chamber was purged with a 50 mL/min flow rate of dry nitrogen. Indium and sapphire disks were used to calibrate the temperature/enthalpy and heat capacity, respectively. The powder was analyzed in non-hermetic standard aluminum pans (TA Instruments, Leatherhead, UK). Samples were heated from 0 °C to 210 °C at 2 °C/min with a modulation of ± 1 °C and a period of 40 s. Data was processed using Universal Analysis 2000 software (TA Instruments, Leatherhead, UK): T_g was reported as the mid-point of inflection in the step change observed in the reverse heat flow signal while crystallization and melting events were recorded in non-reverse and total heat flows.

Thermogravimetric Analysis

TGA experiments were conducted in a TGA Q500 (TA Instruments, Leatherhead, UK) in order to estimate the percentage of residual solvent and moisture content in spray-dried material. The chamber was swept by a 50 mL/min flow rate of dry nitrogen. Samples were set isothermally 5 min at 25 °C and heated to 300 °C at 10 °C/min. Data were processed using the TA instruments software Universal Analysis 2000 software (TA Instruments, Leatherhead, UK).

X-ray Powder Diffraction

The solid state of screened solid dispersions was characterized in XRPD. Analyses were performed on X Bruker AXS D8 Advance (Bruker, Karlsruhe, Germany). Monocrystal silicium holders were used during sample preparation. Analyses on powder were carried out over the range 3.5–30° at a scan speed of 2.5 s/step and a step size of 0.02°. Data was processed using Eva DIFFRAC-SUITE software (Bruker, Karlsruhe, Germany).

XRPD analyses were also conducted in order to monitor the crystallization behavior of the oral liquid formulation. Samplings of 200 µL were taken after 0, 4 and 8 h and were subsequently centrifuged at 8000 rpm during 2 min on 0.45 µm ultrafree centrifugal filter units (Merck Millipore, Burlington, MA, USA). The wet solid filtrate was collected from the filter and analyzed in XRPD over the range 3.5–30° at a scan speed of 0.1 s/step and a step size of 0.02°. Then, a second analysis was conducted on the 'dried' product to evaluate the potential appearance of crystals after water evaporation of the wet solid filtrate.

Polarized Light Microscopy

The observations were performed using a AX10 Zeiss light microscope (Carl Zeiss, Oberkochen, Germany) under polarized light. The samples were observed in the optical resolution ×400. Pictures were collected using Axiocam MRC5 and images were processed using Axiovision 4.0 software (Carl Zeiss, Oberkochen, Germany). The presence of crystallites was determined by the observation of birefractive entities under polarized light.

Raman Spectroscopy

Raman spectroscopy was used to monitor the crystallization behavior of ASD suspension formulation. Analyses were conducted on Raman RXN2 Hybrid Analyzer (Kaiser Optical Systems, Ann Arbor, MI, USA) using a 785 nm laser wavelength in reflexion mode. Spectra were acquired by coupling the analyzer with fiber-optic MR probe with an 1/8" immersion optic. Internal calibration and determination of optimal exposure time were performed prior to analysis. Analyses of both crystalline API and CDP146 ASD suspension in the vehicle of interest were conducted. The immersion optic was inserted in 1 mL of formulation, previously pipetted into a 2 mL HPLC glass vial with PTFE/silicone septa (Waters, Saint-Quentin-en-Yvelines, France). The mixture was magnetically stirred at 350 rpm and spectra were collected every 15 min during 8 h. Measurements were carried out in a black chamber to prevent interference from ambient. The Raman shift of 150–1890 cm^{-1} was examined. Two regions of Raman spectra where crystalline API and freshly prepared ASD suspension were found to display significant differences in peak characteristics, were particularly investigated. Data was obtained with iC Raman software (Kaiser Optical Systems, Ann Arbor, MI, USA) and processed by Matlab R2017b (Mathworks, Natick, MA, USA).

HPLC

Determination of CDP146 content during dissolution tests was performed using HPLC coupled with UV detection. Measurements were conducted on an X Bridge C18 column (Waters, Saint-Quentin-en-Yvelines, France) at 45 °C. The injection volume was fixed at 20 µL and the detection was carried out by UV at 305 nm. The analytical method used a gradient mobile phase composed of a mixture of acetate buffer (pH 4.5) and acetonitrile at a flow rate of 0.8 mL/min. Data were processed by Empower 3 chromatography data software (Waters, Saint-Quentin-en-Yvelines, France). Standard solutions of pure CDP146 were prepared in H_2O/ACN 1:1 (v/v) to cover a calibration linearity over the concentration range of 1–75 µg/mL.

3. Results and Discussion

3.1. Feasibility Evaluation of SDSD Manufacturing (Stage 1)

Screened CDP146-polymer systems were produced by spray-drying (20 mg). Yields ranging from 16–28% were obtained so that sufficient material was collected for subsequent solid state characterization. Therefore, API-polymer combinations were evaluated based upon their ability to form glass solutions after processing at a DL of 40% (w/w). Figure 4 displays the results obtained in the reverse heat flow signal of mDSC and the XRPD patterns of 20 mg ASD batches of CDP146. Glass solutions were obtained for SDSDs of CDP146 made with HPMCP HP50, HPMCAS-LF, Eudragit L100 and Eudragit L100-55. As seen in Figure 4A, the thermograms of these API-polymer systems display a clear T_g, balanced between the T_g of pure components in the blend. No drug melting endotherm was detected in both heat flow and non-reverse signals (data not shown). Additionally, the presence of a large amorphous halo and the absence of Bragg peaks in XRPD pattern confirm the complete amorphization of the drug after processing (Figure 4B). Similar analytic data obtained for the first and the second batch demonstrated that the operating mode of small-scale spray-drying leads to reproducible results. During a 'real' screening, the second batch production can be removed i.e., one single batch of screened solid dispersion (20 mg) can be analyzed both in mDSC and XRPD to minimize API consumption.

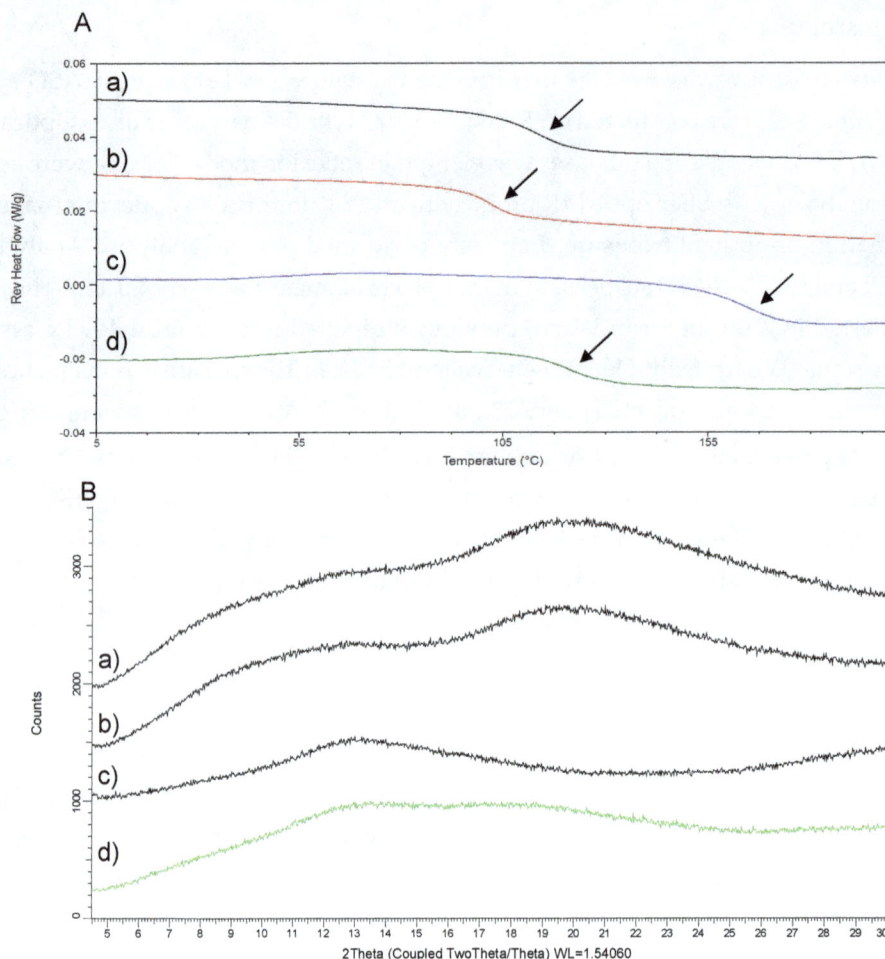

Figure 4. Reverse heat flow signals (**A**) and X-ray powder diffraction (XRPD) patterns (**B**) of 40:60 (*w/w*) CDP146 SDSDs (20 mg) made with HPMCP HP50 (a), HPMCAS-LF (b), Eudragit L100 (c) and Eudragit L100-55 (d).

All tested ASDs were identified as molecularly dispersed glass solutions and can therefore continue in the screening process. At this stage, there is no need to test these API-polymer systems at higher or lower DLs. However, if residual crystallinity is detected for SDSD produced at a DL of 40% (*w/w*), additional experiments at lower DL (e.g., 30% (*w/w*)) would be needed.

In the current case study, preliminary evaluation of CDP146 SDSD miscibility and solid state was not found to discriminate polymers; this can be explained on the basis that CDP146 has a relatively low tendency for recrystallization. According to the classification of Baird et al. (2010) that aims to categorize the crystallization tendency of APIs from undercooled melts, CDP146 was found to belong to the class III group i.e., molecules that display complete amorphization and no recrystallization during a heating/cooling/heating cycle in DSC [35]. Furthermore, the application of the proposed screening strategy in different UCB pharma development projects has demonstrated that the first screening stage allowed realizing a pre-selection of adequate carriers for the SDSD manufacturing of API with higher tendency for recrystallization (data not shown). Preliminary information regarding the API tendency for recrystallization would allow assessing the suitability for ASD as a formulation principle. Nevertheless, a decision regarding the selection of adequate carrier and DL for the development of SDSD cannot be based on the sole criteria of drug–polymer miscibility evaluation. Conduction of dissolution tests is required to assess the "true" performance of ASD to enhance API solubility. Herein, polymer screening would be performed in the second stage of the proposed approach by evaluating the potential of CDP146-polymer glass solutions in terms of solubility enhancement and physical stability upon storage.

As a preliminary step of screening protocol, DCM/EtOH 2:1 (v/v) was identified as the binary solvent mixture of interest for CDP146 SDSD manufacturing. The objective was to keep the same mixture of solvent during the entire duration of the screening protocol because a change in solvent system could impact the final properties of SDSD such as morphology, particle size and solid state [15,36].

3.2. Screening of Polymer and Stabilizer (Stage 2)

Small batches (100 mg) of CDP146 ASDs previously identified as glass solutions were produced by spray-drying. The solid state and miscibility of screened SDSDs was evaluated and results are summarized in Table 2. API-polymer systems were identified as ideal glass solutions and displayed similar T_g value than the respective samples produced at smaller scale. This finding confirms the results obtained during the first stage of the screening strategy and therefore controls the validity of our approach.

Elimination of the process variability factor linked to the choice of the preparation method was achieved by implementing the same manufacturing process (i.e., spray drying) at various scales. This presents the main advantage of our current strategy compared to standard screening methodologies because the generation of 'false negatives and positives' results during the screening phases is minimized and thereby the risk of inappropriate carrier and DL selection is reduced. Analytical results of screened ASD batches produced at 20 and 100 mg scale confirmed that the properties of the produced SDSD are scale-independent.

Table 2. Characterization summary of 40:60 CDP146 ASDs produced by spray-drying (100 mg).

ASD Composition		Yield		Miscibility/Solid State	
Polymer	DL (*w/w*)	Yield (%)	T_g (°C)	T_m (°C)	XRPD Pattern/PLM
HPMCP HP50	40%	68.1	113.5	-	A
HPMCAS-LF	40%	70.9	102.5	-	A
Eudragit L100	40%	71.8	163.4	-	A
Eudragit L100-55	40%	71.7	120.9	-	A

A: amorphous sample characterized by the presence of a large halo in XRPD and the absence of birefringence under PLM observations.

The physical stability of the four CDP146 SDSDs was investigated up to one week under stress and ambient storage conditions. XRPD patterns of 40:60 (w/w) SDSDs of CDP146 stored during one week at 40 °C/75% RH, 25 °C/60% RH and 25 °C dry storage conditions, respectively, are depicted in Figure 5. No evidence of drug recrystallization was reported for the four API-polymer systems upon storage. The absence of both Bragg peaks in XRPD patterns and birefractive crystallites under polarized light observations reveal that the four screened SDSDs were found to maintain their complete amorphous state.

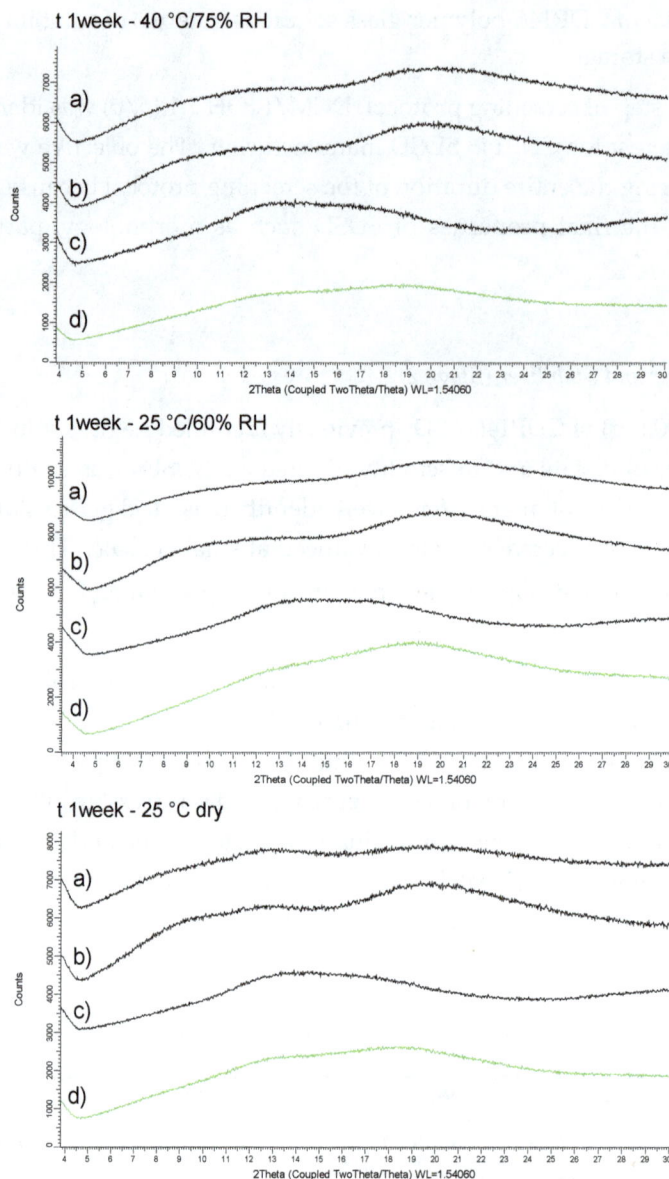

Figure 5. XRPD patterns of 40:60 (w/w) CDP146 SDSDs (100 mg) made with HPMCP HP50 (a), HPMCAS-LF (b), Eudragit L100 (c) and Eudragit L100-55 (d) after 1 week under stress and standard storage conditions.

The four screened polymers i.e., HPMCP HP50, HPMCAS-LF, Eudragit L100 and Eudragit L100-55 were found to have similar potential to inhibit drug crystallization at solid state. This observation correlates well with the relatively high T_g value obtained for 40:60 (w/w) CDP146 SDSDs, detailed in Table 3. Solid dispersion with high T_g generate anti-plasticization effect that reduces the molecular mobility and therefore contributes to the drug stabilization in the amorphous state [37]. At this stage, the assessment of carrier's potential to maintain amorphous state upon storage did not allow discriminating the four carriers. The selection of lead excipient would be conducted based on the dissolution performance of CDP146-polymer systems. Although the duration of the physical stability program did not discriminate API-polymer systems, this study would ensure that solid dispersions will remain physically stable between the manufacturing and the administration phases, which corresponds to an average duration of one week. Results regarding the chemical stability of screened ASDs are not presented in the current case study but would be of interest during Stage 2 [38].

Dissolution performance of API-polymer systems was evaluated at 37 °C in dissolution medium at pH 6.5 with and without stabilizers. At this stage, the generation of supersaturated solution with solubility improvement compared to crystalline drug during a minimum of 4 h is required to maximize in-vivo exposure. This length of time corresponds to the maximum duration of the administration phase during preclinical tests, typically. Dissolution profiles of screened 40:60 (w/w) CDP146 SDSDs in various media are depicted in Figure 6.

As seen in Figure 6a, the four screened ASDs showed a poor solubility enhancement compared to crystalline API which is probably explained by a sudden drug recrystallization in the first seconds of the dissolution testing. This indicates that the presence of a polymer is insufficient and addition of a stabilizer is needed to stabilize the supersaturated solution. Similarly in the presence of 1% (w/v) HPMC (Figure 6b), the dissolution profiles of the four tested SDSDs did not allow generating supersaturation and improving drug solubility, significantly. This invalidates the selection of HPMC as anti-nucleation/stabilizing agent for SDSDs of CDP146.

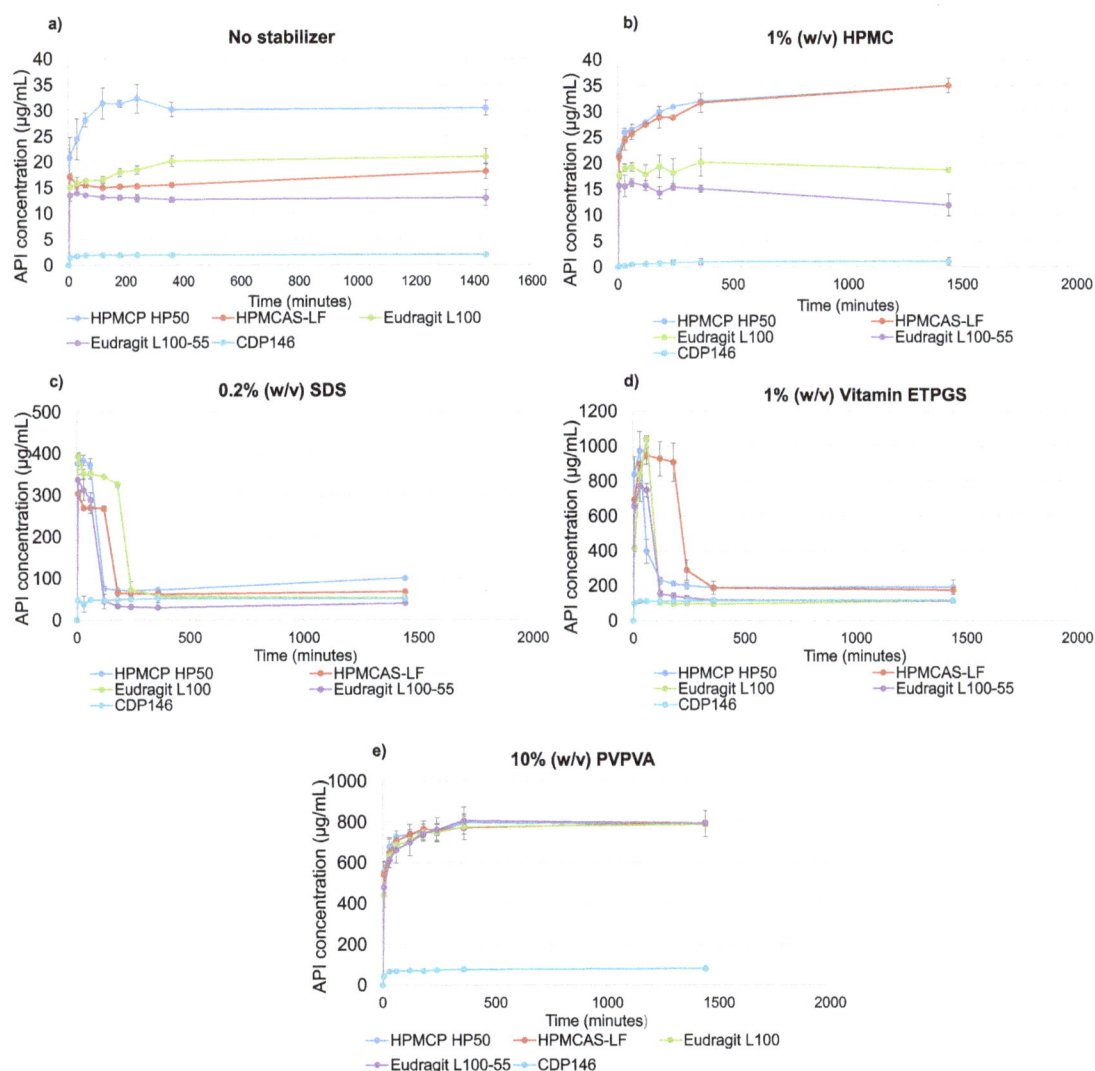

Figure 6. Dissolution profiles of 40:60 (w/w) CDP146 SDSDs (100 mg) and pure crystalline API in 50 mM phosphate buffer (pH 6.5) without stabilizer (**a**) or with 1% (w/v) HPMC (**b**), 0.2% (w/v) SDS (**c**), 1% (w/v) Vitamin ETPGS (**d**) and 10% (w/v) PVPVA (**e**) at an API concentration of 1 mg/mL.

Table 3. Characterization summary and physical stability evaluation of lead CDP146 SDSD produced by spray-drying (1 g).

Lead ASD	Process Considerations		Miscibility/Solid State		Residual Solvent	Physical Stability								
						25 °C/60% RH			40 °C Dry			40 °C/75% RH		
Polymer	DL (w/w)	Yield (%)	T_g (°C)	Tm (°C)	XRPDPattern/PLM	Weight Loss (%)	1 m	2 m	3 m	1 m	2 m	3 m	1 m	2 m	3 m
HPMCAS-LF	40%	88.2	102.5	-	A	0.2	A	A	A	A	A	A	A	A	A

A: amorphous sample characterized by the presence of a large halo in XRPD and the absence of birefringence under PLM observations.

When adding 0.2% (w/v) SDS or 1% (w/v) Vitamin ETPGS in the dissolution medium, the dissolution profiles of the four screened SDSDs of CDP146 were found to generate supersaturation in the first minutes/hours of the tests, as seen in Figure 6c,d. The best performing API-polymer combinations include HPMCAS-LF and Eudragit L100 carriers in dissolution medium containing 1% (w/v) Vitamin ETPGS and 0.2% (w/v) SDS, respectively. These specific ASDs were found to maintain supersaturation up to 3 h corresponding to a solubility improvement of around 720% and 561% after 3 h, respectively. However, recrystallization during dissolution testing characterized by sudden drop in solubility was recorded for all ASDs, as seen in Figure 6c,d. Consequently, the stabilizing potential of SDS and Vitamin ETPGS is not enough to cover the administration phase and alternative stabilizers need to be considered.

Finally, dissolution profiles obtained for all 40:60 (w/w) CDP146 SDSDs in the medium containing 10% (w/v) PVPVA allowed generating and maintaining supersaturation and parachute effect up to 24 h, corresponding to a solubility improvement percentage of around 1000% compared to the crystalline drug. Therefore, PVPVA was found as the best performing stabilizer that allowed sustaining supersaturation generated by 40:60 (w/w) CDP146 SDSDs during a length of time that covers the administration phase. Regarding the selection of adequate carrier, the four screened SDSDs of CDP146 display similar dissolution profiles in the dissolution medium made with 10% (w/v) PVPVA and could be selected, independently. Nevertheless, results obtained in the vehicle made with 1% (w/v) Vitamin ETPGS can be considered as discriminative conditions and confirm that CDP146/HPMCAS-LF 40:60 (w/w) was the only API-polymer combination that reached drug solubility above 900 µg/mL up to 180 min, as seen in Figure 6d. All other ASDs recrystallize during dissolution test before 60 min and lost their solubility enhancement potential, consequently. HPMCAS-LF was found to have a greater potential than other tested carriers in terms of the degree of supersaturation generated and the extent of supersaturation maintenance. Based on these considerations, HPMCAS-LF was selected as adequate carrier for the manufacturing of CDP146 SDSD.

Furthermore, in the case where the interplay between carrier and stabilizer does not allow maintaining supersaturation during a sufficient time to cover the administration phase, two alternatives can be considered: the potential of other stabilizers alone or in combination (e.g., Tween 80, PEG, Soluplus, PVPK15, Docusate, cellulose derivatives ...) can be evaluated and/or considering SDSD with lower DL (e.g., 30% (w/w)) at this stage of the screening approach. Decreasing the DL of solid dispersions is generally known to ease the stabilization of supersaturated solution [18].

3.3. Oral Formulation Development (Stage 3)

A 1 g batch of CDP146/HPMCAS-LF 40:60 (w/w), previously identified as lead API-polymer system was produced by spray-drying. The solid dispersion was characterized in terms of solid state, miscibility and residual solvent content. Results are summarized in Table 3. This SDSD displays a single T_g of around 102 °C in the reverse heat flow of mDSC and the absence of melting and recrystallization process in the non-reverse and total heat flow signals. Large amorphous halo in XRPD pattern confirms the complete drug amorphization after processing. The results obtained in Table 3 correlate well with the properties of CDP146/HPMCAS-LF 40:60 (w/w) generated during the first two stages of the screening approach. This confirms the advantage of the proposed screening strategy compared to standard screening methodologies because limited scale-up effects are observed with this approach and the same manufacturing technology is used during screening and manufacturing stages reducing the need for additional formulation/process development.

Additionally, the physical stability of the lead SDSD of CDP146 was assessed up to three months at 40 °C/75% RH, 40 °C dry storage conditions and 25 °C/60% RH. Results from stability study are summarized in Table 3. Under both ambient and stress conditions, CDP146/HPMCAS-LF was found to maintain complete drug amorphous state during the entire duration of the stability program, which is a good indicator for the long-term stability of the spray-dried material. This helps to gain insight into the shelf life of the product and allows covering drug development up to GLP toxicology studies [8].

Evaluation of long-term stability using Atomic force microscopy (AFM) at this stage of the formulation development can help in the reduction of stability program from months to hours, by detecting phase separation in solid dispersions systems at nanometer scale [39].

In the scope of preclinical studies, lead SDSD of CDP146 was prepared as suspension in a liquid vehicle that contains the stabilizer agent of interest identified during Stage 2 (i.e., 10% (w/v) PVPVA) combined with 1% (w/v) HPC-SSL as a standard suspending agent and 0.1% (w/v) antifoam in 100 mM citrate buffer (pH 4). The influence of the API dose on the stability of the oral liquid formulation was assessed at 1, 10, 30 and 50 mg/mL during 8 h by monitoring drug crystallization in the formulation. The assessment of suspensions stability is a mandatory step before oral administration to animals in order to ensure that no physical change of the ASD has occurred as it can negatively impact drug exposure and lead to misleading interpretation of in-vivo results. XRPD patterns of the wet solid filtrate collected from the oral formulation at t_0, t_{4h} and t_{8h}, are depicted in Figure 7. Results obtained in XRPD reveal that the ASD in suspension remained amorphous in the vehicle and did not convert into its original crystalline state even after 8 h at an API concentration of 50 mg/mL. Similar results were obtained in XRPD after evaporation of the wet solid filtrate, while PLM observations confirm the lack of birefringence of the ASD suspension (data not shown).

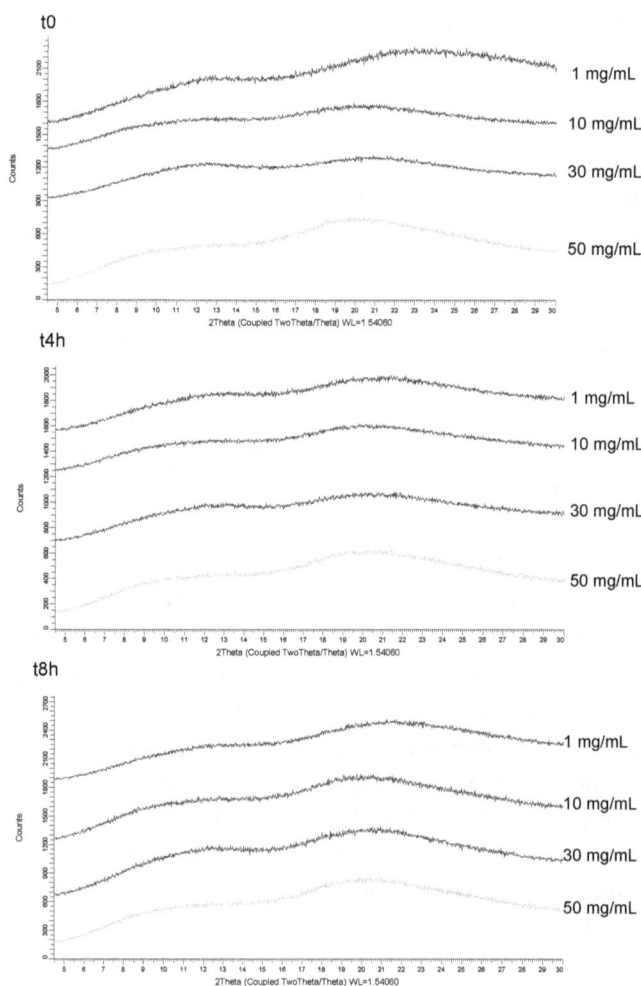

Figure 7. XRPD patterns of the wet solid filtrate collected from the suspension of CDP146/HPMCAS-LF 40:60 (w/w) in 10% (w/v) PVPVA, 1% (w/v) HPC-SSL and 0.1% (w/v) antifoam in 100 mM citrate buffer (pH 4) at 1, 10, 30 and 50 mg/mL.

Figure 8 depicted the Raman spectra of crystalline CDP146 and ASD suspension of CDP146/HPMCAS-LF 40:60 (w/w) prepared at 10 mg/mL and acquired after 0, 4 and 8 h under magnetic stirring (350 rpm). As seen in Figure 8, arrows represented in the Raman spectrum of crystalline API point the characteristic peaks of crystalline CDP146 that displayed significant difference from its amorphous counterpart in a selected region of the Raman Shift. Moreover, the Raman spectra of ASD suspension obtained after 4 and 8 h in the formulation vehicle appear to be identical to the freshly prepared formulation. As no specific peak changes were observed during the run, it is likely that the ASD suspensions remained in the amorphous state throughout the studied time. This provides evidence of the formulation capacity to remain amorphous up to 8 h and confirms the previous results obtained in XRPD and PLM. The aforementioned considerations regarding the stability of the oral formulation confirm the choices made with respect to carrier selection, DL and stabilizer used in the liquid vehicle. Although Raman spectroscopy was used to double-check the results obtained from XRPD and therefore confirms the formulation stability, its application might be optional in order to speed up the oral formulation development process.

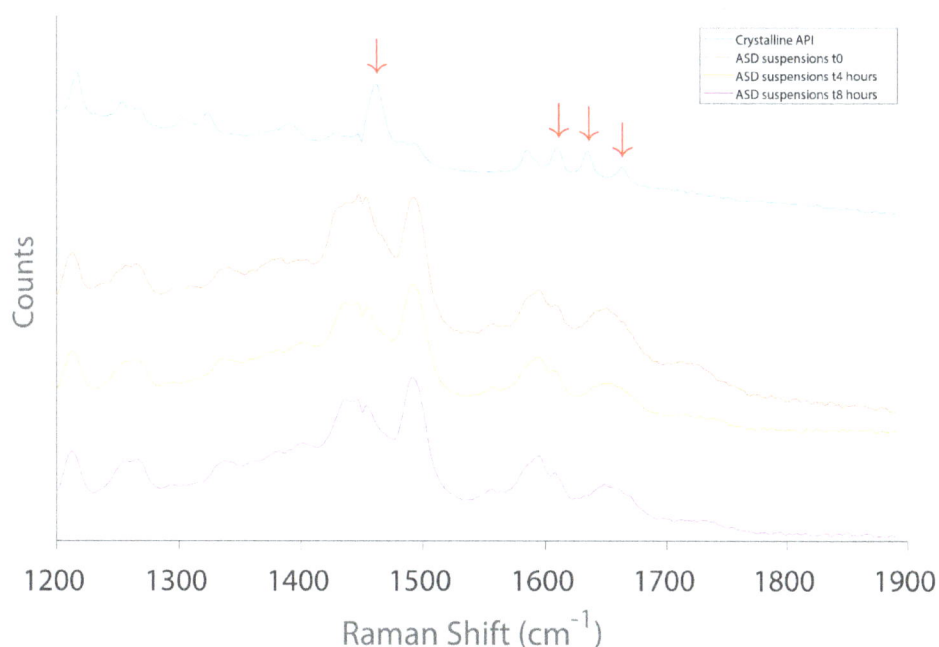

Figure 8. Raman spectra of pure crystalline CDP146 and CDP146/HPMCAS-LF 40:60 (w/w) suspensions (10 mg/mL) recorded at t_0, t_{4h} and t_{8h}.

Since the ASD suspension formulation was found to maintain its amorphous state for longer than the transit time of species used during preclinical studies, the potential of the oral formulation to enhance drug solubility in bio-predictive conditions was evaluated. In this regard, in-vitro dissolution that intended to mimic the gastro-intestinal tract of rat species was conducted as it constituted the most commonly used model during preclinical studies [8]. Dissolution profiles of crystalline drug and oral formulation prepared at various API concentrations in gastric medium and rat intestinal simulated compartments, are depicted in Figure 9. Solubility improvement percentages of oral formulation compared to crystalline drug in gastric and intestinal fluids after 30 and 60 min, respectively, are given in Figure 10. As seen in Figure 9, oral formulation prepared at four different API doses was found to enhance drug solubility, considerably in both gastric and intestinal fluids. Solubility improvement of about 1000% was obtained for oral formulation prepared at 10–50 mg/mL in intestinal compartments. The dissolution profile of each formulation displayed a plateau during the entire duration of the dissolution tests with no recrystallization process. The capacity of the tested oral formulation to maintain supersaturation in intestinal compartment of rat during the absorption window would allow enhancing oral drug bioavailability, considerably. The fact that drug did not recrystallize from supersaturated solution in gastric and first compartment of intestine can be partially attributed to the role of enteric carrier to delay drug release below the pH of polymer hydration. This confirms the great potential of using enteric polymer in the scope of preclinical activities. Despite a dilution factor of 2 between the gastric medium to the intestinal fluid, the solid dispersion formulation was found to display a 'reservoir' effect by recovering high drug solubility in the first minutes of dissolution in each intestinal compartment. Moreover, the different concentrations of supersaturation generated in each of the intestinal compartments, can be attributed to the different compositions of bile salts. As an example, the level of drug concentration reached by the 50 mg/mL formulation was reduced by a factor 2 between the first two intestinal compartments when SIF content was decreased from 35.6 mM to 14 mM. Additionally, no major difference was obtained in the dissolution profile of formulation prepared at 10–50 mg/mL. This can be explained on the basis that at 10 mg/mL, the amorphous solubility is reached in each of the biofluids and increasing API dose to 50 mg/mL cannot exceed this value. Further results generated during in-vivo studies would be necessary to compare the potential of 10–50 mg/mL formulations. Additional tests including drug absorption simulation by a biphasic system can be examined to discriminate formulation prepared at various doses [13]. At this stage, the conduction of dissolution tests in bio-predictive conditions reveals that oral formulation in the API dose range of 1–50 mg/mL was found to fulfill the necessary requirements to be addressed during in-vivo administration studies. In this regard, larger batch production of CDP146/HPMCAS-LF 40:60 (w/w) can be performed to support the preclinical studies.

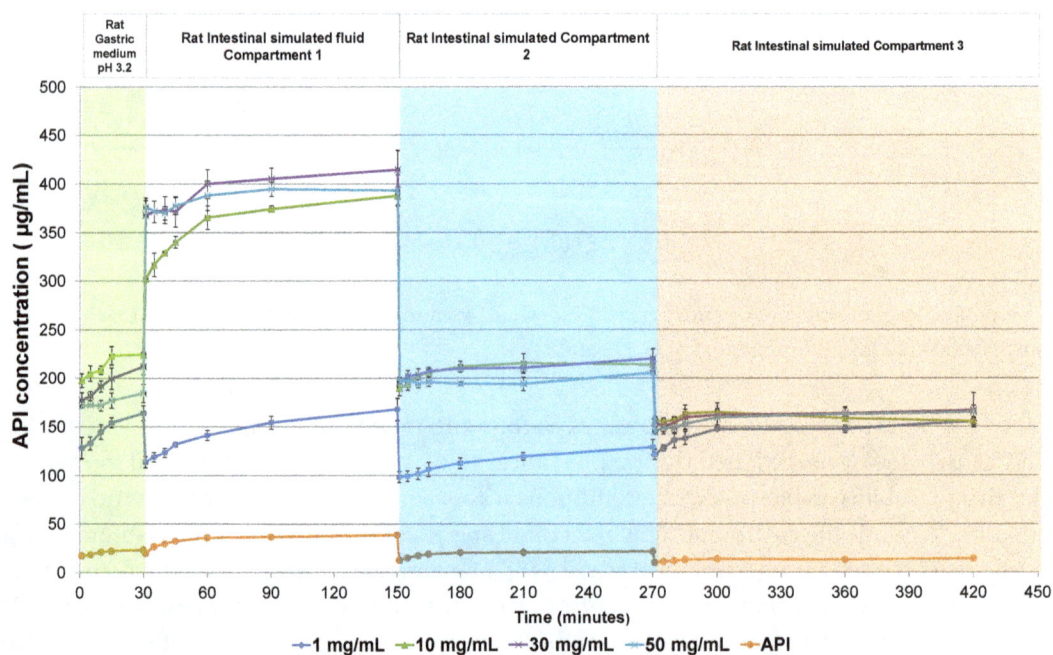

Figure 9. Dissolutions profiles of CDP146/HPMCAS-LF 40:60 (w/w) suspension and pure crystalline API in bio-predictive conditions mimicking gastro-intestinal tract of rat species at an API concentration of 1, 10, 30 and 50 mg/mL.

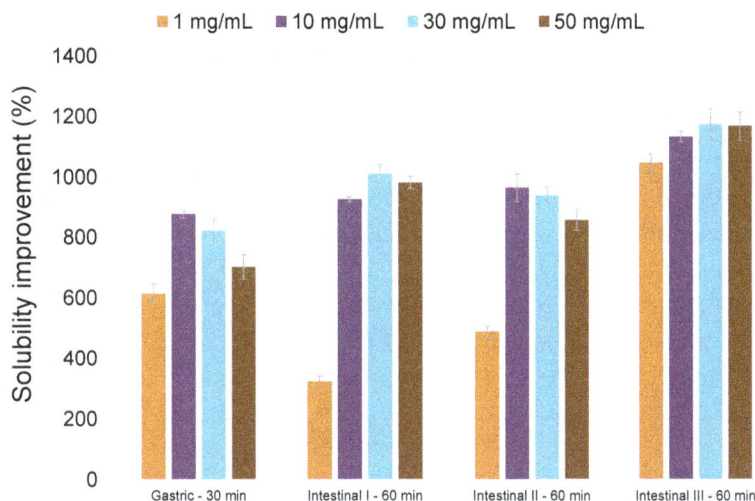

Figure 10. Solubility improvement (%) of CDP146/HPMCAS-LF 40:60 (w/w) suspension compared to crystalline drug after 30 and 60 min in gastric and intestinal fluids, independently.

This novel screening approach developed internally at UCB Pharma has been found to provide a rational selection of polymer and DL prior to the development and manufacturing of SDSD. The proposed three-stage decision protocol has been successfully applied in several projects and respects the development constraints in terms of API consumption and time resources. A maximum amount of 735 mg of API and a duration of 9 days are required in order to screen four polymers and four stabilizers at two different DLs. In the current case study, 600 mg of CDP146 and 9 days were needed from solvent screening stage to the oral formulation optimization.

Additionally, during the traditional ASD pathway development, once the lead API-polymer system has been identified, an additional step including process development using mini spray-dryer is required to finetune optimal DL and identify robust processing and formulation conditions for the manufacturing of SDSD. This transfer stage from screening to mini spray-dryer is basically based on a 'trial and error' approach and requires significant investment in time and API. In a recent study, Wyttenbach et al. (2013) estimated that the traditional ASD solvent casting program using rotary evaporator requires 16 weeks of development time and up to 10 g of API to screen 5 polymers at 2 DLs before the first ASD batch production can be started using mini spray-dryer [18]. In contrast to that, the implementation of spray-drying in a small-scale approach as it occurs for the first time in the proposed strategy allows removing this supplementary stage in ASD development. Herein, the downscaling approach proposed in the current study constituted a more simple and efficient methodology than traditional formulation development, reducing API consumption by a factor 13 and screening/formulation development time by a factor 12.

Contrary to classical ASD development using film casting or quench cooling during the screening phase, the proposed strategy allowed reducing the influence of the preparation method on the polymer and DL selection. Based on experience, it is almost impossible to change the carrier identified during screening phases once the manufacturing phase has started. Results obtained in the current study highlighted that small-scale batches of SDSD generated in the first stage of the screening strategy display similar properties in terms of miscibility, T_g value and solid state compared to larger scale production. This allows to finetune DL selection in the first stage of screening stage and gain insight into the final performance of SDSD.

Particular attention has been paid to propose a screening strategy where only standard analytical equipment were needed, to ensure this approach can be simple enough to be applicable in various pharmaceutical development laboratories. To enable solid state and miscibility characterization of screened SDSDs before and after incubation, the use of mDSC, XRPD and PLM was combined.

Non-sink dissolutions conditions with regard to the crystalline API were performed to assess the solubility enhancement potential of screened SDSDs and the extent of supersaturation.

Although drug–polymer interactions have not been investigated, the authors assume that the results obtained during the physical stability studies and dissolution tests provide valuable information on the polymer's potential to interact with the drug by preventing recrystallization [40]. Additionally, the systematic evaluation of drug–polymer miscibility has given insight into solid dispersion performance and homogeneity i.e., the formation of ideal glass solution is a proof of drug–polymer homogeneity at molecular level. Further studies will focus on adapting this screening approach for the development of ternary SDSDs in which a second polymer/surfactant is added to the ASD blend to improve the solid state stabilization of the amorphous drug as well as the maintenance of supersaturation during dissolution [41,42].

4. Conclusions

The proposed screening approach implements for the first time spray-drying in a methodical small-scale approach for the development of ASD during preclinical activities. This novel screening strategy based on a three-stage decision protocol was verified with CDP146 by evaluating the performance of SDSDs in terms of drug–polymer miscibility, physical stability and in-vitro dissolution. Among the four polymers screened, HPMCAS-LF was found as the adequate carrier to provide physically stable SDSD of CDP146 at 40% (w/w) DL. Best performing stabilizer (10% (w/v) PVPVA) was identified during Stage 2 of the proposed strategy, to help maintain supersaturation during the absorption window of orally administered suspension formulations.

The total duration of the screening and the oral formulation development phases require 9 days and a maximum of 735 mg of API to screen four polymers and four stabilizers at two different DLs. In the current study where the screening protocol was verified with CDP146, only 600 mg of CDP146 and 9 days were needed. In this regard, the proposed screening approach can be classified as a material sparing approach, particularly adapted for the development of SDSDs in the industrial sector. Moreover, the choice of using only standard analytical equipment (e.g., mDSC, XRPD, PLM and TGA) during the screening protocol would ensure wide applicability and facilitate its use to a large number of development groups in the pharmaceutical industry.

Small ASD batches as low as 20 mg were obtained by spray-drying and were representative from larger scale SDSD productions in terms of drug–polymer miscibility and solid state. To this extent, this downscaling approach has never been reported in literature, previously and would allow reducing efforts to correlate information from bench to batch manufacturing. Compared to standard screening methodologies e.g., solvent casting and quench cooling, the proposed screening strategy would improve the prediction accuracy with regards to SDSD properties and performance, resulting in a de-risking and rational selection of appropriate carrier and DL. This is explained on the basis that the process variability factor linked to the choice of the preparation method is minimized. Application of this novel and superior screening approach in UCB projects has replaced previous practices as it demonstrated a straight pathway from screening to manufacturing phases and eased the drug development progress, considerably.

Author Contributions: Conceptualization, A.O., R.C. and P.S.; Methodology, A.O., R.C. and P.S.; Validation, M.A.S. and K.D.; Investigation, A.O.; Resources, F.R., M.A.S. and K.D.; Writing—Original Draft Preparation, A.O. and P.S.; Writing—Review and Editing, A.O., M.A.S. and K.D.; Supervision, F.R., M.A.S. and K.D.; Project Administration, K.D.

Funding: This work is part of the PhD research of A.O. and it was funded by the Product Development department of UCB Pharma.

Acknowledgments: The authors would like to thank the grant from the Product Development department of UCB Pharma and the technical assistance from the solid state characterization group of UCB Pharma. A particular attention was addressed to Ludovic Jeanne and Pedro Durão for their respective help and advice in dissolution tests and Raman experiments assistance, respectively.

Abbreviations

ACN	Acetonitrile
AFM	Atomic force microscopy
API	Active pharmaceutical ingredient
ASD	amorphous solid dispersions
DCM	Dichloromethane
DL	Drug-loading
EtOH	Ethanol
HPLC	High performance liquid chromatography
mDSC	Modulated differential scanning calorimetry
NCE	New chemical entity
PLM	Polarized light microscopy
RH	Relative humidity
SDSD	Spray-dried solid dispersion
SIF	Simulated intestinal fluids
T_g	Glass transition temperature
TGA	Thermogravimetric analysis
T_m	Melting temperature
XRPD	X-ray powder diffraction

References

1. Nieto-Gutierrez, M. Non-clinical assessment requirements. In *Safety and Efficacy of Medicines/Human Medicines Development and Evaluation*; European Medicines Agency: London, UK, 2013.

2. Gad, S.C.; Cassidy, C.D.; Aubert, N.; Spainhour, B.; Robbe, H. Nonclinical vehicle use in studies by multiple routes in multiple species. *Int. J. Toxicol.* **2006**, *25*, 499–521. [CrossRef] [PubMed]

3. Kalepu, S.; Nekkanti, V. Insoluble drug delivery strategies: Review of recent advances and business prospects. *Acta Pharm. Sin. B* **2015**, *5*, 442–453. [CrossRef] [PubMed]

4. Thackaberry, E.A. Vehicle selection for nonclinical oral safety studies. *Expert Opin. Drug Metab. Toxicol.* **2013**, *9*, 1635–1646. [CrossRef] [PubMed]

5. Turner, P.V.; Pekow, C.; Vasbinder, M.A.; Brabb, T. Administration of substances to laboratory animals: Equipment considerations, vehicle selection, and solute preparation. *J. Am. Assoc. Lab. Anim.* **2011**, *50*, 614–627.

6. Kawabata, Y.; Wada, K.; Nakatani, M.; Yamada, S.; Onoue, S. Formulation design for poorly water-soluble drugs based on biopharmaceutics classification system: Basic approaches and practical applications. *Int. J. Pharm.* **2011**, *420*, 1–10. [CrossRef] [PubMed]

7. Vo, C.L.N.; Park, C.; Lee, B.J. Current trends and future perspectives of solid dispersions containing poorly water-soluble drugs. *Eur. J. Pharm. Biopharm.* **2013**, *85*, 799–813. [CrossRef] [PubMed]

8. He, Y.; Ho, C. Amorphous solid dispersions: Utilization and challenges in drug discovery and development. *J. Pharm. Sci.* **2015**, *104*, 3237–3258. [CrossRef] [PubMed]

9. Teja, S.B.; Patil, S.P.; Shete, G.; Patel, S.; Bansal, A.K. Drug-excipient behavior in polymeric amorphous solid dispersions. *J. Excip. Food Chem.* **2013**, *4*, 70–93.

10. Singh, A.; Van den Mooter, G. Spray drying formulation of amorphous solid dispersions. *Adv. Drug Deliv. Rev.* **2016**, *100*, 27–50. [CrossRef] [PubMed]

11. Chen, X.Q.; Stefanski, K.; Shen, H.; Huang, C.; Caporuscio, C.; Yang, W.; Lam, P.; Su, C.; Gudmundsson, O.; Hageman, M. Oral delivery of highly lipophilic poorly water-soluble drugs: Spray-dried dispersions to improve oral absorption and enable high-dose toxicology studies of a p2y1 antagonist. *J. Pharm. Sci.* **2014**, *103*, 3924–3931. [CrossRef] [PubMed]

12. Chiang, P.C.; Ran, Y.; Chou, K.J.; Cui, Y.; Sambrone, A.; Chan, C.; Hart, R. Evaluation of drug load and polymer by using a 96-well plate vacuum dry system for amorphous solid dispersion drug delivery. *AAPS Pharm. Sci. Tech.* **2012**, *13*, 713–722. [CrossRef] [PubMed]

13. Dai, W.G.; Pollock-Dove, C.; Dong, L.C.; Li, S. Advanced screening assays to rapidly identify solubility-enhancing formulations: High-throughput, miniaturization and automation. *Adv. Drug. Deliv. Rev.* **2008**, *60*, 657–672. [CrossRef] [PubMed]

14. Janssens, S.; De Zeure, A.; Paudel, A.; Van Humbeeck, J.; Rombaut, P.; Van den Mooter, G. Influence of preparation methods on solid state supersaturation of amorphous solid dispersions: A case study with itraconazole and eudragit e100. *Pharm. Res.* **2010**, *27*, 775–785. [CrossRef] [PubMed]

15. Shanbhag, A.; Rabel, S.; Nauka, E.; Casadevall, G.; Shivanand, P.; Eichenbaum, G.; Mansky, P. Method for screening of solid dispersion formulations of low-solubility compounds–miniaturization and automation of solvent casting and dissolution testing. *Int. J. Pharm.* **2008**, *351*, 209–218. [CrossRef] [PubMed]

16. Ousset, A.; Meeus, J.; Robin, F.; Schubert, M.A.; Somville, P.; Dodou, K. Comparison of a novel miniaturized screening device with büchi b290 mini spray-dryer for the development of spray-dried solid dispersions (SDSDs). *Processes* **2018**, *6*, 129. [CrossRef]

17. Ousset, A.; Chavez, P.F.; Meeus, J.; Robin, F.; Schubert, M.A.; Somville, P.; Dodou, K. Prediction of phase behavior of spray-dried amorphous solid dispersions: Assessment of thermodynamic models, standard screening methods and a novel atomization screening device with regard to prediction accuracy. *Pharmaceutics* **2018**, *10*, 29. [CrossRef] [PubMed]

18. Wyttenbach, N.; Janas, C.; Siam, M.; Lauer, M.E.; Jacob, L.; Scheubel, E.; Page, S. Miniaturized screening of polymers for amorphous drug stabilization (spads): Rapid assessment of solid dispersion systems. *Eur. J. Pharm. Biopharm.* **2013**, *84*, 583–598. [CrossRef] [PubMed]

19. Parikh, T.; Gupta, S.S.; Meena, A.K.; Vitez, I.; Mahajan, N.; Serajuddin, A.T. Application of film-casting technique to investigate drug-polymer miscibility in solid dispersion and hot-melt extrudate. *J. Pharm. Sci.* **2015**, *104*, 2142–2152. [CrossRef] [PubMed]

20. Overhoff, K.A.; Moreno, A.; Miller, D.A.; Johnston, K.P.; Williams, R.O. Solid dispersions of itraconazole and enteric polymers made by ultra-rapid freezing. *Int. J. Pharm.* **2007**, *336*, 122–132. [CrossRef] [PubMed]

21. Ueda, K.; Higashi, K.; Yamamoto, K.; Moribe, K. The effect of hpmcas functional groups on drug crystallization from the supersaturated state and dissolution improvement. *Int. J. Pharm.* **2014**, *464*, 205–213. [CrossRef] [PubMed]

22. Rowe, R.C.; Sheskey, P.J.; Owen, S.C. *Handbook of Pharmaceutical Excipients*, 5th ed.; Pharmaceutical Press: London, UK, 2006; Volume 5.

23. Patel, R.P.; Patel, M.P.; Suthar, A.M. Spray drying technology: An overview. *Indian J. Sci. Technol.* **2009**, *2*, 44–47.

24. Albers, J.; Matthee, K.; Knop, K.; Kleinebudde, P. Evaluation of predictive models for stable solid solution formation. *J. Pharm. Sci.* **2011**, *100*, 667–680. [CrossRef] [PubMed]

25. Engers, D.; Teng, J.; Jimenez-Novoa, J.; Gent, P.; Hossack, S.; Campbell, C.; Thomson, J.; Ivanisevic, I.; Templeton, A.; Byrn, S.; et al. A solid-state approach to enable early development compounds: Selection and animal bioavailability studies of an itraconazole amorphous solid dispersion. *J. Pharm. Sci.* **2010**, *99*, 3901–3922. [CrossRef] [PubMed]

26. Meng, F.; Trivino, A.; Prasad, D.; Chauhan, H. Investigation and correlation of drug polymer miscibility and molecular interactions by various approaches for the preparation of amorphous solid dispersions. *Eur. J. Pharm. Sci.* **2015**, *71*, 12–24. [CrossRef] [PubMed]

27. Janssens, S.; Van den Mooter, G. Review: Physical chemistry of solid dispersions. *J. Pharm. Pharmacol.* **2009**, *61*, 1571–1586. [CrossRef] [PubMed]

28. Rumondor, A.C.; Stanford, L.A.; Taylor, L.S. Effects of polymer type and storage relative humidity on the kinetics of felodipine crystallization from amorphous solid dispersions. *Pharm. Res.* **2009**, *26*, 2599–2606. [CrossRef] [PubMed]

29. Huang, Y.; Dai, W.G. Fundamental aspects of solid dispersion technology for poorly soluble drugs. *Acta Pharm. Sin. B* **2014**, *4*, 18–25. [CrossRef] [PubMed]

30. Paudel, A.; Worku, Z.A.; Meeus, J.; Guns, S.; Van den Mooter, G. Manufacturing of solid dispersions of poorly water soluble drugs by spray drying: Formulation and process considerations. *Int. J. Pharm.* **2013**, *453*, 253–284. [CrossRef] [PubMed]

31. Baghel, S.; Cathcart, H.; O'Reilly, N.J. Polymeric amorphous solid dispersions: A review of amorphization, crystallization, stabilization, solid-state characterization, and aqueous solubilization of biopharmaceutical classification system class ii drugs. *J. Pharm. Sci.* **2016**, *105*, 2527–2544. [CrossRef] [PubMed]

32. Ormes, J.D.; Zhang, D.; Chen, A.M.; Hou, S.; Krueger, D.; Nelson, T.; Templeton, A. Design of experiments utilization to map the processing capabilities of a micro-spray dryer: Particle design and throughput optimization in support of drug discovery. *Pharm. Dev. Technol.* **2013**, *18*, 121–129. [CrossRef] [PubMed]

33. ProCept. Procept information brochure spray dryer. Available online: http://www.procept.be/spray-dryer-chiller (accessed on 27 August 2018).

34. Sun, D.D.; Wen, H.; Taylor, L.S. Non-sink dissolution conditions for predicting product quality and in vivo performance of supersaturating drug delivery systems. *J. Pharm. Sci.* **2016**, *105*, 2477–2488. [CrossRef] [PubMed]

35. Baird, J.A.; Van Eerdenbrugh, B.; Taylor, L.S. A classification system to assess the crystallization tendency of organic molecules from undercooled melts. *J. Pharm. Sci.* **2010**, *99*, 3787–3806. [CrossRef] [PubMed]

36. Paudel, A.; Van den Mooter, G. Influence of solvent composition on the miscibility and physical stability of naproxen/pvp k 25 solid dispersions prepared by cosolvent spray-drying. *Pharm. Res.* **2012**, *29*, 251–270. [CrossRef] [PubMed]

37. Lin, X.; Hu, Y.; Liu, L.; Su, L.; Li, N.; Yu, J.; Tang, B.; Yang, Z. Physical stability of amorphous solid dispersions: A physicochemical perspective with thermodynamic, kinetic and environmental aspects. *Pharm. Res.* **2018**, *35*, 1–18. [CrossRef] [PubMed]

38. Li, B.; Konecke, S.; Wegiel, L.A.; Taylor, L.S.; Edgar, K.J. Both solubility and chemical stability of curcumin are enhanced by solid dispersion in cellulose derivative matrices. *Carbohydr. Polym.* **2013**, *98*, 1108–1116. [CrossRef] [PubMed]

39. Lauer, M.E.; Siam, M.; Tardio, J.; Page, S.; Kindt, J.H.; Grassmann, O. Rapid assessment of homogeneity and stability of amorphous solid dispersions by atomic force microscopy–from bench to batch. *Pharm. Res.* **2013**, *30*, 2010–2022. [CrossRef] [PubMed]

40. Baghel, S.; Cathcart, H.; O'Reilly, N.J. Theoretical and experimental investigation of drug-polymer interaction and miscibility and its impact on drug supersaturation in aqueous medium. *Eur. J. Pharm. Biopharm.* **2016**, *107*, 16–31. [CrossRef] [PubMed]

41. Prasad, D.; Chauhan, H.; Atef, E. Amorphous stabilization and dissolution enhancement of amorphous ternary solid dispersions: Combination of polymers showing drug-polymer interaction for synergistic effects. *J. Pharm. Sci.* **2014**, *103*, 3511–3523. [CrossRef] [PubMed]

42. Ziaee, A.; Albadarin, A.B.; Padrela, L.; Faucher, A.; O'Reilly, E.; Walker, G. Spray drying ternary amorphous solid dispersions of ibuprofen—An investigation into critical formulation and processing parameters. *Eur. J. Pharm. Biopharm.* **2017**, *120*, 43–51. [CrossRef] [PubMed]

10

Bioinspired Designs, Molecular Premise and Tools for Evaluating the Ecological Importance of Antimicrobial Peptides

Elvis Legala Ongey [1,*] **⬦**, **Stephan Pflugmacher** [2,3] **and Peter Neubauer** [1]

[1] Department of Biotechnology, Technische Universität Berlin, Ackerstraße 76, ACK24,
D-13355 Berlin, Germany; peter.neubauer@tu-berlin.de

[2] Aquatic Ecotoxicology in an Urban Environment, Ecosystems and Environment Research Program, Faculty of Biological and Environmental Sciences, University of Helsinki, Niemenkatu 73, FI-15140 Lahti 2, 00100 Helsinki, Finland; stephan.pflugmacher@helsinki.fi

[3] Korean Institute of Science & Technology Europe, Joint Laboratory of Applied Ecotoxicology, Campus E7 1, 66123 Saarbrücken, Germany

* Correspondence: elvis.ongey2@gmail.com

Abstract: This review article provides an overview of recent developments in antimicrobial peptides (AMPs), summarizing structural diversity, potential new applications, activity targets and microbial killing responses in general. The use of artificial and natural AMPs as templates for rational design of peptidomimetics are also discussed and some strategies are put forward to curtail cytotoxic effects against eukaryotic cells. Considering the heat-resistant nature, chemical and proteolytic stability of AMPs, we attempt to summarize their molecular targets, examine how these macromolecules may contribute to potential environmental risks vis-à-vis the activities of the peptides. We further point out the evolutional characteristics of the macromolecules and indicate how they can be useful in designing target-specific peptides. Methods are suggested that may help to assess toxic mechanisms of AMPs and possible solutions are discussed to promote the development and application of AMPs in medicine. Even if there is wide exposure to the environment like in the hospital settings, AMPs may instead contribute to prevent healthcare-associated infections so long as ecotoxicological aspects are considered.

Keywords: antimicrobial peptides; ecotoxicity; bacteriocins; therapeutic; polyproline helix; membrane disruption

---

1. Introduction

There are many classes of natural compounds, five of which are prevalent in natural product research today, namely: polyketides, alkaloids, terpenoids, ribosomal and non-ribosomal peptides [1], the latter two groups are called antimicrobial peptides (AMPs). AMPs, also known as host defense peptides evolved from ancient times and are an integral component of the innate immune system of most organisms where they function as effector molecules. AMPs may be classified based their biosynthesis mechanism (ribosomal and non-ribosomal), biological sources (bacterial, plants, animal etc.), biological functions (antibacterial, antiviral, antifungal etc.), peptide properties (hydrophobic, amphipathic, cationic etc.), covalent bonding pattern (disulfide bonds, N- to C-termini peptide linkage etc.), 3D structure (alpha-helical, beta-sheet, alpha-beta and non-alpha-beta) and molecular targets (cell surface, and intracellular targeting peptides). Figure 1 presents the 3D structures of some common AMPs from plant and animal sources. AMPs occur naturally in many forms most of which are cationic amphiphilic compounds, constituting evolutional host defense machineries present in different species of all life forms.

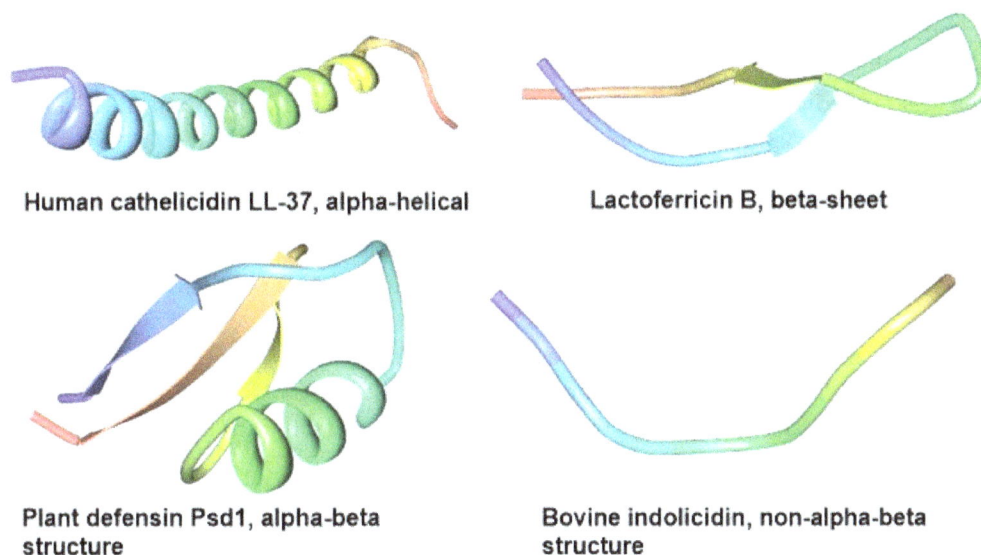

Figure 1. 3D structures of selected AMPs, depicting four structural families based secondary structures found in the compound: alpha, beta, alphabeta and non-alphabeta. Structures were edited with protein workshop using the solution NMR structural data for Human cathelicidin LL-37 (PDB: 2K6O), lactoferricin B (PDB: 1LFC), plant defensin Psd1 (PDB: 1JKZ) and bovine indolicidin (PDB: 1G89).

The fundamental differences that exist between single-cell and multicellular organisms allow them to be targeted differently by AMPs. Some exhibit activities against wide variety of targets such as viruses, bacteria and fungi [2–4]. Others may function beyond the margins of antimicrobials to include disruption of tumour-infected cells [5] as well as modulating organ activity like the cathelicidin AMP which regulates pancreatic islets [6]. Furthermore, rational modifications and the in vivo incorporation of unnatural amino acids into the peptides may further expand the chemical space and provide new diversified functional characteristics [7], including, but not limited to, modulation of chemotaxis, cytokine release and wound healing. Although these modifications may enhance the applicability of the desired compound, little attention is given to the possible effects of such stable molecules on the surrounding environment especially with regards to degradability and the prevention of tolerant bacteria from emerging.

Early studies generally considered the bacterial cytoplasmic membrane as a unique target for AMPs but within the last two decades several reports describing alternative mechanisms of action exist [8–13]. They function over wide pH ranges [14,15], showing extreme stabilities to heat and protease degradation [16–18], and very little or no development of microbial resistances. While these characteristics are generally regarded as attractive features of the peptides, only the latter seems more useful in terms of safety. The fact that AMPs are currently contemplated for potential pharmaceutical use as alternatives to conventional drugs, with a host of them already undergoing clinical trials [19], extensive investigations are required to determine safety of modified analogues and rationally designed synthetic members. AMPs may also be widely implemented in food processing [20]. Most AMPs are obtained from natural origins [21,22], which makes them generally considered as safe for human consumption as opposed to their synthetic counterparts. Interestingly, the market for peptide drugs is increasing steadily as well [23]. However, clinical development and eventually therapeutic application of AMPs are usually thwarted by high manufacturing costs, host toxicity and substandard pharmacokinetic properties which are primarily attributed to their susceptibility to proteolytic inactivation and sustained serum binding in physiological environments [24–27].

Several approaches have been proposed and are currently utilized to improve these challenges created by the intrinsic properties of AMPs [28–31]. In-depth knowledge of structure-activity relationships has enabled the design of synthetic AMP mimics with biocompatible properties, providing another valuable strategy which is also presently employed by many research groups to address some of the drawbacks. Results of these approaches have been reported in many examples like the cationic β-stranded peptide [32], non-membrane-lytic peptides [33], the α-helical OP-145 [34] and the amphipathic helical WR12 and β-sheet D-IK8 peptides [35], which all showed potent antibacterial activities and reduced toxicity to human cells. The quest for new anti-infective compounds is growing over time but information on how to evaluate the ecological effects of these molecules are relatively scarce. The fact that most (if not all) AMPs interact with the lipid bilayer membranes is not a matter to be taken lightly since virtually all organisms contain this component. A disturbance on the bilayer membranes may weaken their integrity and make them more susceptible destruction, such as lipid peroxidation. Moreover, some can even penetrate and interact with intracellular components and as such, artificial AMPs in particular must be evaluated for possible ecotoxicological effects.

Remarkably, some AMPs have structural similarities to well-known toxins like the spider neurotoxin named Cm38 and Cn11, producing considerable toxicity to mammalian cells by themselves [36–38]. It is therefore important to tackle procedures aimed at improving therapeutic qualities of AMPs with caution as novel categories of toxins may evolve in the process. Furthermore, we think that the ability for an AMP to resist heat, protease and chemical inactivation may not only be considered with respect to the benefits those may offer, but also to observe that they may well be difficult to degrade when the need arises. Thus, their investigations must also seek to address some critical feasible queries, which are the possible inactivation/excretion routes and probable side effect if the peptide accumulates in body organs. Perhaps there may be potential ecological effects if the molecules are excreted in their full form. In the present review, we highlight structure-function relationships and mode of action of AMPs that may threaten environmental safety while discussing the use of artificial and/or natural AMPs as templates for rational design of peptidomimetics. We further propose some strategies to reduce cytotoxic effects of AMPs against eukaryotic cells. We also attempt to summarize different molecular targets identified so far, evaluate their possible contributions to environmental instability vis-à-vis the activities of peptides, and suggest methods that may help to assess their ecotoxic mechanisms. Our suggestions are supported by the facts that AMPs may leach via AMP-coated devices, manuring and aquaculture systems, to the surrounding environments; or the peptides may be consumed as drugs or in food (as preservatives) and subsequently excreted into aquatic environments from home reservoirs. However, AMPs are highly potent against pathogenic microbes, targeting multiple cellular macromolecular structures whose constituent building blocks or conformational dynamics vary from species to species and therefore, resistance development is rare. As such, the above phenomena may instead contribute to prevent healthcare-associated infections in hospital settings and food-borne illnesses so long as environmentally friendly species are not targeted.

2. Diverse Sources of AMPs

Genome sequencing and transcriptomic data show that AMPs are ubiquitous in nature, and present in almost all living organisms [39–43], providing defensive roles that significantly protect the host from competing organisms in their respective ecological niches and ensure their survival [44]. Several different AMP families exist (e.g., bacteriocins, defensins etc.), that are isolated from various natural sources with bacterial [39,45], plant [46] and animal [47–49], hosting the majority; while a few are derived from archaea [50], protists [51] and fungi [52]. They may also be derived from chemical synthesis [53]. In the last years the number of newly identified AMPs increased rapidly, supported by the fact that the methods for the isolation, mass detection, sequencing and even structural elucidation have become standard technologies [54]. Wang et al. (2015) reported a total of 2493 registered members (including artificial ones) in the AMP database (APD) at the end of December 2014 [55], 122 natural peptides were isolated in 2015, 86 in 2016, 124 in 2017, adding to 17 new members already reported in 2018 making a total of 2981 compounds hosted by the APD, with well-established sequences and functions. Figure 2 shows a quasi-linear increase in the number of AMPs isolated from natural sources over the last 15 years.

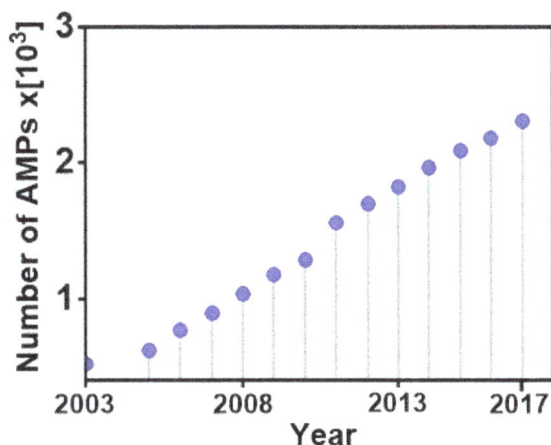

Figure 2. Number of AMPs isolated from natural sources since 2003 (information was extracted from the AMP database (http://aps.unmc.edu/AP).

2.1. Structural Diversity of AMPs from Non-Bacterial Sources

AMPs from plants and animal sources have enormous structural diversity including those described earlier (Figure 1) [56], as well as those illustrated by the examples of EeCentrocin 2 from *Echinus esculentus* [57] and EPrAMP1 from *Echinopsis pachanoi* [37] (Figure 3a,b, respectively). α-helical peptides are usually between 12 and 40 amino acid long and are rich in residues that favour the α-helical conformation like Ala, Leu and Lys. They assume an amphipathic structure when interacting with the membrane [58]. They usually do not contain Cys, but some example like the 11- and 5-kDa peptides purified earlier from guinea pig neutrophils [59] and EeCentrocin 2 (Figure 3a) possesse a unique structural feature by forming an intermolecular disulfide between a heavy chain and a light chain [57]. An additional N-terminal pyroglutamic acid and a C-terminal amidation of the light chain of EeCentrocin 2, as well as the 6-Br-Trp modifications of the heavy chain do not affect its antibacterial function, indicating that these elements may be ascribed to the biostability of the peptide [57].

Contrary to the α-helical peptides, those that adopt the β-sheet conformations contain at least two Cys residues that form between 1 and 5 intramolecular disulfide bonds [60] that stabilize the tertiary structure of the peptides and confer substantial resistance to heat, protease and enzymatic inactivation [61,62]. β-hairpin structures are also common for those containing 2–4 Cys residues e.g., protegrin-1 [63]. A structural motif referred to as the inhibitor cystine knot is an evolutionary conserved feature shared amongst β-sheet peptides as well as the TGF-β/BMP family of regulatory cysteine knot proteins [64]. They provide the conformational correctness that allows the peptides to exhibit diverse biological roles such as antimicrobial, anti-HIV, insecticidal, protease inhibition and G-protein-coupled receptors regulatory activities [62,65–68]. The representative example of EPrAMP1 (Figure 3b) has three disulfide bridges involving (i) Cys1–Cys17, (ii) Cys8–Cys23 and (iii) Cys16–Cys33 disulfide bonds. The interconnecting backbones of (i) and (ii) constitute a ring that impregnates (iii), yielding a structural arrangement that stabilizes three strands of β-sheet covering residues 7–8, 22–26 and 30–34 [37]. The disulfide bonds and stabilized secondary structure contribute extensively to the overall tertiary folded structure which has a flat, disc-shaped appearance.

BnPRP1 from *Brassica napus* (Figure 3c) like many other proline-rich AMPs (PrAMPs) forms random coils with little amount of α-helix composition that engage in a non-lytic modes of bacterial inactivation [69]. Since proline is incompatible with α-helical or β-sheet conformation, its frequent occurrence in a polypeptide sequence causes a conformational rearrangement that forces the molecule to adopt the polyproline II (PPII) helical structure [70–72] and ample evidence suggest that the PPII conformation may be the biologically active form for all PrAMP [72–79].

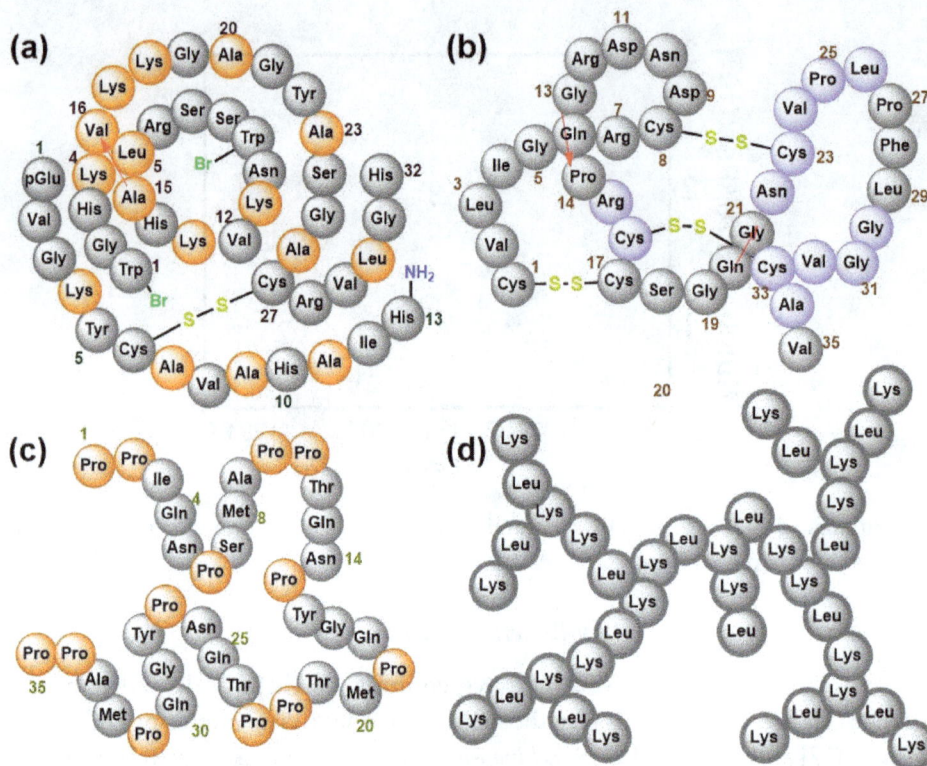

Figure 3. Diversified schematic structures of natural and artificial AMPs. (**a**) EeCentrocin 2 is an α-helical heterodimeric peptide with a heavy and a light chain connected via a disulfide bridge (helix-stabilizing residues are indicated in light brown). (**b**) EPrAMP1 has three disulfide bridges and three strands of beta-sheet (shown in violet). (**c**) BnPRP1 is a proline-rich peptide. (**d**) G3KL is a tree-like synthetic polymer composing of alternating residues of lysine and leucine. Red arrows indicate direction of crossing in the peptide chain.

The PP-II helix is an extended polypeptide structure which is arranged such that it consists of three amino acid residues per turn [80], and it is however, not the only component required to produce antimicrobial activity as Guzmán et al. (2013) showed, that the PPII-like secondary structure of proline homopeptides alone is not enough to elicit bacterial inhibitory effects. This demonstrated the distorting effects of the cyclic side chain of proline that forms a rigid conformation in PrAMPs which may constraint flexible movement at the membrane interface that is necessary to enable the peptide to adopt different structural forms while interacting with the membrane [81].

Studies show that synthetic peptides that are predominantly composed of Lys residues also fold into PPII helix in aqueous solution [72,78], and AMPs with such amino acids composition can interact with bacterial membranes and eventually penetrate into the cell [82,83]. Other studies also revealed that odd-numbered residues of Lysine homopeptides elicit full growth inhibition of Gram-positive and Gram-negative bacteria [72,78]. However, the PPII helix does not seem to apply to the biologically active dendritic topology of G3KL (Figure 3d) whose alternating residues of lysine and leucine produces tree-like branches that kill Gram-negative strains, exhibiting low toxicity to red blood cells [84].

Rationally designed AMPs like the G3KL, IK12 [85] and K4R2-Nal2-S1 [86], mostly target the cell membranes since the functional relationships with this component have been investigated extensively. Although the killing mechanisms of some of the newly identified peptides are not yet investigated, the fact that TLN-58 derived from eccrine sweat upregulates interleukins especially IL-8 [20] suggests that its mode of action may involve chemotaxis and peptide receptor–like induction of angiogenesis which may be used in therapeutic procedures involving mesenchymal stem cells for the treatment of diseases like stroke and spinal cord injury [28]. Similarly EeCentrocins are rich in hydrophobic and positively charged amino acids, hence they contain significant cationicity and hydrophobicity that are necessary to form an amphipathic structure that may enable the peptides to act on the membranes of Gram-positive bacteria because the hydrophilic portion enables interaction with the polar heads, while the hydrophobic regions interact with the hydrophobic core of the lipid bilayer membrane [57]. Summarily, majority of AMPs from sources other than bacteria kill mostly Gram positive bacteria except for a few like G3KL, Thaulin-1 from *Pleurodema thaul* [87], BnPRP1, *Mj*Pen-II from *Marsupenaeus japonicus* [15] and Scolopendin from *Scolopendra subspinipes mutilans* [88] which are able to kill Gram negative and/or other microorganisms. Moreover, some function beyond microbial inhibition/killing e.g., K4R2-Nal2-S1 may be used to treat cancer [86] and TLN-58 for immune modulation [20] as described above.

Summarily, we have seen that a wide variety of structural motifs exist in eukaryotic AMPs (and rationally designed peptides), but they possess an amphipathic structure that is a common feature to all of them. This feature enables them to bind and interact at the lipid bilayer membrane interface. The fact that most of these peptides interact with the lipid bilayer membranes is particularly concerning since such disturbance on the membranes may weaken their strength and render the cells more prone to lysis. Moreover, some AMPs (mostly from plants and insects) have the ability to penetrate the membrane and interact with intracellular processes and as such, this must be kept in mind when modifying or designing a new molecule to ensure its relevance and safety.

2.2. Structural Diversity of AMPs from Bacterial Sources

AMPs produced by bacteria are generally called ribosomal or non-ribosomal peptides based on their biosynthesis mechanism. Those that are ribosomally synthesized are generally referred to as bacteriocins. Bacteriocins are defined as "a group of proteinaceous substances produced at ribosomal level, having multifunctional properties whose antimicrobial activities are concentration-dependent [89]". This definition largely eliminate the general consideration that they are amphipathic in nature and possessing an overall positive charge, because anionic AMPs such as subtilosin A do exist [90]. Bacteriocins are prevalent amongst all species of bacteria especially the lactic acid bacteria (LAB). They are grouped into three main classes namely; post-translationally modified bacteriocins (class I), unmodified bacteriocins (class II) and bacteriolysin (class III) [91]. Bacteriocins usually inactivate their targets via membrane disruption or by forming pores, or even terminate cell division by targeting and dissociating lipid II which serves as a precursor molecule during bacterial cell wall synthesis [91].

Research has demonstrated that amongst the different families of AMPs, bacteriocins may be used as alternatives to conventional antibiotics based on their diverse structural characteristics and remarkable potencies against drug-resistant bacteria strains [45]. Class I bacteriocins are more interesting with respect to the diverse structural forms present in this group. A subclass referred to as lasso peptides possess a characteristic ring formed via an amide bond between the first residue of the core peptide and a negatively charged core residue at positions +7, +8 or +9; after which the ring then embodies the linear C-terminus of the sequence [1,91,92]. Additional modifications such as intramolecular disulfide bridges like in the case of sviceucin (Figure 4a) from *Streptomyces sviceus* [93,94] are also possible. Such structural arrangement confers high stability to the peptides and hence they may be used as peptide scaffolds [91].

Cyclic bacteriocins are also modified peptides that contain a head-to-tail peptide bond linkage (involving condensation of the N- and C-termini) to generate the cyclic structure of the molecules [95]. All members possess α-helices of similar sizes that fold into a tertiary structure having a central pore surrounded by a compact globular bundle comparable to the saposin folds [96–98]. A good example is carnocyclin A (Figure 4b) from *Carnobacterium maltaromaticum* [99]. Furthermore, glycocins are a group of bacteriocins with one or more residues in the peptide chain linked to a carbohydrate moeity [1]. Sublancin 168 (Figure 4c) is an example of a glycocin from *Bacillus subtilis* with a β-S-linked glucose moiety [100,101]. Another group of bacteriocins called the sactipeptides contain sulphur-to-α-carbon linkages [1,90]. Extensive studies performed with subtilosin A (an example of this class) from *B. subtilis* [102] show that the carbon-sulfur linkages and hairpins are common structural elements [95,103,104]. Subtilosin A has three sulfur-to-α-carbon cross-linkages (Figure 4d) and demonstrate wide activity spectrum against a variety of bacterial strains [90,105]. Overall, the occurrence of these natural structural features, posttranscriptional modifications and unusual amino acids make the peptides more stable and effective as anti-infective agents.

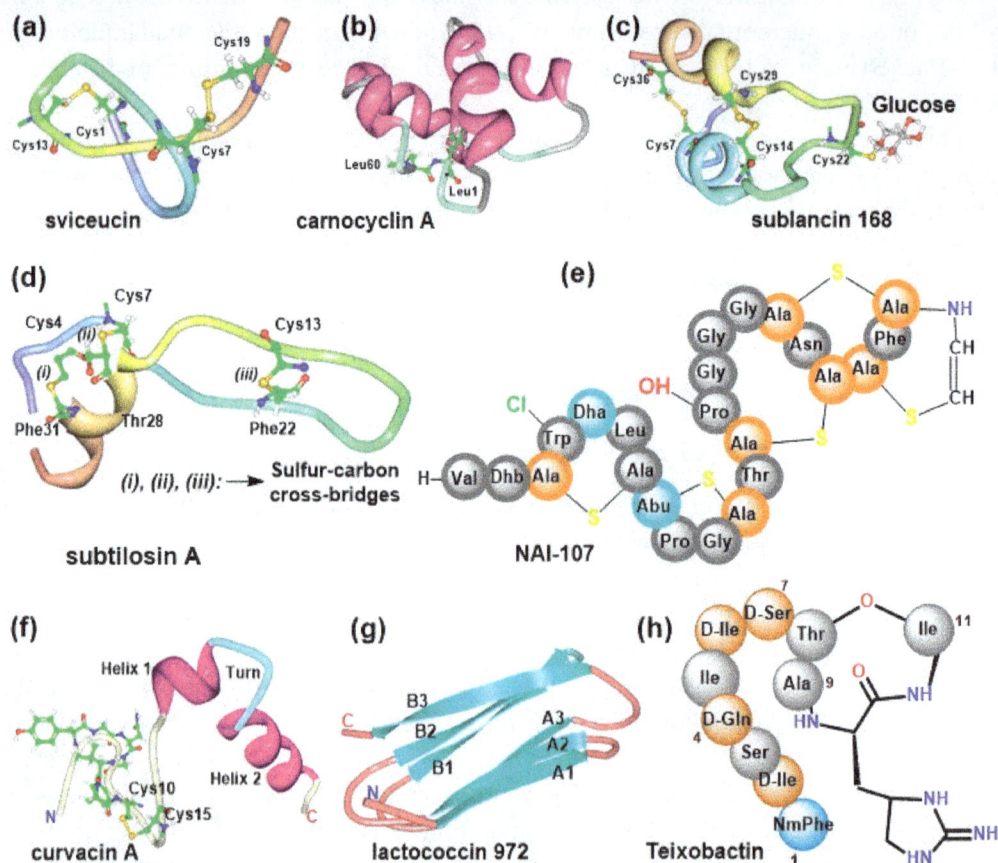

Figure 4. Structure of selected peptides from bacterial sources. (**a**) Lasso peptides sviceucin, showing two intramolecular disulfide bridges. (**b**) Circular peptide carnocyclin A, showing N- to C-terminal peptidyl linkage between Leu1 and Leu60. (**c**) Glycocin peptide sublancin 168, showing a glucose moiety linked to Cys22 and two intramolecular disulfide bridges. (**d**) Sactipeptides subtilosin A, showing the coordination of the sulfur-α-carbon bridges. (**e**) NAI-107 has 5 intramolecular thioether cross-linkages, additional 5-chloro-trypthopan, mono-/bis-hydroxylated proline and a c-terminal aminovinylcysteine. (**f**) Pediocin-like curvacin A, showing the N-terminal YGNGVXC conserved motif, the N-terminal intramolecular disulfide bridge between to Cys10 and Cys15, and the distinct C-terminal helical region. (**g**) Non-pediocin-like single-peptide lactococcin 972. (**h**) Non-ribosomally synthesized peptide teixobactin compose of four D-amino acids, enduracididine and an N-terminal methylphenylalanine. Structures were edited with protein workshop using the solution NMR structural data for each molecule.

Class I bacteriocins, also referred to as lantibiotics are ribosomally synthesized and comprise of non-proteinogenic amino acids and cross-linkages formed between dehydrated side chains of threonine/serine and the sulfhydryl group of cysteine. An example is NAI-107 (Figure 4e) from

Microbispora sp. [106] where additional modifications such as hydroxylation of proline, halogenation of Trp and aminovinylcysteine also exist. Unnatural amino acid and thioether rings are prevalent in the different classes of lantibiotic [107,108] while hydroxylation, halogenation [57,106,109,110], and even therapeutically relevant moieties like *N*-glycosylation [111] are rarely present in a few examples. The posttranslational modifications in lantibiotics make them more resistant to protease degradation [112] and also accord them limited conformational freedom which confers target specificity [113]. The rigid conformational flexibilities facilitate high biological activities with very low minimal inhibitory concentrations (MICs) against wide variety of infections ranging from antimicrobial to antiallodynic effects [114].

Pediocin-like bacteriocins are heat-stable and are produced by a variety of LAB [115]. Their N-terminus has an overall positive charge, a disulfide bridge formed between two cysteine residues and a conserved YGNGVXC consensus motif (Figure 4f), which may be actively involved in target recognition and the killing process [115,116]. The disulfide bridge may play a stability role and not necessary directly involved in the killing process since its replacement by hydrophobic interaction did not abolish the activity of leucocin A [117]. An unmodified bacteriocin like the heat-labile Lactococcin 972 (Figure 4g) has two three-stranded antiparallel β-sheets that fold into a β-sandwich to confer stability [118].

The presence of unnatural amino acids in peptides revolutionize their overall activities against multidrug-resistant microbes with very low MIC [119,120]. Teixobactin (Figure 4h) is a non-bacteriocin peptide with interesting chemical constitution including four D-amino acids, enduracididine, an N-terminal methylphenylalanine and a thioesterase ring formed between Thr8 and Ile11 [121]. These features provide resilience and target-specific properties to most non-ribosomally synthesized peptides including vancomycin, bacitracin and valinomycin making them therapeutically more interesting.

It is worthy to note that altering the features that are responsible for activity or stability like hydrophobicity, α-helices, β-strands and unnatural amino acids may help to improve the therapeutic qualities of AMPs but may also produce negative effects on the desired functions. For instance, D-amino acids is important in enhancing biostability but its coexistence with L-amino acids tend to form special structural motifs that may be responsible for non-specificity and cytotoxicity [122]. However, altering these motifs in most cases result in drastic decrease in activity [123]. Meanwhile suboptimal structural arrangement of the peptide may take credit for such eventualities, it may be prudent to rethink on making these peptides more specific to make them safe for human consumption and ecofriendly to other organisms.

3. General and Specific Modes of Action of AMPs

Some reviews analyzed the different modes of action of AMPs and explained how bacteria may develop resistances against them by modifying their cell surfaces to sequester or repel the peptide, secreting proteases that inactivate them, producing transmembrane efflux pumps, forming biofilms and secreting molecules that may trap the AMP and inhibit their activities [9,124]. Although theoretical analyses of the pharmacodynamic differences between AMPs and conventional antibiotic with regards to their propensities to illicit resistance evolution show low probabilities for AMPs [125], extensive knowledge on the different molecular targets and their responses to AMPs' interaction is required to fully understand and prevent these situations. Widespread opinions hold that most antibacterial peptides engage in membrane interactive mechanisms to inactivate their targets. However, this general believe has gradually faded away over the last two decades as numerous studies have identified different molecular targets (Table 1). Most AMPs exhibit conformational amphipathicity at the bacterial membrane interface to enhance electrostatic interactions with the negatively charged surface [126,127]. Irrespective of an AMP's killing mechanism, the peptide may adopt a different conformation at the level of bilayer membrane to facilitate its activity. α-helical AMPs for example usually permeabilize the cytoplasmic membrane into subcellular compartments to interrupt essential cellular pathways [128].

A model by Sánchez-Barrena et al. describes the interactions between α-helical AMP and the lipid bilayer. As illustrated in Figure 5 (grey-shaded region), two protomeric units of the bacteriocin AS-48 interact via their hydrophobic and polar helices to produce two dimeric forms. The free-state dimeric form (I) targets the membrane and undergoes a transition from dimeric form (I) to the second dimeric form (II) at the membrane's surface. Their non-polar regions are then buried into the hydrophobic core of the phospholipid bilayer while the polar helices interact with the polar heads [129]. Additionally, an earlier model described how cationic peptides cross the lipopolysaccharides (LPS) of Gram negative bacteria into the periplasm and subsequently engage the cytoplasmic membrane [130]. The simultaneous interaction and disruption of membrane bilayer may be achieved in different ways. Three well-established methods of how AMPs perform these actions include barrel-stave pore, carpet, and toroidal pore mechanisms [131,132] as illustrated in Figure 5. At low concentrations some AMPs, mainly PrAMPs, stereoselectively diffuse into the cell via the membrane protein SbmA to interfere with intracellular pathways by binding to molecular components such as DNA and RNA as well as cytoplasmic and membrane-bound proteins [70,132]. However, they may also nonspecifically invade the lipid bilayer at high concentrations (Figure 5).

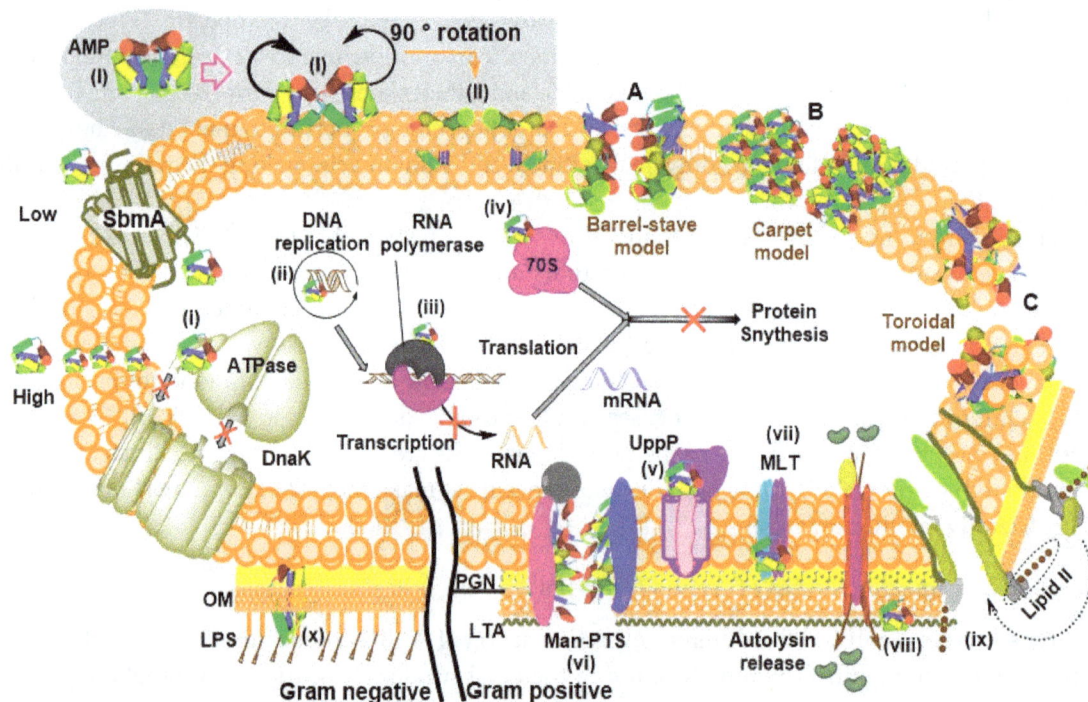

Figure 5. Membrane penetration mechanisms and mode of action of AMPs. Shaded region illustrates a structural model of the molecular interaction of an AMP with the phospholipid bilayer. **A,** Barrel-stave pore membrane disruption mechanism where the peptides line the hollow pore, and are oriented parallel to the phospholipid chains. **B,** Carpet mechanism where the peptides have a detergent-like effect on the membrane. **C,** Toroidal pore where the lumen of the pore constitutes a mixture of peptide and phospholipids resulting from perpendicular insertion of the peptides in the bilayer. Non-invasive mechanisms of AMPs include binding to: (**i**) DnaK, (**ii**) duplex DNA helices (**iii**) RNA polymerase, (**iv**) 70S ribosome, (**v**) undecaprenyl pyrophosphate phosphatase (UppP), (**vi**) mannose phosphotransferase system (Man-PTS), (**vii**) maltose transporter (MLT), (**viii**) Lipoteichoic acid (LTA), (**ix**) lipid II, inhibiting cell wall biosynthesis, and (**x**) LPS. The abbreviations PGN, peptidoglycan; OM, outer membrane.

Conceivably, the binding of AMPs to lipid bilayer are purposefully driven by the negatively charged surfaces of bacteria cells, contributed by the predominance of teichoic acids at the cell surface of Gram-positive [133] and the LPS of the outer membrane of Gram negative bacteria [134]. However, other opinions argue that sustained interaction at the outer membrane interface may constrain the effectiveness of AMP by decreasing the active concentration that finally arrives the cytoplasmic membrane where bactericidal activity is actually observed [135]. Furthermore, PrAMPs constitute the group of peptides that do not destroy the membranes, but engage in non-lytic inhibitory approaches against microbes via distinct molecular mechanisms involving cell penetration and intracellular localization [70,136–138]. PrAMPs may also interact and/or bind to LPS of Gram negative bacteria which initiates a conformational change whose rate is dependent on the structural properties of the compound [139].

Table 1. Characterized AMP targets and their killing mechanisms.

Target Molecule	Killing Method	Examples	Reference
MLT	Efflux of intracellular and/or influx of extracellular solutes	Garvicin ML	[140]
Man-PTS	Efflux of intracellular and/or influx of extracellular solutes	Pediocin-like bacteriocins, Lactococcin A, microcin E492	[73,141]
UppP	Disrupts cell-wall synthesis	Lactococcin G and Enterocin 1071	[10]
MBM	Prevent proteolytic breakdown of a misfolded protein	LsbB	[13,142]
70S ribosome	Inhibit protein synthesis	Bac7$_{(1-35)}$, insect-derived PrAMPs	[143,144]
RPol	Inhibit transcription by obstructing RNA polymerase activity	Microcin J25, Capistruin	[145,146]
DnaK	Inhibit ATPase activity	Pyrrhocoricin, Bac7 (PrAMPs)	[137,147,148]
LTA	Release of autolysin	RTD2 and Pep5	[149]
Lipid II	Inhibit cell wall biosynthesis, pore formation	nisin	[150]
LPS	Restrict LPS binding to CD14+ cells and hence prevent fatal septic shock syndrome Interact with AMP and enable folding	Human cathelicidin LL-37 Indolicidin, magainin 2, cecropin A, esculentin-derived AMP, pyrrhocoricin	[12,33,137,139,151,152]
DNA/RNA	Inhibiting DNA replication	Indolicidin, Buforin II, tachyplesin, RR4	[11,153,154]

Abbreviations: MBM, Membrane-bound metallopeptidase; RPol, RNA polymerase.

Non-lytic peptides are obviously interesting to investigate further to identify additional properties that enable them to perform their functions. Some may also combine membrane disruption and cytoplasmic genomic DNA binding which further facilitates cell death [155]. The physiological responses of organisms when attacked by an AMP through various activity targets are described in Table 1, citing an overview of well-characterized examples.

4. Potential Applications and Accompanying Challenges

AMPs have a wide range of possible uses including therapeutic, template for creating new drugs and in medical devices; largely ascribed to their ability to elicit antimicrobial activity over a wide spectrum at low MICs. They bind specific targets, exhibit little endotoxic effects, act synergistically with conventional antibiotics, and display negligible tendencies to develop resistances [156]. Comprehensive reports describing therapeutic successes of AMPs with reference to the number of patents approved or applied for since 2003 were recently published [157,158]. These articles described the universal trends and approaches implemented in rational design of novel peptides and techniques used to decipher and evaluate possible routes of biological activity. Some loopholes such as susceptibility of the peptides to host protease inactivation and in vivo toxicity were also highlighted as associated factors that limit effective therapeutic applicability [158].

A variety of potential medical applications like the treatment of bacterial biofilms and associated complications [159], implementations in ectopic therapeutic operations, synergistic action in combination with conventional antibiotics against multidrug-resistant pathogens, and their use as building blocks for rational peptide drug design to overcome therapeutic challenges [160], were reviewed recently. Different AMP-containing formulation strategies have been considered to resolve the problem of chemical or biological inactivation of the drug molecule and also reduce adverse effects, thereby enhancing their potencies and safety [161]. Typical applicable examples in biomedical science like the potential use of cathelicidin-overexpressing bacteria to treat inflammatory bowel disease, taking advantage of its antifibrogenic effects in models of colitis, is possible [162]. In fact, endogenous AMP production has been suggested as an ideal approach for multiple disease treatment in humans and animals [127]. Furthermore, epithelial tissue repair, treatment of wound infections and promoting wound healing, that are chiefly inspired by the immune stimulatory properties of some AMPs are also attainable [163].

The generation of antimicrobial surfaces on medical devices is an interesting area for both researchers and medical practitioners especially for implant therapy. Different immobilization techniques exist [164] to create antimicrobial surfaces that are modified to leach out anti-infective agents onto the surface of the material or the surface itself is designed to possess bactericidal properties, thereby preventing contamination and reducing disease burdens from healthcare-associated infections [165,166]. Additionally, a plausible way to fight biofilm-related infections in clinical settings is to coat the abiotic surfaces of medical implantable devices with multifunctional AMPs that remain stable over prolonged periods, to supply anti-infective functions and/or prevent microbes from sticking to the device [156,167]. AMPs may be used in peptide surface coating, biosensors and detection, and nanoparticle-based drug delivery [9]; e.g., in microfluidic chip where the peptides were coated via cysteinyl interactions to a gold surface and used to specifically detect varied species of bacteria [168]. Low sample consumption in such experiments is an added advantage of surface covalent tethering of AMPs [32]. Interestingly, this strategy may also be used to identify possible mechanisms of action since only membrane disruptive peptides may easily elicit significant activity when immobilized. This may further reduce costs of pre-clinical evaluation with respect to amount of the product required for studies and hence encourage investments in this direction.

Tethering AMPs to solid surfaces via physical or chemical means may be compromised by the peptide's disorientation, reduced flexibility, limited surface density of reactive groups, coupling conditions and steric hindrances, which may affect final biological activity [169,170]. Perhaps it is also difficult to obtain biomolecular structures of surface immobilized peptides. The physical immobilization technique may have some downsides that circumvent its extension to medical devices namely; short-term antibacterial effect and the leaching of antibacterial agents with potential environmental toxicity that may also encourage development of microbial resistances [171–173]. The same scenario could also be observed if AMPs were to be applied in disinfectants that are mostly used in hospital environments. It is conceivable that tethering AMPs to abiotic surfaces would require biostable, physically and chemically resistant molecules, which require huge capital and intellectual investments to achieve. Although realizing such a project may be an attractive venture opportunity, potential actors mostly feel apprehensive about the outcome.

5. The Paradox Surrounding Artificial AMPs and Semisynthetic Derivatives

Efforts to develop artificial antimicrobials have grown over time as scientists try to resolve the challenges of antimicrobial resistances. Although, this strategy allows for flexibility in designing active candidates, unaddressed concerns that may hinder progress in this direction seem likely to have a direct link to limited information that is available on their pharmacological properties. Poor intrinsic therapeutic qualities of AMPs such as biostability, solubility and bioavailability under physiological conditions, are amongst the strategic factors that restrict their clinical applications as drugs. Synthetic mimics are mostly inspired by the natural compounds' abilities to kill multidrug-resistant pathogens at very high potency, while guaranteeing enhanced pharmacological properties like low MIC and low toxicity [119]. In general, both peptidic and non-peptidic synthetic variants have been inspired by the amphiphilicity of natural AMPs since numerous studies have identified this structural feature to be responsible for their functions. Many interesting molecules with significant functional properties have been produced such as AMPs with a hydrophobic center, flanked by two cationic regions [32] and K4R2-Nal2-S1 that possesses both antibacterial and anticancer activities [86].

The huge conformational flexibility of artificial peptides may cause them to be less specific thereby facilitating interactions with a wide range of targets and eventually producing side effects and unfavourable immunogenic responses [25]. As an alternative solution, semisynthetic modifications of naturally produced peptides may be used, which are efficiently produced in a bioprocess, but chemically or enzymatically modified afterwards [174]. Variants of deoxyactagardine B [175,176] and nisin [6] are such examples of how the clinical value of natural AMPs can be increased by the use of such combined strategies. Moreover, semi-synthesis is a greener process and produces higher yields within a shorter timeframe than total synthesis. Given that natural AMPs show little adverse effects and very low median effective dose, both in vitro and in vivo, in comparison to conventional antibiotics [45], it may be helpful to utilize their backbones as templates rather than creating entirely new synthetic peptides that may provoke unexpected side reactions. This can also be achieved by tackling modular approaches via the use of specific incorporated non-canonical amino acids into the peptide chain that warrant modifications via click chemistry [7,177]. Unnatural amino acids would expand the chemical reactivity space within a peptide and thus create room for enhancing biological activities as well as diversifying its applications [7,178].

Furthermore, the costs of developing a new peptide may be an argument for starting with a natural one which already has some kind of selectable biological activity. As an example, dendritic peptides like the G3KL described earlier are easier to produce and generally have a relatively simple structure [179]. Their stability enable them to be used in several applications including antimicrobial and tumor-targeting functions [180]. However, care must be taken when considering them as drug candidates since an example like the G3KL possesses structural features that are analogous to antibodies, which consequently may provoke undesired immunogenic responses. The fact that they can self-assemble into helical pores [181] may also increase their toxicity to higher organisms preceding insertion of the hydrophobic regions into the lipid bilayer membrane. Attention must be drawn to the fact that this is just one of many structural features that may result from an artificial peptide design. Even more worrying is also the fact that some of the features (e.g., PPII helix) allow interaction and membrane translocation of the molecules. Paradoxically, there exists a plethora of research supporting the design and use of artificial peptides as alternative drug candidates. We are of the view that utilizing natural AMPs as backbones in semisynthetic processes is an effective way to design novel compounds and to develop lower-cost production processes that are amenable to economically feasible industrial applications. Moreover, having a natural backbone is advantageous in that the properties of the new molecule may not deviate very much from the original one, and therefore its safety limits would not be narrowed.

6. Controlling the Unspecificity of AMPs

This section focusses on possible structural and molecular bases of unspecificity since details of the kind of conformational transitions that a peptide adopts at the bilayer membrane are subjects still under investigation to decipher the molecular mechanisms of toxicity. Analyzing the physicochemical parameters that influence attraction of a peptide to the cytoplasmic membranes of both bacterial and eukaryotic cells, may be very helpful in therapeutic considerations once a correlation with a biological assays is established. Some AMPs that have significant bactericidal activity profiles also display higher levels of hemolytic activities like the recent cases of EPrAMP1 and EeCentrocins [37,57]. Methods such as adding D- and fluorinated amino acids into the core peptides to restrict targeting of host cells have been discussed earlier [182]. However, substituting residues for D-amino acid or proline in respective AMPs considerably reduced their amphiphilicity and/or helicity, decreased binding affinities to cell membranes as well as bactericidal activity [183,184]. A similar approach was used earlier to reduce cytotoxicity of AMPs marked by eukaryotic cell membrane damage [185]. Therefore a compromise must be anticipated between the desired biological effect and the overall applicability of the final product.

The structural motifs of the non-lytic PrAMP may be interesting for rational design or modifications of already existing peptides to improve their activities and reduce toxicity to eukaryotic cells. A comparison between the cytotoxic activities of Pro, Lys and Arg homopeptides with increasing peptide chain lengths showed a trend with proline consistently displaying lower cytotoxicity [72]. Nonetheless, little is known about the interactions of specific groups or the PPII helical conformation of PrAMPs with eukaryotic cells. A recent publication described a couple of methods that may be used to investigate bacterial membrane permeabilization and localization of PrAMPs in the cytoplasm where they interfere with cellular functions [186]. The review postulated a variety of means to generate data that would eventually enhance the design of potent antimicrobial agents, however, the molecular description of how the peptides translocate across the cell membrane that could perhaps have strengthened these suggestions are scarcely available in current literature. Nevertheless, a recent study by Tossi's group showed that human LL-37 forms covalently linked hexamers at higher concentrations and also demonstrated a strong correlation between the type of oligomerization and antimicrobial activity, as well as nonspecific disruption of target [187]. Prior to this work, already Johansson et al. (1998) had established a model that described the dependence of the formation of α-helices and the concentration of a peptide to the following oligomerization. The authors recognized the hydrophobic effect of the oligomers as the driving force behind the conformational rearrangement [188].

Although it was suggested that disrupting helix formation may be a conceivable means of mitigating cytotoxicity of AMPs [189,190], it would not be logical to proceed as such since the approach also decreased the anti-infective properties of the compounds. Both cytotoxicity and antimicrobial activity of an AMP are equally important during therapeutic evaluation and therefore it is necessary to first consider the physiological environment where it will act and how much potency is desired to tune the peptide to achieve maximum clinical effects. Moreover, the presence of α-helices and β-strands in a peptide, combined with increased cationicity and amphipathicity leads to improved antibacterial effects. On the contrast, reducing its charge or hydrophobicity and amphipathicity results in simultaneous decrease in potency and cytotoxicity [28,128,191,192]. Schmidtchen and colleagues discussed how hydrophobic modifications of AMPs may provide alternative means of addressing these issues by supplying information on how to correlate physicochemical observations to biological realities [193]. Although it is unclear why an AMP like EeCentrocin 2 is highly haemolytic, engineering the peptide to reduce its hydrophobicity at the helix hydrophobic face may significantly decrease its cytotoxicity, though at the expense of antimicrobial activity [182].

The positions and types of hydrophobic residues distribution play a key role in the antimicrobial activity of an AMP and have therefore enabled the rational design of a few compounds with potent activities [184,194]. For example, it was reported that the addition of β-naphthylalanine to the C-

or N-terminus of an AMP induces higher cytotoxicity [195], while incorporating positive charged residues like lysine and arginine to the N- and/or C-terminus reduced toxicity to human red blood cells and human fibroblasts [86,196]. Interestingly, incorporating a bulkier hydrophobic group into an inactive chymotrypsin-resistant human LL-37 peptide revived its anti-MRSA properties and also played an additional role by recruiting monocytes to the infection site [197].

Finally, AMPs function synergistically with conventional antibiotics [198,199] and as such, coupling the antibiotic molecule to the peptide via chemical means may help to improve stability and limit likelihood of microbial resistance by (i) offering biological and physicochemical resistance to the peptide without altering the peptide chain and (ii) multiple killing mechanisms by the conjugated compounds which may allow for lower MICs incapable of eliciting toxicity to host cells or development of resistances by the targeted organisms. This type of modification has already been reported where a diaminoalkane chain and a 3,5-dichlorobenzylamine group were coupled to the C-terminus of deoxyactagardine B to produce NVB302 and NVB333 [175,176], both having very good pharmacokinetic/pharmacodyanamic profiles [27]. Nevertheless, the complexity and cost of producing each component, as well as deciding at which position to incorporate the drug molecule to the peptide chain are some of the questions that extensive research in this area may help to resolve.

7. Molecular Premise for Evaluating the Ecotoxicity of AMPs

Generally, AMPs especially those of class I bacteriocins, as well as unnatural amino acids containing members have complicated structures that are not easily degraded via natural enzymatic processes. They also have high resistance to heat and chemical inactivation which may prevent degradation of the compounds both in vitro and in vivo. Whether these properties represent potential environmental risk factors remains an open question. We try to address this question by discussing some molecular interactions that draw attention towards the topic. First and foremost, AMPs may leach out from AMP-coated devices, manuring and in aquaculture to the surrounding environments. If consumed in food and animal feed (as preservatives) or as therapeutic drugs, they may be released into the wastewater effluent from home reservoirs.

Proposing a methodology to evaluate cellular targets for AMPs and the mechanisms of their action is technically challenging and risky because of the complexity of their killing mechanism which may involve more than one target, and thus require sophisticated methodological approaches. Nowadays, several methods have been developed for that purpose ranging from phenotype and metabolite profiling, to microscopic and biophysical studies using artificial membranes, different types of hemolytic assays, endotoxin-release assays etc. Since optimal assay conditions may vary depending on the expected outcomes, integrative approaches that incorporate short-term and long-term perturbations by a compound on the environment would be effective in toxicity screening. However, before evaluating toxic mechanisms like genotoxicity, oxidative stress responses, ATP leakage, nucleic acids binding etc., demographic endpoints like organism's survival, growth inhibition, motility, population changes and reproduction must have shown clear indications [200] that ascertain the ecotoxicity risk of an AMP. A summary of standard tests that are routinely used to assess the environmental risks of chemicals, including details of environmental species, exposure and test endpoints are described elsewhere [200,201]. Meanwhile present ecotoxicological evaluation focus predominantly on nanoparticles and other industrial chemicals that are occasionally leached to the environment, attention has rarely been given to AMPs despite structural similarities of some members to unfriendly toxins [36–38]. We discuss here some aspects of AMPs' killing mechanisms that directly or indirectly interrupt survival, growth or reproduction, and examine how these events may factor into potential environmental risks and how they may be assessed.

7.1. Cell Wall

Like vancomycin and isoniazid, AMPs such as polybia-MPI, G3KL, EeCentrocin 1 and 2 and indolicidin kill their targets by disrupting the cell wall [57,84,202,203]. Cellulosic or chitinic multilayered cell walls are common in fungi, algae and higher plants while bacteria contain Lipoteichoic acid (LTA) and lipopolysaccharides (LPS). These structures constitute defensive barriers that when compromised may result in deleterious consequences. Although unspecific disruption of cell wall may be considered as a potential threat, LPS distinguish prokaryotic cell envelopes from those of eukaryotes by having lower anionic charge and high cholesterol levels [204]. Since some AMPs elicit antimicrobial activities via LPS [12,33,137,139,151,152] and because of its ubiquitous presence in microorganisms, the LPS layer may be a specific target to treat infections. An acute toxicity evaluation of environmentally friendly microbes that possess this unique feature may be performed using the luminescent bacterium *Vibrio fischeri*. Gram staining, SR2200 dye [205] and Lugol's solution [206] may be used in conjunction with transmission and/or scanning electron microscopy to investigate the status of the cell wall.

7.2. Lipid Bilayer Membrane and Pore Formation

The size, cationic charge and amphipathic nature allow interactions and subsequent insertion of AMPs into the lipid bilayer membrane to form pores via several mechanisms described as 'carpet', 'barrel-stave' or 'toroidal-pore' [132]. Pore-forming AMPs constitute an integral part of the pathogenic microbial virulence arsenal [207]. Epithelial barriers are usually compromised by pore-forming toxins secreted by proliferating bacterial pathogens that help to modulate or disrupt the host immune system, producing cellular responses such as changes in ion concentrations and membrane repairs [208]. Reports show that cytotoxicity to mammalian cells is observed at elevated concentrations of AMP, plausibly via apoptotic mechanisms of cell death [209]. Although AMPs can perform their desired function at suboptimal concentrations, it is necessary to be able to evaluate their effects in a broad range since the peptide may accumulate to build concentrations that exceed safety limits. For example EeCentrocin 2 has an unexplained high hemolytic activity [57], which may apply to other AMPs as well. Their abilities to nonspecifically damage eukaryotic cell membranes drives the need for ecotoxicity evaluation. This is because indiscriminate disruption of the cell membrane could constitute an adverse condition that limit the proliferation of non-target organisms. Hemolytic assays such as the lactate dehydrogenase activity assay may be used to assess hemolysis while methods like the anilinonaphthalene-8-sulfonic acid uptake [210] or the dye leakage assay [211] may be used to measure concentration-dependent membrane disruption.

7.3. Nucleic Acid Binding or Damage

Stereoselective diffusion across the plasma membrane into the cell is a common phenomenon exhibited by non-lytic peptides like the PrAMPs [70,132]. The hypotheses that translocated AMPs can inhibit enzymatic activity, nucleic acids or protein syntheses are supported by a few studies [11,145,146,153,154]. Interruption of intracellular pathways may in fact be a bigger problem since it cannot be easily detected. CM15 is an example of AMP that induces oxidative stress in *Escherichia coli* [212]. Oxidative stress produces reactive oxygen species that may damage DNA resulting in slow development and low production yields of plants [213] and death of fungal cells [214]. The possibilities that these events might have only long-term effects on the affected organisms should be considered with extreme caution. Therefore, it is necessary to evaluate the extent to which AMPs interact with nucleic acids so that their effects can be better controlled. In plants, oxidative stress responses and other physiological changes in photosynthetic pigment, enzymes activity and lipid peroxidation may be measured as described elsewhere [215–217]. Techniques such as CellROX Green or Amplex Red oxidation assays [214] may be used to evaluate similar situations in smaller microbes. AMPs may bind cytoplasmic genomic DNA to facilitate cell death [155]. The Comet assay has proven to be a sensitive, rapid and reliable tool for assessing genotoxicity [218–220]. It is also important to investigate the specific molecular interactions that facilitate these events in order to establish methods to control them.

7.4. Membrane Transporters and Receptors

So far, MLT, Man-PTS, UppP and MBM have been identified as targets for AMPs activity. These transporters/receptors are important cellular components that enable their smooth functioning. Their interactions with AMPs [for example Garvicin ML with MLT [140] or Lactococcin G with UppP [10]] may be suicidal to the cells since inhibition of the membrane-located receptor may disrupt transportation of sugar or cell wall synthesis. Furthermore, the interaction of LsbB with Membrane-bound metallopeptidase [13] can cause a lot of complication due to accumulation of a misfolded proteins (that would have perhaps been degraded by the MBM) leading to septic shock. We believe that membrane transporters may also function as a docking site for the peptide or that they may be permeable to the molecules, allowing them to cross the membrane and attack other yet to be identified intracellular targets. The identification of the UppP and the metallopeptidase receptors, open new avenues to suggest that the heterogeneous structures of lanthipeptides for example, may have different targets and different killing mechanisms that are not yet known [221].

Sugar transport across the cell membrane may be assessed using rudimentary approaches that measure sugars uptake by cells. Flow cytometry or fluorimetry or liquid scintillation counting may be used in conjunction with a fluorescent sugar analogue like the 2-[N-(7-nitrobenz-2-oxa-1,3-diazol-4-yl) amino]-2-deoxy-D-glucose (2-NBDG) to measure sugar transport across the cell membrane.

The ToxTracker assay [222] which has been extended to identify differences in cellular responses to DNA damage [223] may be used to assess protein misfolding and oxidative stress.

7.5. Chaperones

Apidaecin, pyrrhocoricin and drosocin are PrAMPs that displayed defined interactions with *E. coli* DnaK [224]. However, inactive pyrrhocoricin analogue together with cecropin A or magainin 2 which are membrane-active AMPs did not show any inhibition of this macromolecule [147], indicating structural specificity. The binding of the peptides to this chaperone inhibits its ATPase activity resulting in accumulation of non-functional misfolded proteins [225]. Since all living organisms depend the smooth functioning of the heat shock proteins (chaperones), it makes sense to evaluate the potential effects of AMPs against different environmental species. The ToxTracker assay mentioned above may be used to sense protein misfolding that may result from likely inactivation of the chaperone system by an AMP. However, extensive sequence variation at various domains of the macromolecules in different species makes it possible to design a peptide that would specifically inhibit a target organism, eliminating cross-reactivity that may trigger adverse reactions to the host or facilitate development of resistances.

7.6. RNA polymerase and 70S Ribosomes

Bac7$_{(1-35)}$, and other insect-derived PrAMPs were shown to bind or interact with 70S ribosomes [143,144] while Microcin J25 and Capistruin interacted RNA polymerase [145,146]. In all the reported cases, gene transcription or translation was blocked in the presence of peptide. Structural and biochemical data show that interaction of PrAMPs with the ribosome occur within the exit tunnel where the peptide binds with a reverse orientation and prevent nascent polypeptide chain from entering the elongation phase of translation [79]. Inhibition of transcription and translation can directly affect survival, growth or reproduction. The anti-infective agents acting as inhibitors of these processes obliges further investigations to identify if they can in fact cause significant damages to the ecosystem, but again these macromolecular complexes have dissimilar structural features which serve as a plus in target-specific peptidomimetic drug design.

8. Conclusions

Several screening methods have enabled isolation and characterization of novel antimicrobial peptides both from natural and synthetic sources. Special features are required in the peptides for them to perform the desired functions, provide resilience and target specificities that make them therapeutically interesting. Although the market situation for AMPs like Bacitracin, Polymyxin and Fuzeon® have encouraging records, there is no doubt that AMPs face a lot of developmental challenges ranging from production to clinical development. These obstacles are conflicting with the numerous academic publications that appear every year to argue the potentials of these biomolecules as alternative drug targets. Perhaps better understanding of the mode of action, target molecules or complex, and mechanism of host protection may further improve the current situation and reduce time and capital investments which may be frustrating at best in the event of an unsuccessful venture. The solution to these challenges must be multifaceted in nature. This may include, amongst others, utilizing natural AMPs as backbones in rational semisynthetic desins to improve their therapeutic qualities and engineering the peptides to reduce toxicity to host cells, or increase their activities.

Membrane interactive models like the toroidal pore formation, carpet and barrel-stave pore have allowed the possibilities to evaluate how AMPs affect bacteria based on their conformational flexibilities and nature of the lipids in the bilayer and thus, understanding the molecular interconnectivities of the peptide-target interactions may greatly facilitate the creation of new molecules using the current ones as templates. Analysing the molecular bases of targeting intracellular components is also important to identify the types and nature of interactions involved, which may provide information on how to develop peptides with superior potencies and the propensity to escape bacterial resistances. Meanwhile suboptimal structural arrangement in the peptides may result in drastic decrease in activity, it may be useful to design peptides that are more target-specific to make them safe for human consumption and ecofriendly to other organisms.

Nevertheless, natural AMPs show high potency against pathogenic microbes, targeting multiple cellular macromolecular structures whose constituent building blocks or conformational dynamics vary from species to species and therefore, resistance development is rare. As such, even if there is wide exposure to the environment like in the hospital settings, AMPs may instead contribute to prevent healthcare-associated infections in hospital settings and food-borne illnesses so long as environmentally friendly species are not targeted.

Author Contributions: Conceptualization, P.N. and S.P.; Resources, E.L.O.; Data Curation, E.L.O.; Writing-Original Draft Preparation, E.L.O.; Writing-Review & Editing, E.L.O. and P.N.; Supervision, P.N. and S.P.; Funding Acquisition, P.N.

Funding: This work was supported by the Deutsche Forschungsgemeinschaft (DFG) within the framework of the German Initiative for Excellence (EXC 314). OEL obtained a grant from the Graduate School Scholarship Programme, 2014 (57034101) of the German Academic Exchange Service (DAAD).

Acknowledgments: This work is part of the Cluster of Excellence "Unifying Concepts in Catalysis" coordinated by the Technische Universität Berlin and its graduate school, Berlin International Graduate School of Natural Sciences and Engineering (BIGNSE). PN and OEL are thankful for the support of this program. We acknowledge support by the German Research Foundation and the Open Access Publication Fund of TU Berlin.

References

1. Arnison, P.G.; Bibb, M.J.; Bierbaum, G.; Bowers, A.A.; Bugni, T.S.; Bulaj, G.; Camarero, J.A.; Campopiano, D.J.; Challis, G.L.; Clardy, J.; et al. Ribosomally synthesized and post-translationally modified peptide natural products: Overview and recommendations for a universal nomenclature. *Nat. Prod. Rep.* **2013**, *30*, 108–160. [CrossRef] [PubMed]

2. Cruz, J.; Ortiz, C.; Guzman, F.; Fernandez-Lafuente, R.; Torres, R. Antimicrobial peptides: Promising compounds against pathogenic microorganisms. *Curr. Med. Chem.* **2014**, *21*, 2299–2321. [CrossRef] [PubMed]

3. Van Compernolle, S.; Smith, P.B.; Bowie, J.H.; Tyler, M.J.; Unutmaz, D.; Rollins-Smith, L.A. Inhibition of HIV infection by caerin 1 antimicrobial peptides. *Peptides* **2015**, *71*, 296–303. [CrossRef] [PubMed]

4. Delattin, N.; De Brucker, K.; De Cremer, K.; Cammue, B.; Thevissen, K. Antimicrobial peptides as a strategy to combat fungal biofilms. *Curr. Top. Med. Chem.* **2017**, *17*, 604–612. [CrossRef] [PubMed]

5. Gaspar, D.; Veiga, A.S.; Castanho, M.A. From antimicrobial to anticancer peptides. *A review.* **2013**, *4*, 294.

6.   Koopmans, T.; Wood, T.M.; Hart, P.; Kleijn, L.H.; Hendrickx, A.P.; Willems, R.J.; Breukink, E.; Martin, N.I. Semisynthetic lipopeptides derived from nisin display antibacterial activity and lipid II binding on par with that of the parent compound. *J. Am. Chem. Soc.* **2015**, *137*, 9382–9389. [CrossRef] [PubMed]

7.   Baumann, T.; Nickling, J.H.; Bartholomae, M.; Buivydas, A.; Kuipers, O.P.; Budisa, N. Prospects of in vivo incorporation of noncanonical amino acids for the chemical diversification of antimicrobial peptides. *Front. Microbiol.* **2017**, *8*, 124. [CrossRef] [PubMed]

8.   Omardien, S.; Brul, S.; Zaat, S.A. Antimicrobial activity of cationic antimicrobial peptides against gram-positives: Current progress made in understanding the mode of action and the response of bacteria. *Front. Cell Dev. Biol.* **2016**, *4*, 111. [CrossRef] [PubMed]

9.   Joo, H.-S.; Fu, C.-I.; Otto, M. Bacterial strategies of resistance to antimicrobial peptides. *Philos. Trans. R. Soc. B* **2016**, *371*, 20150292. [CrossRef] [PubMed]

10.   Kjos, M.; Oppegård, C.; Diep, D.B.; Nes, I.F.; Veening, J.W.; Nissen-Meyer, J.; Kristensen, T. Sensitivity to the two-peptide bacteriocin lactococcin G is dependent on UppP, an enzyme involved in cell-wall synthesis. *Mol. Microbiol.* **2014**, *92*, 1177–1187. [CrossRef] [PubMed]

11.   Ghosh, A.; Kar, R.K.; Jana, J.; Saha, A.; Jana, B.; Krishnamoorthy, J.; Kumar, D.; Ghosh, S.; Chatterjee, S.; Bhunia, A. Indolicidin targets duplex DNA: Structural and mechanistic insight through a combination of spectroscopy and microscopy. *ChemMedChem* **2014**, *9*, 2052–2058. [CrossRef] [PubMed]

12.   Ghosh, A.; Bera, S.; Shai, Y.; Mangoni, M.L.; Bhunia, A. NMR structure and binding of esculentin-1a (1–21) NH 2 and its diastereomer to lipopolysaccharide: Correlation with biological functions. *Biochim. Biophys. Acta (BBA)-Biomembr.* **2016**, *1858*, 800–812. [CrossRef] [PubMed]

13.   Miljkovic, M.; Uzelac, G.; Mirkovic, N.; Devescovi, G.; Diep, D.B.; Venturi, V.; Kojic, M. LsbB bacteriocin interacts with the third transmembrane domain of the YvjB receptor. *Appl. Environ. Microbiol.* **2016**, *82*, 5364–5374. [CrossRef] [PubMed]

14.   Chan, Y.S.; Ng, T.B. Northeast red beans produce a thermostable and pH-stable defensin-like peptide with potent antifungal activity. *Cell Biochem. Biophys.* **2013**, *66*, 637–648. [CrossRef] [PubMed]

15.   An, M.-Y.; Gao, J.; Zhao, X.-F.; Wang, J.-X. A new subfamily of penaeidin with an additional serine-rich region from kuruma shrimp (*Marsupenaeus japonicus*) contributes to antimicrobial and phagocytic activities. *Dev. Comp. Immunol.* **2016**, *59*, 186–198. [CrossRef] [PubMed]

16.   Ebbensgaard, A.; Mordhorst, H.; Overgaard, M.T.; Nielsen, C.G.; Aarestrup, F.M.; Hansen, E.B. Comparative evaluation of the antimicrobial activity of different antimicrobial peptides against a range of pathogenic bacteria. *PLoS ONE* **2015**, *10*, e0144611. [CrossRef] [PubMed]

17.   Miao, J.; Guo, H.; Ou, Y.; Liu, G.; Fang, X.; Liao, Z.; Ke, C.; Chen, Y.; Zhao, L.; Cao, Y. Purification and characterization of bacteriocin F1, a novel bacteriocin produced by *Lactobacillus paracasei* subsp. *tolerans* FX-6 from Tibetan kefir, a traditional fermented milk from Tibet. *China. Food Control* **2014**, *42*, 48–53.

18.   Svenson, J.; Stensen, W.; Brandsdal, B.-O.; Haug, B.E.; Monrad, J.; Svendsen, J.S. Antimicrobial peptides with stability toward tryptic degradation. *Biochemistry* **2008**, *47*, 3777–3788. [CrossRef] [PubMed]

19.   Greber, K.E.; Dawgul, M. Antimicrobial peptides under clinical trials. *Curr. Top. Med. Chem.* **2017**, *17*, 620–628. [CrossRef] [PubMed]

20.   Murakami, M.; Masuda, K.; Utsunomiya, R.; Shiraishi, K.; Mori, H.; Tohyama, M.; Sayama, K. TLN-58, newly discovered hCAP18 processing form found in the lesion vesicle of palmoplantar pustulosis. *J. Dermatol. Sci.* **2016**, *84*, e116. [CrossRef]

21.   Craik, D.J.; Fairlie, D.P.; Liras, S.; Price, D. The future of peptide-based drugs. *Chem. Biol. Drug Des.* **2013**, *81*, 136–147. [CrossRef] [PubMed]

22.   Newman, D.J.; Cragg, G.M. Natural products as sources of new drugs from 1981 to 2014. *J. Nat. Prod.* **2016**, *79*, 629–661. [CrossRef] [PubMed]

23.   Fosgerau, K.; Hoffmann, T. Peptide therapeutics: Current status and future directions. *Drug Discov. Today* **2015**, *20*, 122–128. [CrossRef] [PubMed]

24.   Oyston, P.; Fox, M.; Richards, S.; Clark, G. Novel peptide therapeutics for treatment of infections. *J. Med. Microbiol.* **2009**, *58*, 977–987. [CrossRef] [PubMed]

25.   Vlieghe, P.; Lisowski, V.; Martinez, J.; Khrestchatisky, M. Synthetic therapeutic peptides: Science and market. *Drug Discov. Today* **2010**, *15*, 40–56. [CrossRef] [PubMed]

26. Slootweg, J.C.; Liskamp, R.M.; Rijkers, D.T. Scalable purification of the lantibiotic nisin and isolation of chemical/enzymatic cleavage fragments suitable for semi-synthesis. *J. Pept. Sci.* **2013**, *19*, 692–699. [CrossRef] [PubMed]

27. Ongey, E.L.; Yassi, H.; Pflugmacher, S.; Neubauer, P. Pharmacological and pharmacokinetic properties of lanthipeptides undergoing clinical studies. *Biotechnol. Lett.* **2017**, *39*, 473–482. [CrossRef] [PubMed]

28. Hou, Y.; Ryu, C.H.; Jun, J.; Kim, S.M.; Jeong, C.H.; Jeun, S.-S. IL-8 enhances the angiogenic potential of human bone marrow mesenchymal stem cells by increasing vascular endothelial growth factor. *Cell Biol. Int.* **2014**, *38*, 1050–1059. [CrossRef] [PubMed]

29. Field, D.; Cotter, P.D.; Hill, C.; Ross, R. Bioengineering lantibiotics for therapeutic success. *Front. Microbiol.* **2015**, *6*, 1363. [CrossRef] [PubMed]

30. Escano, J.; Smith, L. Multipronged approach for engineering novel peptide analogues of existing lantibiotics. *Expert Opin. Drug Discov.* **2015**, *10*, 857–870. [CrossRef] [PubMed]

31. Field, D.; Cotter, P.D.; Ross, R.P.; Hill, C. Bioengineering of the model lantibiotic nisin. *Bioengineered* **2015**, *6*, 187–192. [CrossRef] [PubMed]

32. Rapsch, K.; Bier, F.F.; Tadros, M.; von Nickisch-Rosenegk, M. Identification of antimicrobial peptides and immobilization strategy suitable for a covalent surface coating with biocompatible properties. *Bioconjug. Chem.* **2014**, *25*, 308–319. [CrossRef] [PubMed]

33. Bera, S.; Ghosh, A.; Sharma, S.; Debnath, T.; Giri, B.; Bhunia, A. Probing the role of proline in the antimicrobial activity and lipopolysaccharide binding of indolicidin. *J. Colloid Interface Sci.* **2015**, *452*, 148–159. [CrossRef] [PubMed]

34. Malanovic, N.; Leber, R.; Schmuck, M.; Kriechbaum, M.; Cordfunke, R.A.; Drijfhout, J.W.; de Breij, A.; Nibbering, P.H.; Kolb, D.; Lohner, K. Phospholipid-driven differences determine the action of the synthetic antimicrobial peptide OP-145 on Gram-positive bacterial and mammalian membrane model systems. *Biochim. Biophys. Acta (BBA)-Biomembr.* **2015**, *1848*, 2437–2447. [CrossRef] [PubMed]

35. Mohamed, M.F.; Abdelkhalek, A.; Seleem, M.N. Evaluation of short synthetic antimicrobial peptides for treatment of drug-resistant and intracellular *Staphylococcus aureus*. *Sci. Rep.* **2016**, *6*, 29707. [CrossRef] [PubMed]

36. Ovchinnikova, T.V.; Balandin, S.V.; Aleshina, G.M.; Tagaev, A.A.; Leonova, Y.F.; Krasnodembsky, E.D.; Men'shenin, A.V.; Kokryakov, V.N. Aurelin, a novel antimicrobial peptide from jellyfish *Aurelia aurita* with structural features of defensins and channel-blocking toxins. *Biochem. Biophys. Res. Commun.* **2006**, *348*, 514–523. [CrossRef] [PubMed]

37. Aboye, T.L.; Strömstedt, A.A.; Gunasekera, S.; Bruhn, J.G.; El-Seedi, H.; Rosengren, K.J.; Göransson, U. A Cactus-Derived Toxin-Like Cystine Knot Peptide with Selective Antimicrobial Activity. *ChemBioChem* **2015**, *16*, 1068–1077. [CrossRef] [PubMed]

38. Dueñas-Cuellar, R.A.; Kushmerick, C.; Naves, L.A.; Batista, I.F.; Guerrero-Vargas, J.A.; Pires, O.R., Jr.; Fontes, W.; Castro, M.S. Cm38: A new antimicrobial peptide active against *Klebsiella pneumoniae* is homologous to Cn11. *Protein Pep. Lett.* **2015**, *22*, 164–172.

39. Hassan, M.; Kjos, M.; Nes, I.; Diep, D.; Lotfipour, F. Natural antimicrobial peptides from bacteria: Characteristics and potential applications to fight against antibiotic resistance. *J. Appl. Microbiol.* **2012**, *113*, 723–736. [CrossRef] [PubMed]

40. Avitabile, C.; Capparelli, R.; Rigano, M.; Fulgione, A.; Barone, A.; Pedone, C.; Romanelli, A. Antimicrobial peptides from plants: Stabilization of the γ core of a tomato defensin by intramolecular disulfide bond. *J. Pept. Sci.* **2013**, *19*, 240–245. [CrossRef] [PubMed]

41. Carter, V.; Underhill, A.; Baber, I.; Sylla, L.; Baby, M.; Larget-Thiery, I.; Zettor, A.; Bourgouin, C.; Langel, Ü.; Faye, I. Killer bee molecules: Antimicrobial peptides as effector molecules to target sporogonic stages of Plasmodium. *PLoS Pathog.* **2013**, *9*, e1003790. [CrossRef] [PubMed]

42. Lehrer, R.I. Evolution of antimicrobial peptides: A view from the cystine chapel. In *Antimicrobial Peptides and Innate Immunity*; Springer: New Yok, NY, USA, 2013; pp. 1–27.

43. Boman, H. Antibacterial peptides: Basic facts and emerging concepts. *J. Intern. Med.* **2003**, *254*, 197–215. [CrossRef] [PubMed]

44. Guaní-Guerra, E.; Santos-Mendoza, T.; Lugo-Reyes, S.O.; Terán, L.M. Antimicrobial peptides: General overview and clinical implications in human health and disease. *Clin. Immunol.* **2010**, *135*, 1–11. [CrossRef] [PubMed]

45. Cotter, P.D.; Ross, R.P.; Hill, C. Bacteriocins—A viable alternative to antibiotics? *Nat. Rev. Microbiol.* **2013**, *11*, 95–105. [CrossRef] [PubMed]

46. Goyal, R.K.; Mattoo, A.K. Plant antimicrobial peptides. In *Host Defense Peptides and Their Potential as Therapeutic Agents*; Springer: New Yok, NY, USA, 2016; pp. 111–136.

47. Bhat, Z.; Kumar, S.; Bhat, H.F. Bioactive peptides of animal origin: A review. *J. Food Sci. Technol.* **2015**, *52*, 5377–5392. [CrossRef] [PubMed]

48. Kamali Alamdari, E.; Ehsani, M. Antimicrobial peptides derived from milk: A review. *J. Food Biosci. Technol.* **2017**, *7*, 49–56.

49. Théolier, J.; Fliss, I.; Jean, J.; Hammami, R. MilkAMP: A comprehensive database of antimicrobial peptides of dairy origin. *Dairy Sci. Technol.* **2014**, *94*, 181–193. [CrossRef]

50. Besse, A.; Peduzzi, J.; Rebuffat, S.; Carre-Mlouka, A. Antimicrobial peptides and proteins in the face of extremes: Lessons from archaeocins. *Biochimie* **2015**, *118*, 344–355. [CrossRef] [PubMed]

51. Fan, X.; Bai, L.; Zhu, L.; Yang, L.; Zhang, X. Marine algae-derived bioactive peptides for human nutrition and health. *J. Agric. Food Chem.* **2014**, *62*, 9211–9222. [CrossRef] [PubMed]

52. Matejuk, A.; Leng, Q.; Begum, M.; Woodle, M.; Scaria, P.; Chou, S.; Mixson, A. Peptide-based antifungal therapies against emerging infections. *Drugs Future* **2010**, *35*, 197. [CrossRef] [PubMed]

53. Fjell, C.D.; Hiss, J.A.; Hancock, R.E.; Schneider, G. Designing antimicrobial peptides: Form follows function. *Nat. Rev. Drug Discov.* **2012**, *11*, 37–51. [CrossRef] [PubMed]

54. Haney, E.F.; Mansour, S.C.; Hancock, R.E. Antimicrobial Peptides: An Introduction. *Methods Mol. Biol.* **2017**, *1548*, 3–22. [PubMed]

55. Wang, G.; Mishra, B.; Lau, K.; Lushnikova, T.; Golla, R.; Wang, X. Antimicrobial peptides in 2014. *Pharmaceuticals* **2015**, *8*, 123–150. [CrossRef] [PubMed]

56. Nguyen, L.T.; Haney, E.F.; Vogel, H.J. The expanding scope of antimicrobial peptide structures and their modes of action. *Trends Biotechnol.* **2011**, *29*, 464–472. [CrossRef] [PubMed]

57. Solstad, R.G.; Li, C.; Isaksson, J.; Johansen, J.; Svenson, J.; Stensvåg, K.; Haug, T. Novel Antimicrobial Peptides EeCentrocins 1, 2 and EeStrongylocin 2 from the Edible Sea Urchin *Echinus esculentus* Have 6-Br-Trp Post-Translational Modifications. *PLoS ONE* **2016**, *11*, e0151820. [CrossRef] [PubMed]

58. Takahashi, D.; Shukla, S.K.; Prakash, O.; Zhang, G. Structural determinants of host defense peptides for antimicrobial activity and target cell selectivity. *Biochimie* **2010**, *92*, 1236–1241. [CrossRef] [PubMed]

59. Yomogida, S.; Nagaoka, I.; Yamashita, T. Purification of the 11-and 5-kDa antibacterial polypeptides from guinea pig neutrophils. *Arch. Biochem. Biophys.* **1996**, *328*, 219–226. [CrossRef] [PubMed]

60. Tossi, A.; Sandri, L. Molecular diversity in gene-encoded, cationic antimicrobial polypeptides. *Curr. Pharm. Des.* **2002**, *8*, 743–761. [CrossRef] [PubMed]

61. Silverman, A.P.; Kariolis, M.S.; Cochran, J.R. Cystine-knot peptides engineered with specificities for αIIbβ3 or αIIbβ3 and αvβ3 integrins are potent inhibitors of platelet aggregation. *J. Mol. Recognit.* **2011**, *24*, 127–135. [CrossRef] [PubMed]

62. Molesini, B.; Treggiari, D.; Dalbeni, A.; Minuz, P.; Pandolfini, T. Plant cystine-knot peptides: Pharmacological perspectives. *Br. J. Clin. Pharmacol.* **2017**, *83*, 63–70. [CrossRef] [PubMed]

63. Mani, R.; Tang, M.; Wu, X.; Buffy, J.; Waring, A.; Sherman, M.; Hong, M. Membrane-bound dimer structure of a β-hairpin antimicrobial peptide from rotational-echo double-resonance solid-state NMR. *Biochemistry* **2006**, *45*, 8341–8349. [CrossRef] [PubMed]

64. Schwarz, E. Cystine knot growth factors and their functionally versatile proregions. *Biol. Chem.* **2017**, *398*, 1295–1308. [CrossRef] [PubMed]

65. Pallaghy, P.K.; Norton, R.S.; Nielsen, K.J.; Craik, D.J. A common structural motif incorporating a cystine knot and a triple-stranded β-sheet in toxic and inhibitory polypeptides. *Protein Sci.* **1994**, *3*, 1833–1839. [CrossRef] [PubMed]

66. Chiche, L.; Heitz, A.; Gelly, J.-C.; Gracy, J.; Chau, P.T.; Ha, P.T.; Hernandez, J.-F.; Le-Nguyen, D. Squash inhibitors: From structural motifs to macrocyclic knottins. *Curr. Protein Pept. Sci.* **2004**, *5*, 341–349. [CrossRef] [PubMed]

67. Daly, N.L.; Craik, D.J. Bioactive cystine knot proteins. *Curr. Opin. Chem. Biol.* **2011**, *15*, 362–368. [CrossRef] [PubMed]

68. Göransson, U.; Burman, R.; Gunasekera, S.; Strömstedt, A.A.; Rosengren, K.J. Circular proteins from plants and fungi. *J. Biol. Chem.* **2012**, *287*, 27001–27006. [CrossRef] [PubMed]

69. Cao, H.; Ke, T.; Liu, R.; Yu, J.; Dong, C.; Cheng, M.; Huang, J.; Liu, S. Identification of a novel proline-rich antimicrobial peptide from *Brassica napus*. *PLoS ONE* **2015**, *10*, e0137414. [CrossRef] [PubMed]

70. Scocchi, M.; Tossi, A.; Gennaro, R. Proline-rich antimicrobial peptides: Converging to a non-lytic mechanism of action. *Cell. Mol. Life Sci.* **2011**, *68*, 2317–2330. [CrossRef] [PubMed]

71. Rucker, A.L.; Creamer, T.P. Polyproline II helical structure in protein unfolded states: Lysine peptides revisited. *Protein Sci.* **2002**, *11*, 980–985. [PubMed]

72. Guzmán, F.; Marshall, S.; Ojeda, C.; Albericio, F.; Carvajal-Rondanelli, P. Inhibitory effect of short cationic homopeptides against Gram-positive bacteria. *J. Pept. Sci.* **2013**, *19*, 792–800. [CrossRef] [PubMed]

73. Bieler, S.; Silva, F.; Soto, C.; Belin, D. Bactericidal activity of both secreted and nonsecreted microcin E492 requires the mannose permease. *J. Bacteriol.* **2006**, *188*, 7049–7061. [CrossRef] [PubMed]

74. Cabiaux, V.; Agerberths, B.; Johansson, J.; Homble, F.; Goormaghtigh, E.; Ruysschaert, J.M. Secondary structure and membrane interaction of PR-39, a Pro+ Arg-rich antibacterial peptide. *Eur. J. Biochem.* **1994**, *224*, 1019–1027. [CrossRef] [PubMed]

75. Raj, P.A.; Edgerton, M. Functional domain and poly-L-proline II conformation for candidacidal activity of bactenecin 5. *FEBS Lett.* **1995**, *368*, 526–530. [PubMed]

76. Kuriakose, J.; Hernandez-Gordillo, V.; Nepal, M.; Brezden, A.; Pozzi, V.; Seleem, M.N.; Chmielewski, J. Targeting intracellular pathogenic bacteria with unnaturalproline-rich peptides: Coupling antibacterial activity with macrophage penetration. *Angew. Chem.* **2013**, *125*, 9846–9849. [CrossRef]

77. Nepal, M.; Thangamani, S.; Seleem, M.N.; Chmielewski, J. Targeting intracellular bacteria with an extended cationic amphiphilic polyproline helix. *Org. Biomol. Chem.* **2015**, *13*, 5930–5936. [CrossRef] [PubMed]

78. Carvajal-Rondanelli, P.; Aróstica, M.; Marshall, S.H.; Albericio, F.; Álvarez, C.A.; Ojeda, C.; Aguilar, L.F.; Guzmán, F. Inhibitory effect of short cationic homopeptides against Gram-negative bacteria. *Amino Acids* **2016**, *48*, 1445–1456. [CrossRef] [PubMed]

79. Rios, A.C.; Moutinho, C.G.; Pinto, F.C.; Del Fiol, F.S.; Jozala, A.; Chaud, M.V.; Vila, M.M.D.C.; Teixeira, J.A.; Balcão, V.M. Alternatives to overcoming bacterial resistances: State-of-the-art. *Microbiol. Res.* **2016**, *191*, 51–80. [CrossRef] [PubMed]

80. Kay, B.K.; Williamson, M.P.; Sudol, M. The importance of being proline: The interaction of proline-rich motifs in signaling proteins with their cognate domains. *FASEB J.* **2000**, *14*, 231–241. [CrossRef] [PubMed]

81. Russell, A.L.; Kennedy, A.M.; Spuches, A.M.; Venugopal, D.; Bhonsle, J.B.; Hicks, R.P. Spectroscopic and thermodynamic evidence for antimicrobial peptide membrane selectivity. *Chem. Phys. Lipids* **2010**, *163*, 488–497. [CrossRef] [PubMed]

82. Ruzza, P.; Biondi, B.; Marchiani, A.; Antolini, N.; Calderan, A. Cell-penetrating peptides: A comparative study on lipid affinity and cargo delivery properties. *Pharmaceuticals* **2010**, *3*, 1045–1062. [CrossRef] [PubMed]

83. Wadhwani, P.; Reichert, J.; Bürck, J.; Ulrich, A.S. Antimicrobial and cell-penetrating peptides induce lipid vesicle fusion by folding and aggregation. *Eur. Biophys. J.* **2012**, *41*, 177–187. [CrossRef] [PubMed]

84. Pires, J.; Siriwardena, T.N.; Stach, M.; Tinguely, R.; Kasraian, S.; Luzzaro, F.; Leib, S.L.; Darbre, T.; Reymond, J.-L.; Endimiani, A. In vitro activity of the novel antimicrobial peptide dendrimer G3KL against multidrug-resistant *Acinetobacter baumannii* and *Pseudomonas aeruginosa*. *Antimicrob. Agents Chemother.* **2015**, *59*, 7915–7918. [CrossRef] [PubMed]

85. Kumaresan, V.; Bhatt, P.; Ganesh, M.-R.; Harikrishnan, R.; Arasu, M.; Al-Dhabi, N.A.; Pasupuleti, M.; Marimuthu, K.; Arockiaraj, J. A novel antimicrobial peptide derived from fish goose type lysozyme disrupts the membrane of *Salmonella enterica*. *Mol. Immunol.* **2015**, *68*, 421–433. [CrossRef] [PubMed]

86. Chu, H.-L.; Yip, B.-S.; Chen, K.-H.; Yu, H.-Y.; Chih, Y.-H.; Cheng, H.-T.; Chou, Y.-T.; Cheng, J.-W. Novel antimicrobial peptides with high anticancer activity and selectivity. *PLoS ONE* **2015**, *10*, e0126390. [CrossRef] [PubMed]

87. Marani, M.M.; Perez, L.O.; de Araujo, A.R.; Plácido, A.; Sousa, C.F.; Quelemes, P.V.; Oliveira, M.; Gomes-Alves, A.G.; Pueta, M.; Gameiro, P.; et al. Thaulin-1: The first antimicrobial peptide isolated from the skin of a Patagonian frog *Pleurodema thaul* (Anura: Leptodactylidae: Leiuperinae) with activity against *Escherichia coli*. *Gene* **2016**, *605*, 70–80. [CrossRef] [PubMed]

88. Lee, W.; Hwang, J.-S.; Lee, D.G. A novel antimicrobial peptide, scolopendin, from *Scolopendra subspinipes mutilans* and its microbicidal mechanism. *Biochimie* **2015**, *118*, 176–184. [CrossRef] [PubMed]

89. Chikindas, M.L.; Weeks, R.; Drider, D.; Chistyakov, V.A.; Dicks, L.M. Functions and emerging applications of bacteriocins. *Curr. Opin. Biotechnol.* **2018**, *49*, 23–28. [CrossRef] [PubMed]

90. Mathur, H.; C Rea, M.; D Cotter, P.; Hill, C.; Paul Ross, R. The sactibiotic subclass of bacteriocins: An update. *Curr. Protein Pept. Sci.* **2015**, *16*, 549–558. [CrossRef] [PubMed]

91. Alvarez-Sieiro, P.; Montalbán-López, M.; Mu, D.; Kuipers, O.P. Bacteriocins of lactic acid bacteria: Extending the family. *Appl. Microbiol. Biotechnol.* **2016**, *100*, 2939–2951. [CrossRef] [PubMed]

92. Hegemann, J.D.; Zimmermann, M.; Xie, X.; Marahiel, M.A. Lasso peptides: An intriguing class of bacterial natural products. *Acc. Chem. Res.* **2015**, *48*, 1909–1919. [CrossRef] [PubMed]

93. Li, Y.; Ducasse, R.; Zirah, S.; Blond, A.; Goulard, C.; Lescop, E.; Giraud, C.; Hartke, A.; Guittet, E.; Pernodet, J.-L.; et al. Characterization of sviceucin from Streptomyces provides insights into enzyme exchangeability and disulfide bond formation in lasso peptides. *ACS Chem.Biol.* **2015**, *10*, 2641–2649. [CrossRef] [PubMed]

94. Kersten, R.D.; Yang, Y.-L.; Xu, Y.; Cimermancic, P.; Nam, S.-J.; Fenical, W.; Fischbach, M.A.; Moore, B.S.; Dorrestein, P.C. A mass spectrometry–guided genome mining approach for natural product peptidogenomics. *Nat. Chem. Biol.* **2011**, *7*, 794–802. [CrossRef] [PubMed]

95. Maqueda, M.; Sánchez-Hidalgo, M.; Fernández, M.; Montalbán-López, M.; Valdivia, E.; Martínez-Bueno, M. Genetic features of circular bacteriocins produced by Gram-positive bacteria. *FEMS Microbiol. Rev.* **2008**, *32*, 2–22. [CrossRef] [PubMed]

96. Montalbán-López, M.; Sánchez-Hidalgo, M.; Cebrián, R.; Maqueda, M. Discovering the bacterial circular proteins: Bacteriocins, cyanobactins, and pilins. *J. Biol. Chem.* **2012**, *287*, 27007–27013. [CrossRef] [PubMed]

97. Acedo, J.Z.; van Belkum, M.J.; Lohans, C.T.; McKay, R.T.; Miskolzie, M.; Vederas, J.C. Solution structure of acidocin B, a circular bacteriocin produced by *Lactobacillus acidophilus* M46. *Appl. Environ. Microbiol.* **2015**, *81*, 2910–2918. [CrossRef] [PubMed]

98. Himeno, K.; Rosengren, K.J.; Inoue, T.; Perez, R.H.; Colgrave, M.L.; Lee, H.S.; Chan, L.Y.; Henriques, S.T.; Fujita, K.; Ishibashi, N. Identification, characterization, and three-dimensional structure of the novel circular bacteriocin, enterocin NKR-5-3B, from *Enterococcus faecium*. *Biochemistry* **2015**, *54*, 4863–4876. [CrossRef] [PubMed]

99. Martin-Visscher, L.A.; van Belkum, M.J.; Garneau-Tsodikova, S.; Whittal, R.M.; Zheng, J.; McMullen, L.M.; Vederas, J.C. Isolation and characterization of carnocyclin A, a novel circular bacteriocin produced by *Carnobacterium maltaromaticum* UAL307. *Appl. Environ. Microbiol.* **2008**, *74*, 4756–4763. [CrossRef] [PubMed]

100. Paik, S.H.; Chakicherla, A.; Hansen, J.N. Identification and characterization of the structural and transporter genes for, and the chemical and biological properties of, sublancin 168, a novel lantibiotic produced by *Bacillus subtilis* 168. *J. Biol. Chem.* **1998**, *273*, 23134–23142. [CrossRef] [PubMed]

101. Garcia De Gonzalo, C.V.; Zhu, L.; Oman, T.J.; Van Der Donk, W.A. NMR structure of the S-linked glycopeptide sublancin 168. *ACS Chem. Biol.* **2014**, *9*, 796–801. [CrossRef] [PubMed]

102. Babasaki, K.; Takao, T.; Shimonishi, Y.; Kurahashi, K. Subtilosin A, a new antibiotic peptide produced by *Bacillus subtilis* 168: Isolation, structural analysis, and biogenesis. *J. Biochem.* **1985**, *98*, 585–603. [CrossRef] [PubMed]

103. Murphy, K.; O'Sullivan, O.; Rea, M.C.; Cotter, P.D.; Ross, R.P.; Hill, C. Genome mining for radical SAM protein determinants reveals multiple sactibiotic-like gene clusters. *PLoS ONE* **2011**, *6*, e20852. [CrossRef] [PubMed]

104. Kawulka, K.; Sprules, T.; McKay, R.T.; Mercier, P.; Diaper, C.M.; Zuber, P.; Vederas, J.C. Structure of Subtilosin A, an Antimicrobial Peptide from *Bacillus s ubtilis* with Unusual Posttranslational Modifications Linking Cysteine Sulfurs to α-Carbons of Phenylalanine and Threonine. *J. Am. Chem. Soc.* **2003**, *125*, 4726–4727. [CrossRef] [PubMed]

105. Montalban-Lopez, M.; Sanchez-Hidalgo, M.; Valdivia, E.; Martinez-Bueno, M.; Maqueda, M. Are bacteriocins underexploited? Novel applications for old antimicrobials. *Curr. Pharm. Biotechnol.* **2011**, *12*, 1205–1220. [CrossRef] [PubMed]

106. Castiglione, F.; Lazzarini, A.; Carrano, L.; Corti, E.; Ciciliato, I.; Gastaldo, L.; Candiani, P.; Losi, D.; Marinelli, F.; Selva, E. Determining the structure and mode of action of microbisporicin, a potent lantibiotic active against multiresistant pathogens. *Chem. Biol.* **2008**, *15*, 22–31. [CrossRef] [PubMed]

107. McIntosh, J.A.; Donia, M.S.; Schmidt, E.W. Ribosomal peptide natural products: Bridging the ribosomal and nonribosomal worlds. *Nat. Prod. Rep.* **2009**, *26*, 537–559. [CrossRef] [PubMed]

108. Dischinger, J.; Basi Chipalu, S.; Bierbaum, G. Lantibiotics: Promising candidates for future applications in health care. *Int. J. Med. Microbiol.* **2014**, *304*, 51–62. [CrossRef] [PubMed]

109. Castiglione, F. A novel lantibiotic acting on bacterial cell wall synthesis produced by the uncommon actinomycete *Planomonospora* sp. *Biochemistry* **2007**, *46*, 5884–5895. [CrossRef] [PubMed]

110. Cruz, J.C.S.; Iorio, M.; Monciardini, P.; Simone, M.; Brunati, C.; Gaspari, E.; Maffioli, S.I.; Wellington, E.; Sosio, M.; Donadio, S. Brominated variant of the lantibiotic NAI-107 with enhanced antibacterial potency. *J. Nat. Prod.* **2015**, *78*, 2642–2647. [CrossRef] [PubMed]

111. Iorio, M.; Sasso, O.; Maffioli, S.I.; Bertorelli, R.; Monciardini, P.; Sosio, M.; Bonezzi, F.; Summa, M.; Brunati, C.; Bordoni, R. A glycosylated, labionin-containing lanthipeptide with marked antinociceptive activity. *ACS Chem. Biol.* **2013**, *9*, 398–404. [CrossRef] [PubMed]

112. Rink, R.; Arkema-Meter, A.; Baudoin, I.; Post, E.; Kuipers, A.; Nelemans, S.; Akanbi, M.H.J.; Moll, G. To protect peptide pharmaceuticals against peptidases. *J. Pharmacol. Toxicol. Methods* **2010**, *61*, 210–218. [CrossRef] [PubMed]

113. Goto, Y.; Okesli, A.E.; van der Donk, W.A. Mechanistic studies of Ser/Thr dehydration catalyzed by a member of the LanL lanthionine synthetase family. *Biochemistry* **2011**, *50*, 891–898. [CrossRef] [PubMed]

114. Repka, L.M.; Chekan, J.R.; Nair, S.K.; van der Donk, W.A. Mechanistic understanding of lanthipeptide biosynthetic enzymes. *Chem. Rev.* **2017**, *117*, 5457–5520. [CrossRef] [PubMed]

115. Cui, Y.; Zhang, C.; Wang, Y.; Shi, J.; Zhang, L.; Ding, Z.; Qu, X.; Cui, H. Class IIa bacteriocins: Diversity and new developments. *Int. J. Mol. Sci.* **2012**, *13*, 16668–16707. [CrossRef] [PubMed]

116. Perez, R.H.; Zendo, T.; Sonomoto, K. Novel bacteriocins from lactic acid bacteria (LAB): Various structures and applications. *Microb. Cell Fact.* **2014**, *13*, S3. [CrossRef] [PubMed]

117. Sit, C.S.; Lohans, C.T.; van Belkum, M.J.; Campbell, C.D.; Miskolzie, M.; Vederas, J.C. Substitution of a conserved disulfide in the type IIa bacteriocin, leucocin A, with L-leucine and L-serine residues: Effects on activity and three-dimensional structure. *ChemBioChem* **2012**, *13*, 35–38. [CrossRef] [PubMed]

118. Turner, D.L.; Lamosa, P.; Rodríguez, A.; Martínez, B. Structure and properties of the metastable bacteriocin Lcn972 from *Lactococcus lactis*. *J. Mol. Struct.* **2013**, *1031*, 207–210. [CrossRef]

119. Azmi, F.; Skwarczynski, M.; Toth, I. Towards the development of synthetic antibiotics: Designs inspired by natural antimicrobial peptides. *Curr. Med. Chem.* **2016**, *23*, 4610–4624. [CrossRef] [PubMed]

120. Khara, J.S.; Priestman, M.; Uhía, I.; Hamilton, M.S.; Krishnan, N.; Wang, Y.; Yang, Y.Y.; Langford, P.R.; Newton, S.M.; Robertson, B.D. Unnatural amino acid analogues of membrane-active helical peptides with anti-mycobacterial activity and improved stability. *J. Antimicrob. Chemother.* **2016**, *71*, 2181–2191. [CrossRef] [PubMed]

121. Ling, L.L.; Schneider, T.; Peoples, A.J.; Spoering, A.L.; Engels, I.; Conlon, B.P.; Mueller, A.; Schäberle, T.F.; Hughes, D.E.; Epstein, S. A new antibiotic kills pathogens without detectable resistance. *Nature* **2015**, *517*, 455–459. [CrossRef] [PubMed]

122. Feng, Z.; Xu, B. Inspiration from the mirror: D-amino acid containing peptides in biomedical approaches. *Biomol. Concepts* **2016**, *7*, 179–187. [CrossRef] [PubMed]

123. Papo, N.; Oren, Z.; Pag, U.; Sahl, H.-G.; Shai, Y. The consequence of sequence alteration of an amphipathic α-helical antimicrobial peptide and its diastereomers. *J. Biol. Chem.* **2002**, *277*, 33913–33921. [CrossRef] [PubMed]

124. Guilhelmelli, F.; Vilela, N.; Albuquerque, P.; Derengowski, L.d.S.; Silva-Pereira, I.; Kyaw, C.M. Antibiotic development challenges: The various mechanisms of action of antimicrobial peptides and of bacterial resistance. **2013**. [CrossRef] [PubMed]

125. Zhang, L.-J.; Gallo, R.L. Antimicrobial peptides. *Curr. Biol.* **2016**, *26*, R14–R19. [CrossRef] [PubMed]

126. Bechinger, B.; Gorr, S.-U. Antimicrobial peptides mechanisms of action and resistance. *J. Dent. Res.* **2016**, *6*, 254–260. [CrossRef] [PubMed]

127. Freund, S.; Jung, G.; Gutbrod, O.; Foikers, G.; Gibbons, W.A.; Allgaier, H.; Werner, R. The solution structure of the lantibiotic gallidermin. *Biopolymers* **1991**, *31*, 803–811. [CrossRef] [PubMed]

128. Tossi, A.; Sandri, L.; Giangaspero, A. Amphipathic, α-helical antimicrobial peptides. *Pept. Sci.* **2000**, *55*, 4–30. [CrossRef]

129. Sánchez-Barrena, M.; Martnez-Ripoll, M.; Gálvez, A.; Valdivia, E.; Maqueda, M.; Cruz, V.; Albert, A. Structure of bacteriocin AS-48: From soluble state to membrane bound state. *J. Mol. Biol.* **2003**, *334*, 541–549. [CrossRef] [PubMed]

130. Epand, R.M.; Vogel, H.J. Diversity of antimicrobial peptides and their mechanisms of action. *Biochim. Biophys. Acta (BBA)-Biomembr.* **1999**, *1462*, 11–28. [CrossRef]

131. Melo, M.N.; Ferre, R.; Castanho, M.A. Antimicrobial peptides: Linking partition, activity and high membrane-bound concentrations. *Nat. Rev. Microbiol.* **2009**, *7*, 245–250. [CrossRef] [PubMed]

132. Brogden, K.A. Antimicrobial peptides: Pore formers or metabolic inhibitors in bacteria? *Nat. Rev. Microbiol.* **2005**, *3*, 238–250. [CrossRef] [PubMed]

133. Brown, S.; Santa Maria, J.P., Jr.; Walker, S. Wall teichoic acids of gram-positive bacteria. *Annu. Rev. Microbiol.* **2013**, *67*, 313–336. [CrossRef] [PubMed]

134. Makin, S.A.; Beveridge, T.J. The influence of A-band and B-band lipopolysaccharide on the surface characteristics and adhesion of *Pseudomonas aeruginosa* to surfaces. *Microbiology* **1996**, *142*, 299–307. [CrossRef] [PubMed]

135. Lohner, K. Membrane-active antimicrobial peptides as template structures for novel antibiotic agents. *Curr. Top. Med. Chem.* **2017**, *17*, 508–519. [CrossRef] [PubMed]

136. Scocchi, M.; Mardirossian, M.; Runti, G.; Benincasa, M. Non-membrane permeabilizing modes of action of antimicrobial peptides on bacteria. *Curr. Top. Med. Chem.* **2016**, *16*, 76–88. [CrossRef] [PubMed]

137. Otvos, L., Jr. Antibacterial peptides isolated from insects. *J. Pept. Sci.* **2000**, *6*, 497–511. [CrossRef]

138. Gennaro, R.; Zanetti, M.; Benincasa, M.; Podda, E.; Miani, M. Pro-rich antimicrobial peptides from animals: Structure, biological functions and mechanism of action. *Curr. Pharm. Des.* **2002**, *8*, 763–778. [CrossRef] [PubMed]

139. Avitabile, C.; D'Andrea, L.D.; Romanelli, A. Circular dichroism studies on the interactions of antimicrobial peptides with bacterial cells. *Sci. Rep.* **2014**, *4*, 4293. [CrossRef] [PubMed]

140. Gabrielsen, C.; Brede, D.A.; Hernández, P.E.; Nes, I.F.; Diep, D.B. The maltose ABC transporter in Lactococcus lactis facilitates high-level sensitivity to the circular bacteriocin garvicin ML. *Antimicrob. Agents Chemother.* **2012**, *56*, 2908–2915. [CrossRef] [PubMed]

141. Diep, D.B.; Skaugen, M.; Salehian, Z.; Holo, H.; Nes, I.F. Common mechanisms of target cell recognition and immunity for class II bacteriocins. *Proc. Natl. Acad. Sci. USA* **2007**, *104*, 2384–2389. [CrossRef] [PubMed]

142. Uzelac, G.; Kojic, M.; Lozo, J.; Aleksandrzak-Piekarczyk, T.; Gabrielsen, C.; Kristensen, T.; Nes, I.F.; Diep, D.B.; Topisirovic, L. A Zn-dependent metallopeptidase is responsible for sensitivity to LsbB, a class II leaderless bacteriocin of *Lactococcus lactis subsp. lactis* BGMN1-5. *J. Bacteriol.* **2013**, *195*, 5614–5621. [CrossRef] [PubMed]

143. Mardirossian, M.; Grzela, R.; Giglione, C.; Meinnel, T.; Gennaro, R.; Mergaert, P.; Scocchi, M. The host antimicrobial peptide Bac7 1-35 binds to bacterial ribosomal proteins and inhibits protein synthesis. *Chem. Biol.* **2014**, *21*, 1639–1647. [CrossRef] [PubMed]

144. Krizsan, A.; Volke, D.; Weinert, S.; Sträter, N.; Knappe, D.; Hoffmann, R. Insect-derived proline-rich antimicrobial peptides kill bacteria by inhibiting bacterial protein translation at the 70 S ribosome. *Angew. Chem. Int. Ed.* **2014**, *53*, 12236–12239. [CrossRef] [PubMed]

145. Mukhopadhyay, J.; Sineva, E.; Knight, J.; Levy, R.M.; Ebright, R.H. Antibacterial peptide microcin J25 inhibits transcription by binding within and obstructing the RNA polymerase secondary channel. *Mol. Cell* **2004**, *14*, 739–751. [CrossRef] [PubMed]

146. Kuznedelov, K.; Semenova, E.; Knappe, T.A.; Mukhamedyarov, D.; Srivastava, A.; Chatterjee, S.; Ebright, R.H.; Marahiel, M.A.; Severinov, K. The antibacterial threaded-lasso peptide capistruin inhibits bacterial RNA polymerase. *J. Mol. Biol.* **2011**, *412*, 842–848. [CrossRef] [PubMed]

147. Kragol, G.; Lovas, S.; Varadi, G.; Condie, B.A.; Hoffmann, R.; Otvos, L. The antibacterial peptide pyrrhocoricin inhibits the ATPase actions of DnaK and prevents chaperone-assisted protein folding. *Biochemistry* **2001**, *40*, 3016–3026. [CrossRef] [PubMed]

148. Scocchi, M.; Lüthy, C.; Decarli, P.; Mignogna, G.; Christen, P.; Gennaro, R. The proline-rich antibacterial peptide Bac7 binds to and inhibits in vitro the molecular chaperone DnaK. *Int. J. Pept. Res. Ther.* **2009**, *15*, 147–155. [CrossRef]

149. Wilmes, M.; Stockem, M.; Bierbaum, G.; Schlag, M.; Götz, F.; Tran, D.Q.; Schaal, J.B.; Ouellette, A.J.; Selsted, M.E.; Sahl, H.-G. Killing of staphylococci by θ-defensins involves membrane impairment and activation of autolytic enzymes. *Antibiotics* **2014**, *3*, 617–631. [CrossRef] [PubMed]

150. Bierbaum, G.; Sahl, H.G. Lantibiotics: Mode of action, biosynthesis and bioengineering. *Curr. Pharm. Biotechnol.* **2009**, *10*, 2–18. [CrossRef] [PubMed]

151. Nagaoka, I.; Hirota, S.; Niyonsaba, F.; Hirata, M.; Adachi, Y.; Tamura, H.; Tanaka, S.; Heumann, D. Augmentation of the lipopolysaccharide-neutralizing activities of human cathelicidin CAP18/LL-37-derived antimicrobial peptides by replacement with hydrophobic and cationic amino acid residues. *Clin. Diagn. Lab. Immunol.* **2002**, *9*, 972–982. [CrossRef] [PubMed]

152. Bociek, K.; Ferluga, S.; Mardirossian, M.; Benincasa, M.; Tossi, A.; Gennaro, R.; Scocchi, M. Lipopolysaccharide phosphorylation by the waay kinase affects the susceptibility of *Escherichia coli* to the human antimicrobial peptide LL-37. *J. Biol. Chem.* **2015**, *290*, 19933–19941. [CrossRef] [PubMed]

153. Park, C.B.; Kim, H.S.; Kim, S.C. Mechanism of action of the antimicrobial peptide buforin II: Buforin II kills microorganisms by penetrating the cell membrane and inhibiting cellular functions. *Biochem. Biophys. Res. Commun.* **1998**, *244*, 253–257. [CrossRef] [PubMed]

154. Masuda, R.; Dazai, Y.; Mima, T.; Koide, T. Structure–Activity Relationships and Action Mechanisms of Collagen-like Antimicrobial Peptides. *Pept. Sci.* **2017**, *108*. [CrossRef] [PubMed]

155. Miao, J.; Zhou, J.; Liu, G.; Chen, F.; Chen, Y.; Gao, X.; Dixon, W.; Song, M.; Xiao, H.; Cao, Y. Membrane disruption and DNA binding of *Staphylococcus aureus* cell induced by a novel antimicrobial peptide produced by *Lactobacillus paracasei subsp. tolerans* FX-6. *Food Control* **2016**, *59*, 609–613. [CrossRef]

156. Costa, F.; Carvalho, I.F.; Montelaro, R.C.; Gomes, P.; Martins, M.C.L. Covalent immobilization of antimicrobial peptides (AMPs) onto biomaterial surfaces. *Acta Biomater.* **2011**, *7*, 1431–1440. [CrossRef] [PubMed]

157. Kosikowska, P.; Lesner, A. Antimicrobial peptides (AMPs) as drug candidates: A patent review (2003–2015). *Expert Opin. Ther. Pat.* **2016**, *26*, 689–702. [CrossRef] [PubMed]

158. Kang, H.-K.; Kim, C.; Seo, C.H.; Park, Y. The therapeutic applications of antimicrobial peptides (AMPs): A patent review. *J. Microbiol.* **2017**, *55*, 1–12. [CrossRef] [PubMed]

159. Strempel, N.; Strehmel, J.; Overhage, J. Potential application of antimicrobial peptides in the treatment of bacterial biofilm infections. *Curr. Pharm. Des.* **2015**, *21*, 67–84. [CrossRef] [PubMed]

160. Mylonakis, E.; Podsiadlowski, L.; Muhammed, M.; Vilcinskas, A. Diversity, evolution and medical applications of insect antimicrobial peptides. *Philos. Trans. R. Soc. B* **2016**, *371*, 20150290. [CrossRef] [PubMed]

161. Nordström, R.; Malmsten, M. Delivery systems for antimicrobial peptides. *Adv. Colloid Interface Sci.* **2017**, *242*, 17–34. [CrossRef] [PubMed]

162. Leake, I. IBD: Cathelicidin can reverse intestinal fibrosis in models of colitis. *Nat. Rev. Gastroenterol. Hepatol.* **2015**, *12*, 3. [CrossRef] [PubMed]

163. Otvos, L., Jr.; Ostorhazi, E. Therapeutic utility of antibacterial peptides in wound healing. *Expert Rev. Anti Infect. Ther.* **2015**, *13*, 871–881. [CrossRef] [PubMed]

164. Alves, D.; Olívia Pereira, M. Mini-review: Antimicrobial peptides and enzymes as promising candidates to functionalize biomaterial surfaces. *Biofouling* **2014**, *30*, 483–499. [CrossRef] [PubMed]

165. Fang, B.; Jiang, Y.; Nüsslein, K.; Rotello, V.M.; Santore, M.M. Antimicrobial surfaces containing cationic nanoparticles: How immobilized, clustered, and protruding cationic charge presentation affects killing activity and kinetics. *Colloids Surf. B. Biointerfaces* **2015**, *125*, 255–263. [CrossRef] [PubMed]

166. Muller, M.; MacDougall, C.; Lim, M. Antimicrobial surfaces to prevent healthcare-associated infections: A systematic review. *J. Hosp. Infect.* **2016**, *92*, 7–13. [CrossRef] [PubMed]

167. Salwiczek, M.; Qu, Y.; Gardiner, J.; Strugnell, R.A.; Lithgow, T.; McLean, K.M.; Thissen, H. Emerging rules for effective antimicrobial coatings. *Trends Biotechnol.* **2014**, *32*, 82–90. [CrossRef] [PubMed]

168. Lillehoj, P.B.; Kaplan, C.W.; He, J.; Shi, W.; Ho, C.-M. Rapid, electrical impedance detection of bacterial pathogens using immobilized antimicrobial peptides. *J. Lab. Autom.* **2014**, *19*, 42–49. [CrossRef] [PubMed]

169. Onaizi, S.A.; Leong, S.S. Tethering antimicrobial peptides: Current status and potential challenges. *Biotechnol. Adv.* **2011**, *29*, 67–74. [CrossRef] [PubMed]

170. Bagheri, M.; Beyermann, M.; Dathe, M. Immobilization reduces the activity of surface-bound cationic antimicrobial peptides with no influence upon the activity spectrum. *Antimicrob. Agents Chemother.* **2009**, *53*, 1132–1141. [CrossRef] [PubMed]

171. Shalev, T.; Gopin, A.; Bauer, M.; Stark, R.W.; Rahimipour, S. Non-leaching antimicrobial surfaces through polydopamine bio-inspired coating of quaternary ammonium salts or an ultrashort antimicrobial lipopeptide. *J. Mater. Chem.* **2012**, *22*, 2026–2032. [CrossRef]

172. Murata, H.; Koepsel, R.R.; Matyjaszewski, K.; Russell, A.J. Permanent, non-leaching antibacterial surfaces—2: How high density cationic surfaces kill bacterial cells. *Biomaterials* **2007**, *28*, 4870–4879. [CrossRef] [PubMed]

173. Ferreira, L.; Zumbuehl, A. Non-leaching surfaces capable of killing microorganisms on contact. *J. Mater. Chem.* **2009**, *19*, 7796–7806. [CrossRef]

174. Goodwin, D.; Simerska, P.; Toth, I. Peptides as therapeutics with enhanced bioactivity. *Curr. Med. Chem.* **2012**, *19*, 4451–4461. [CrossRef] [PubMed]

175. Dawson, M.J.; Appleyard, A.N.; Bargallo, J.C.; Wadman, S.N. Actagardine Derivatives, and Pharmaceutical Use Thereof. U.S. Patent WO 2,010,082,019 A1, 22 July 2010.

176. Boakes, S.; Weiss, W.J.; Vinson, M.; Wadman, S.; Dawson, M.J. Antibacterial activity of the novel semisynthetic lantibiotic NVB333 in vitro and in experimental infection models. *J. Antibiot.* **2016**, *69*, 850–857. [CrossRef] [PubMed]

177. Dieterich, D.C.; Lee, J.J.; Link, A.J.; Graumann, J.; Tirrell, D.A.; Schuman, E.M. Labeling, detection and identification of newly synthesized proteomes with bioorthogonal non-canonical amino-acid tagging. *Nat. Protoc.* **2007**, *2*, 532–540. [CrossRef] [PubMed]

178. Cox, V.E.; Gaucher, E.A. Molecular evolution directs protein translation using unnatural amino acids. *Curr. Protoc. Chem. Biol.* **2015**, 223–228.

179. Sadler, K.; Tam, J.P. Peptide dendrimers: Applications and synthesis. *Rev. Mol. Biotechnol.* **2002**, *90*, 195–229. [CrossRef]

180. Pini, A.; Falciani, C.; Bracci, L. Branched peptides as therapeutics. *Curr. Protein Pept. Sci.* **2008**, *9*, 468–477. [CrossRef] [PubMed]

181. Percec, V.; Dulcey, A.E.; Balagurusamy, V.S.; Miura, Y.; Smidrkal, J.; Peterca, M.; Nummelin, S.; Edlund, U.; Hudson, S.D.; Heiney, P.A. Self-assembly of amphiphilic dendritic dipeptides into helical pores. *Nature* **2004**, *430*, 764–768. [CrossRef] [PubMed]

182. Matsuzaki, K. Control of cell selectivity of antimicrobial peptides. *Biochim. Biophys. Acta (BBA)-Biomembr.* **2009**, *1788*, 1687–1692. [CrossRef] [PubMed]

183. Ringstad, L.; Schmidtchen, A.; Malmsten, M. Effects of single amino acid substitutions on peptide interaction with lipid membranes and bacteria–variants of GKE21, an internal sequence from human LL-37. *Colloids Surf. Physicochem. Eng. Asp.* **2010**, *354*, 65–71. [CrossRef]

184. Andrushchenko, V.V.; Vogel, H.J.; Prenner, E.J. Interactions of tryptophan-rich cathelicidin antimicrobial peptides with model membranes studied by differential scanning calorimetry. *Biochim. Biophys. Acta (BBA)-Biomembr.* **2007**, *1768*, 2447–2458. [CrossRef] [PubMed]

185. Giangaspero, A.; Sandri, L.; Tossi, A. Amphipathic α helical antimicrobial peptides. *Eur. J. Biochem.* **2001**, *268*, 5589–5600. [CrossRef] [PubMed]

186. Benincasa, M.; Runti, G.; Mardirossian, M.; Gennaro, R.; Scocchi, M. Methods for elucidating the mechanism of action of proline-rich and other non-lytic antimicrobial peptides. *Methods Mol. Biol.* **2017**, *1548*, 283–295. [PubMed]

187. Xhindoli, D.; Pacor, S.; Guida, F.; Antcheva, N.; Tossi, A. Native oligomerization determines the mode of action and biological activities of human cathelicidin LL-37. *Biochem. J.* **2014**, *457*, 263–275. [CrossRef] [PubMed]

188. Johansson, J.; Gudmundsson, G.H.; Rottenberg, M.E.; Berndt, K.D.; Agerberth, B. Conformation-dependent antibacterial activity of the naturally occurring human peptide LL-37. *J. Biol. Chem.* **1998**, *273*, 3718–3724. [CrossRef] [PubMed]

189. Zelezetsky, I.; Pacor, S.; Pag, U.; Papo, N.; Shai, Y.; Sahl, H.-G.; Tossi, A. Controlled alteration of the shape and conformational stability of α-helical cell-lytic peptides: Effect on mode of action and cell specificity. *Biochem. J.* **2005**, *390*, 177–188. [CrossRef] [PubMed]

190. Pasupuleti, M.; Walse, B.R.; Svensson, B.; Malmsten, M.; Schmidtchen, A. Rational design of antimicrobial C3a analogues with enhanced effects against Staphylococci using an integrated structure and function-based approach. *Biochemistry* **2008**, *47*, 9057–9070. [CrossRef] [PubMed]

191. Mojsoska, B.; Zuckermann, R.N.; Jenssen, H. Structure-activity relationship study of novel peptoids that mimic the structure of antimicrobial peptides. *Antimicrob. Agents Chemother.* **2015**, *59*, 4112–4120. [CrossRef] [PubMed]

192. Zhong, G.; Cheng, J.; Liang, Z.C.; Xu, L.; Lou, W.; Bao, C.; Ong, Z.Y.; Dong, H.; Yang, Y.Y.; Fan, W. Short synthetic β-sheet antimicrobial peptides for the treatment of multidrug-resistant *Pseudomonas aeruginosa* burn wound infections. *Adv. Healthc. Mater.* **2017**, *6*. [CrossRef] [PubMed]

193. Schmidtchen, A.; Pasupuleti, M.; Malmsten, M. Effect of hydrophobic modifications in antimicrobial peptides. *Adv. Colloid Interface Sci.* **2014**, *205*, 265–274. [CrossRef] [PubMed]

194. Jiang, Z.; Vasil, A.I.; Gera, L.; Vasil, M.L.; Hodges, R.S. Rational Design of α-Helical Antimicrobial Peptides to Target Gram-negative Pathogens, Acinetobacter baumannii and Pseudomonas aeruginosa: Utilization of Charge,'Specificity Determinants', Total Hydrophobicity, Hydrophobe Type and Location as Design Parameters to Improve the Therapeutic Ratio. *Chem. Biol. Drug Des.* **2011**, *77*, 225–240. [PubMed]

195. Chu, H.-L.; Yu, H.-Y.; Yip, B.-S.; Chih, Y.-H.; Liang, C.-W.; Cheng, H.-T.; Cheng, J.-W. Boosting salt resistance of short antimicrobial peptides. *Antimicrob. Agents Chemother.* **2013**, *57*, 4050–4052. [CrossRef] [PubMed]

196. Yin, L.M.; Edwards, M.A.; Li, J.; Yip, C.M.; Deber, C.M. Roles of hydrophobicity and charge distribution of cationic antimicrobial peptides in peptide-membrane interactions. *J. Biol. Chem.* **2012**, *287*, 7738–7745. [CrossRef] [PubMed]

197. Wang, G.; Hanke, M.L.; Mishra, B.; Lushnikova, T.; Heim, C.E.; Chittezham Thomas, V.; Bayles, K.W.; Kielian, T. Transformation of human cathelicidin LL-37 into selective, stable, and potent antimicrobial compounds. *ACS Chem. Biol.* **2014**, *9*, 1997–2002. [CrossRef] [PubMed]

198. Naghmouchi, K.; Le Lay, C.; Baah, J.; Drider, D. Antibiotic and antimicrobial peptide combinations: Synergistic inhibition of *Pseudomonas fluorescens* and antibiotic-resistant variants. *Res. Microbiol.* **2012**, *163*, 101–108. [CrossRef] [PubMed]

199. Nuding, S.; Frasch, T.; Schaller, M.; Stange, E.F.; Zabel, L.T. Synergistic effects of antimicrobial peptides and antibiotics against *Clostridium difficile*. *Antimicrob. Agents Chemother.* **2014**, *58*, 5719–5725. [CrossRef] [PubMed]

200. Crane, M.; Handy, R.D.; Garrod, J.; Owen, R. Ecotoxicity test methods and environmental hazard assessment for engineered nanoparticles. *Ecotoxicology* **2008**, *17*, 421. [CrossRef] [PubMed]

201. Bour, A.; Mouchet, F.; Silvestre, J.; Gauthier, L.; Pinelli, E. Environmentally relevant approaches to assess nanoparticles ecotoxicity: A review. *J. Hazard. Mater.* **2015**, *283*, 764–777. [CrossRef] [PubMed]

202. Wang, K.; Yan, J.; Dang, W.; Liu, X.; Chen, R.; Zhang, J.; Zhang, B.; Zhang, W.; Kai, M.; Yan, W. Membrane active antimicrobial activity and molecular dynamics study of a novel cationic antimicrobial peptide polybia-MPI, from the venom of *Polybia paulista*. *Peptides* **2013**, *39*, 80–88. [CrossRef] [PubMed]

203. Lee, D.G.; Kim, H.K.; Am Kim, S.; Park, Y.; Park, S.-C.; Jang, S.-H.; Hahm, K.-S. Fungicidal effect of indolicidin and its interaction with phospholipid membranes. *Biochem. Biophys. Res. Commun.* **2003**, *305*, 305–310. [CrossRef]

204. Bahar, A.A.; Ren, D. Antimicrobial peptides. *Pharmaceuticals* **2013**, *6*, 1543–1575. [CrossRef] [PubMed]

205. Musielak, T.J.; Schenkel, L.; Kolb, M.; Henschen, A.; Bayer, M. A simple and versatile cell wall staining protocol to study plant reproduction. *Plant Reprod.* **2015**, *28*, 161–169. [CrossRef] [PubMed]

206. Bartnicki-Garcia, S.; Nickerson, W.J. Isolation, composition, and structure of cell walls of filamentous and yeast-like forms of *Mucor rouxii*. *Biochim. Biophys. Acta* **1962**, *58*, 102–119. [CrossRef]

207. Los, F.C.; Randis, T.M.; Aroian, R.V.; Ratner, A.J. Role of pore-forming toxins in bacterial infectious diseases. *Microbiol. Mol. Biol. Rev.* **2013**, *77*, 173–207. [CrossRef] [PubMed]

208. Dal Peraro, M.; Van Der Goot, F.G. Pore-forming toxins: Ancient, but never really out of fashion. *Nat. Rev. Microbiol.* **2016**, *14*, 77–92. [CrossRef] [PubMed]

209. Bacalum, M.; Radu, M. Cationic antimicrobial peptides cytotoxicity on mammalian cells: An analysis using therapeutic index integrative concept. *Int. J. Pept. Res. Ther.* **2015**, *21*, 47–55. [CrossRef]

210. Slavík, J. Anilinonaphthalene sulfonate as a probe of membrane composition and function. *Biochim. Biophys. Acta (BBA)-Rev. Biomembr.* **1982**, *694*, 1–25. [CrossRef]

211. Ramamoorthy, A.; Thennarasu, S.; Tan, A.; Lee, D.-K.; Clayberger, C.; Krensky, A.M. Cell selectivity correlates with membrane-specific interactions: A case study on the antimicrobial peptide G15 derived from granulysin. *Biochim. Biophys. Acta (BBA)-Biomembr.* **2006**, *1758*, 154–163. [CrossRef] [PubMed]

212. Choi, H.; Yang, Z.; Weisshaar, J.C. Single-cell, real-time detection of oxidative stress induced in *Escherichia coli* by the antimicrobial peptide CM15. *Proc. Natl. Acad. Sci. USA* **2015**, *112*, E303–E310. [CrossRef] [PubMed]

213. Manova, V.; Gruszka, D. DNA damage and repair in plants–from models to crops. *Front. Plant Sci.* **2015**, *6*, 885. [CrossRef] [PubMed]

214. Helmerhorst, E.J.; Troxler, R.F.; Oppenheim, F.G. The human salivary peptide histatin 5 exerts its antifungal activity through the formation of reactive oxygen species. *Proc. Natl. Acad. Sci. USA* **2001**, *98*, 14637–14642. [CrossRef] [PubMed]

215. Pflugmacher, S.; Kwon, K.-S.; Baik, S.; Kim, S.; Kühn, S.; Esterhuizen-Londt, M. Physiological responses of *Cladophora glomerata* to cyanotoxins: A potential new phytoremediation species for the Green Liver Systems. *Toxicol. Environ. Chem.* **2016**, *98*, 241–259. [CrossRef]

216. Vilvert, E.; Contardo-Jara, V.; Esterhuizen-Londt, M.; Pflugmacher, S. The effect of oxytetracycline on physiological and enzymatic defense responses in aquatic plant species *Egeria densa*, *Azolla caroliniana*, and *Taxiphyllum barbieri*. *Toxicol. Environ. Chem.* **2017**, *99*, 104–116. [CrossRef]

217. Pflugmacher, S. Promotion of oxidative stress in the aquatic macrophyte *Ceratophyllum demersum* during biotransformation of the cyanobacterial toxin microcystin-LR. *Aquat. Toxicol.* **2004**, *70*, 169–178. [CrossRef] [PubMed]

218. Dhawan, A.; Anderson, D. *The Comet Assay in Toxicology*; Royal Society of Chemistry: Cambridge, UK, 2016; Volume 30.

219. de Lapuente, J.; Lourenço, J.; Mendo, S.A.; Borràs, M.; Martins, M.G.; Costa, P.M.; Pacheco, M. The Comet assay and its applications in the field of ecotoxicology: A mature tool that continues to expand its perspectives. *Front. Genet.* **2015**, *6*, 180. [CrossRef] [PubMed]

220. Frenzilli, G.; Bean, T.; Lyons, B. The application of the Comet assay in aquatic environments. *Comet Assay Toxicol.* **2016**, *30*, 354.

221. Cotter, P.D. An 'Upp'-turn in bacteriocin receptor identification. *Mol. Microbiol.* **2014**, *92*, 1159–1163. [CrossRef] [PubMed]

222. Hendriks, G.; Atallah, M.; Morolli, B.; Calléja, F.; Ras-Verloop, N.; Huijskens, I.; Raamsman, M.; van de Water, B.; Vrieling, H. The ToxTracker assay: Novel GFP reporter systems that provide mechanistic insight into the genotoxic properties of chemicals. *Toxicol. Sci.* **2011**, *125*, 285–298. [CrossRef] [PubMed]

223. Hendriks, G.; Derr, R.S.; Misovic, B.; Morolli, B.; Calléja, F.M.; Vrieling, H. The extended ToxTracker assay discriminates between induction of DNA damage, oxidative stress, and protein misfolding. *Toxicol. Sci.* **2015**, *150*, 190–203. [CrossRef] [PubMed]

224. Otvos, L., Jr.; O, I.; Rogers, M.E.; Consolvo, P.J.; Condie, B.A.; Lovas, S.; Bulet, P.; Blaszczyk-Thurin, M. Interaction between heat shock proteins and antimicrobial peptides. *Biochemistry* **2000**, *39*, 14150–14159. [CrossRef] [PubMed]

225. Mashaghi, A.; Bezrukavnikov, S.; Minde, D.P.; Wentink, A.S.; Kityk, R.; Zachmann-Brand, B.; Mayer, M.P.; Kramer, G.; Bukau, B.; Tans, S.J. Alternative modes of client binding enable functional plasticity of Hsp70. *Nature* **2016**, *539*, 448–451. [CrossRef] [PubMed]

11

Characterization of the Lytic Capability of a LysK-Like Endolysin, Lys-phiSA012, Derived from a Polyvalent *Staphylococcus aureus* Bacteriophage

Jumpei Fujiki [1],[†] (ID), **Tomohiro Nakamura** [1],[†], **Takaaki Furusawa** [1], **Hazuki Ohno** [1], **Hiromichi Takahashi** [1], **Junya Kitana** [1], **Masaru Usui** [2], **Hidetoshi Higuchi** [3], **Yasunori Tanji** [4] (ID), **Yutaka Tamura** [2],[5] and **Hidetomo Iwano** [1],[*] (ID)

[1]   Laboratory of Biochemistry, School of Veterinary Medicine, Rakuno Gakuen University, Ebetsu 069-8501, Japan; j-fujiki@rakuno.ac.jp (J.F.); tomohiro-tobi-@hotmail.co.jp (T.N.); s21441012@stu.rakuno.ac.jp (T.F.); leafmoon-0812@honey.ocn.ne.jp (H.O.); l3ump_fnch@yahoo.co.jp (H.T.); s21361043@stu.rakuno.ac.jp (J.K.)

[2]   Laboratory of Food Microbiology and Food Safety, School of Veterinary Medicine, Rakuno Gakuen University, Ebetsu 069-8501, Japan; usuima@rakuno.ac.jp (M.U.); tamuray@rakuno.ac.jp (Y.T.)

[3]   Laboratory of Veterinary Hygiene, School of Veterinary Medicine, Rakuno Gakuen University, Ebetsu 069-8501, Japan; higuchi@rakuno.ac.jp

[4]   Department of Bioengineering, Tokyo Institute of Technology, Yokohama 226-8502, Japan; ytanji@bio.titech.ac.jp

[5]   Center for Veterinary Drug Development, Rakuno Gakuen University, Ebetsu 069-8501, Japan

[*]   Correspondence: h-iwano@rakuno.ac.jp

[†]   These authors contributed equally to this paper.

Abstract: Antibiotic-resistant bacteria (ARB) have spread widely and rapidly, with their increased occurrence corresponding with the increased use of antibiotics. Infections caused by *Staphylococcus aureus* have a considerable negative impact on human and livestock health. Bacteriophages and their peptidoglycan hydrolytic enzymes (endolysins) have received significant attention as novel approaches against ARB, including *S. aureus*. In the present study, we purified an endolysin, Lys-phiSA012, which harbors a cysteine/histidine-dependent amidohydrolase/peptidase (CHAP) domain, an amidase domain, and a SH3b cell wall binding domain, derived from a polyvalent *S. aureus* bacteriophage which we reported previously. We demonstrate that Lys-phiSA012 exhibits high lytic activity towards staphylococcal strains, including methicillin-resistant *S. aureus* (MRSA). Analysis of deletion mutants showed that only mutants possessing the CHAP and SH3b domains could lyse *S. aureus*, indicating that lytic activity of the CHAP domain depended on the SH3b domain. The presence of at least 1 mM Ca^{2+} and 100 μM Zn^{2+} enhanced the lytic activity of Lys-phiSA012 in a turbidity reduction assay. Furthermore, a minimum inhibitory concentration (MIC) assay showed that the addition of Lys-phiSA012 decreased the MIC of oxacillin. Our results suggest that endolysins are a promising approach for replacing current antimicrobial agents and may contribute to the proper use of antibiotics, leading to the reduction of ARB.

Keywords: antibiotic resistant; multidrug resistant; antimicrobial agent; phage therapy; bacteriophage; endolysin; staphylococci; *Staphylococcus aureus*

1. Introduction

Antibiotic-resistant bacteria (ARB) have spread rapidly worldwide and are an important global health issue. ARB often result from the inappropriate use of antibiotics [1–3] and the occurrence of ARB is correlated with the amount of antibiotics used [4]. In the United States, about half of antibiotics are used to treat humans annually and the other half to treat livestock and for other agricultural applications [5]. Notably, antibiotics are administered to livestock for not only preventive and therapeutic approaches against infectious diseases, but also to improve growth [6]. Annual worldwide veterinary antibiotics (VA) use is now 10^5–10^6 tones [7,8]. Several reports have suggested that antibiotics are used more heavily in livestock than in humans and VAs may be the largest source of ARB [9–11]. Indeed, transmission of ARB, such as methicillin-resistant *Staphylococcus aureus* (MRSA), by veterinary staff in contact with ARB carrier animals, and the potential role of the farm environment in the spread of ARB, have been reported [12–16], suggesting the environmental transfer of ARB from animals to humans.

ARBs that exhibit resistance to more than three classes of antibiotics are called multidrug-resistant bacteria (MDR). *Staphylococcus aureus*, an ESKAPE pathogen (*Enterococcus faecium, Staphylococcus aureus, Klebsiella pneumoniae, Acinetobacter baumanii, Pseudomonas aeruginosa* and *Enterobacter* spp.), is frequently isolated from clinical samples and is considered the major MDR. *S. aureus* has a considerable negative impact on human and veterinary medicine because the treatment of antibiotic-resistant *S. aureus*, including MRSA infections, are complicated due to the bacterium's multiple antibiotic-resistant mechanisms. In the veterinary field, mastitis caused by *S. aureus* negatively impacts milk production, leading to an economic loss of more than $100 million annually in the United States and Japan [17,18]. *S. aureus* also is the most common pathogen causing chronic mastitis [19]. Furthermore, MRSA is spreading in hospitalized patients [20]. According to World Health Organization (WHO) reports, patients with MRSA are estimated to be 64% more likely to die compared with patients with non-resistant infections. A study by Lord O'Neill and colleagues, commissioned by the United Kingdom government, estimated that ARB would cause 10 million deaths each year by 2050 and will become a bigger risk than cancer [21,22]. Therefore, we face an unprecedented challenge from the emergence of ARB such as MRSA and MDR *P. aeruginosa*, putting humans and livestock at great risk. A novel alternative antimicrobial strategy is thus urgently required. Bacteriophages and bacteriophage enzyme-based approaches have potential as alternative tools for overcoming infectious diseases caused by ARB [23,24].

Phage therapy, an alternative to classical antibiotic therapy, is receiving significant attention because bacteriophages are the most abundant organisms and infect bacteria specifically [24,25]. This allows their rapid and simple isolation from the environment and clinical application to kill pathogenic bacteria. We previously demonstrated that phage therapy is effective for treating equine keratitis caused by *P. aeruginosa* [26] and the lysis of antibiotic-resistant *P. aeruginosa* [27]. We also reported the isolation of a bacteriophage, phiSA012, and its wide host range towards various *S. aureus* strains [28] and its effective lytic capacity in a mouse mastitis model caused by *S. aureus* [29]. Challenges in the use of phage therapy have also been reported, such as the occurrence of phage-resistant bacteria, and horizontal gene transfer leading to increased bacterial virulence [30,31].

Endolysins are peptidoglycan hydrolytic enzymes produced by bacteriophages and cleave cell wall peptidoglycan. Endolysins can thus target bacteria at the last stage of the lytic cycle using mechanisms different from those of antibiotics, and show cell lysis activity toward ARB such as *S. aureus* [23] and *P. aeruginosa* [32] in the absence of horizontal gene transfer. Interestingly, bacteria are unlikely to develop resistance towards endolysins [33,34] because endolysins may cleave peptidoglycan sites essential for bacterial survival, and bacteriophages have developed highly efficient enzymes through evolution [35–37]. In addition, endolysins affect persisters, which are dormant bacteria showing high tolerance to antibiotics, and biofilms [38,39], and can be engineered to readily fuse with functional peptides [37]. Taken together, endolysins have enormous potential as a flexible tool for combatting ARB.

S. aureus bacteriophage endolysins such as Lys-phiK, Lys-GH15 and Lys-phiTwort have been isolated and investigated [40–42]. These endolysins are multidomain enzymes composed of a cysteine, histidine dependent amidohydrolase/peptidase (CHAP) domain at the N-terminus, an amidase (AMID) domain and a SH3b cell wall binding domain at the C-terminus and demonstrate high lytic activity toward *S. aureus*. The lytic efficacy and immune response of Lys-GH15 in vivo was previously reported [41,43]. In addition, the structures of three individual domains of Lys-GH15 were determined [44]. Notably, Lys-phiK is regarded as one of the best-characterized endolysins [23] and reveals a broad antimicrobial spectrum toward staphylococci isolated clinically from bovine and human [40]. It was reported that the Lys-phiK CHAP domain plays a critical role in the lysis of live staphylococcus and that lysis depends on the SH3b domain [45]. The crystal structure of the CHAP domain has been determined [46]. However, the properties of Lys-phiK related endolysins are not fully characterized. The aim of the present study was to demonstrate the possible preventive and therapeutic utility of efficient endolysins for clinical applications. To this end, we isolated and purified Lys-phiSA012, which has high amino acid sequence similarity with Lys-phiK, and studied the properties of Lys-phiSA012 lytic activity.

2. Materials & Methods

2.1. Bacterial Strains

Bacterial strains used in the turbidity reduction assays, minimum inhibitory concentration (MIC) assay, and minimum bactericidal concentration (MBC) assay, are summarized in Table 1. The staphylococcal and streptococcal strains were grown at 37 °C with aeration in lysogeny broth (LB) containing 2% tryptone (Difco, Detroit, MI, USA), 0.5% yeast extract (Difco) and Tod-Hewitt broth (THB) (Kanto Kagaku, Tokyo, Japan). *Escherichia coli* DH5α and BL21(DE3) (Takara, Otsu, Japan) were grown at 37 °C with aeration in LB medium for all subcloning. When needed, 100 µg/mL ampicillin was added to the LB medium (final concentration).

Table 1. Staphylococcal and streptococcal strains.

Bacterial Strains	Name	References and Remarks				
Staphylococcus aureus	SA003	Synnott, A.J. et al. [28], Iwano, H. et al. [29]				
Staphylococcus pseudointermedius	StaP001					
Staphylococcus haemolyticus	StaH001	Field isolates identified by their 16s ribosomal RNA sequences.				
Streptococcus agalactiae	StrA001					
		Scc *mec*	MLST	spa type	Antimicrobial-resistance pattern	Refarences
MRSA	MRSA 2007-13	II	NT	t002	MPIPC, GM, KM, EM, OTC, ERFX	Ishihara, K. et al. [47]
	MRSA 2007-28	II	NT	t1265	MPIPC, KM, EM,	
	MRSA 2007-57	IV	NT	t008	MPIPC, GM, KM, EM	
	MRSA 2007-93	II	NT	t062	MPIPC, KM, EM, OTC, CP, ERFX	
	MRSA VC39 Vet-1	IV	ST380	t021	MPIPC, SM, KM, GM, EM	Ishihara, K. et al. [48]
	MRSA VC50 Vet-1	IV	ST30	t1852	MPIPC, KM, GM, EM, CPFX	

MPIPC; oxacillin (breakpoint, 4 µg/mL), GM; gentamicin (16 µg/mL), KM; kanamycin (64 µg/mL), EM; erythromycin (8 µg/mL), OTC; oxytetracyclin (32 µg/mL), ERFX; enrofloxacin (4 µg/mL), CP; chloramphenicol (32 µg/mL) SM; streptomycin (64 µg/mL), CPFX; ciprofloxacin (4 µg/mL). Breakpoints were adopted according to the Clinical and Laboratory Standards Institute guidelines [49].

2.2. Bacteriophage and Genome Analysis

We previously reported the isolation of phiSA012 from a sewage treatment plant located in Tokyo (Japan) [28]. The genomic sequence of phiSA012 was published (NC_023573.1) and the endolysin amino acid sequence is available (YP_009006722). Protein sequence analysis and classification of Lys-phiSA012 were performed using InterPro to predict the domain architecture. The DNA of phiSA012 was isolated as described by Synnott et al. using a plate assay and centrifuged in polyethylene glycol 6000-NaCl [28]. PhiSA012 was then incubated in SNET buffer (400 µg/mL ProteinaseK (Takara), 20 mM Tris-HCl, 400 mM NaCl, 1% SDS, 5 mM EDTA) at 55 °C overnight, phiSA012 DNA was extracted using phenol and chloroform, then purified by ethanol precipitation.

2.3. Purification of Lys-phiSA012 Recombinant Protein

The extracted phiSA012 DNA was used for subcloning of Lys-phiSA012. The endolysin gene was amplified with the primers Lys012-1Fw and Lys012-495Rv, as shown in Table 2. The amplified fragment was purified and subcloned into pGEX-6P-2 (GE, Buckinghamshire, UK) encoding a glutathione S-transferase (GST)-tag sequence at the C-terminal using an In-Fusion HD cloning kit (Clontech, Palo Alto, CA, USA), then the plasmid encoding Lys-phiSA012, pGEX-Lys012WT, was constructed. All subcloning was performed in *E. coli* DH5α. Plasmid construct accuracy was confirmed by DNA sequence analysis using a Big Dye Terminator V3.1 cycle sequencing kit (Applied Biosystems, Foster City, CA, USA) and an Applied Biosystems 3130 Genetic Analyzer. The cloned gene expression was performed as described elsewhere [45,50] with slight modifications. In brief, the plasmid was used to transform *E. coli* BL21(DE3) and expression of the endolysin gene was induced by the addition of 0.1 mM isopropyl-β-thiogalactopyranoside (final concentration) (Nacalai Tesque, Kyoto, Japan). Cells were incubated with shaking overnight at 25 °C in a BIO-SHAKER BR-40LF (Taitec, Saitama, Japan). After centrifugation at $2300 \times g$ for 5 min at 4 °C, the supernatant was removed and 50 mM Tris-HCl, 1 M $MgCl_2$ and 10% NP-40 (Wako, Osaka, Japan) were added to the pellet and the mixture was sonicated using a Bioruptor UCD-200 (Cosmo Bio, Tokyo, Japan). The mixture was centrifuged at $16,000 \times g$ for 30 min at 4 °C, then the supernatant containing soluble protein was purified using Econo-Pac® disposable chromatography columns (Bio-Rad Laboratories, Inc., Hercules, CA, USA) packed with glutathione Sepharose 4B (GE). The identity and concentration of the expressed protein was confirmed by sodium dodecyl sulfate polyacrylamide gel electrophoresis (SDS-PAGE). The obtained Lys-phiSA012 was stored at −30 °C until use.

Table 2. Plasmids and primers.

Plasmids	Protein Produced (Amino Acids)	Forward Primes	Reverse Primers	Recipient Vectors
pGEX-Lys012WT	1-495	Lys012-1Fw	Lys012-495Rv	pGEX-6P-2
pGEX-Lys012Δmt1	161-495	Lys012-161Fw	Lys012-495Rv	pGEX-6P-2
pGEX-Lys012Δmt2	1-221, 390-495	1-221; Lys012-1Fw	1-221; Lys012-Δmt2Rv	pGEX-6P-2
		390-495; Lys012-Δmt2Fw	390-495; Lys012-495Rv	
		Overwrap; Lys012-1Fw	Overwrap; Lys012-495Rv	
pGEX-Lys012Δmt2′	1-221	Lys012-1Fw	Lys012-221Rv	pGEX-6P-2
pGEX-Lys012Δmt3	1-408	Lys012-1Fw	Lys012-408Rv	pGEX-6P-2
pGEX-Lys012Δmt4	386-495	Lys012-386Fw	Lys012-495Rv	pGEX-6P-2
pGEX-Lys012Δmt5	161-408	Lys012-161Fw	Lys012-408Rv	pGEX-6P-2
pGEX-Lys012Δmt6	1-187	Lys012-1Fw	Lys012-187Rv	pGEX-6P-2

Primers	Sequences
Lys012-1Fw	5′-<u>TCCCCAGGAATTCCC</u>ATGGCTAAGACTCAAGCAGA-3′
Lys012-161Fw	5′-TCCCCAGGAATTCCCATGATACCTGTAAAAGCAGGAA-3′
Lys012-386Fw	5′-TCCCCAGGAATTCCCATGACAAGTAGCGCA-3′
Lys012-187Rv	5′-CGCTCCAGTCGACCCCTATTTCTTTTTAGGTGCAG-3′
Lys012-221Rv	5′-CGCTCGAGTCGACCCCTATGAAGAACGACCTGC-3′
Lys012-408Rv	5′-CGCTAGTCGACCCCTAAGTTCCGTACTGGTTC-3′
Lys012-495Rv	5′-<u>CGCTCGAGTCGACCCC</u>TACTTGAATACTCCCCAGG-3′
Lys012-Δmt2Fw	5′-CACAACGATGCAGGTCGTTCTTCAAGTACACCGGCAACTAGACCAGTTAC-3′
Lys012-Δmt2Rv	5′-GTAACTGGTCTAGTTGCCGGTGTACTTGAAGAACGACCTGCATCGTTGTG-3′

Sequences complementary to linearized pGEX-6P-2 for In-fusion cloning are underlined.

2.4. Generation of Domain(s) Deletion Mutants

pGEX-Lys012WT was used for the construction of seven deletion mutant plasmids encoding a single domain or multiple domains of endolysin. Certain fragments of gene for Lys-phiSA012 were amplified with the primers summarized in Table 2. To construct pGEX-Lys012Δmt2, two amplified fragments, corresponding to amino acids 1–221 and 390–495, were used for overwrap PCR using Lys012-1Fw and Lys012-495Rv primers. The amplified fragments were subcloned into pGEX-6P-2 and each protein was purified as described above.

2.5. Turbidity Reduction Assays

The lytic activity of Lys-phiSA012 and each deletion mutant protein was assessed using turbidity reduction assays as described by Becker et al. [45] and Son et al. [51], with some modifications. In brief, staphylococcal strains and streptococcal strains were grown in LB medium or THB medium at 37 °C to an OD_{600} of 1.0. Each culture was centrifuged at $2300\times g$ for 5 min at 4 °C and the cells were resuspended in $2\times$ LB medium, then stored on ice until use. Turbidity reduction assays were initiated by adding the same amount of purified Lys-phiSA012 or each domain(s) deletion mutant, then the OD_{600} value was monitored using a plate reader (Sunrise Rainbow Thermos RC, TECAN Austria GmbH, Salzburg, Austria). To evaluate the effect of Ca^{2+} and Zn^{2+} on endolysin lytic activity, SA003 was prepared as described above. After centrifugation at $2300\times g$ for 5 min at 4 °C, the cells were resuspended in TBS (50 mM Tris-HCl, 138 mM NaCl, 2.7 mM KCl) buffer with $CaCl_2$ (0 μM, 1 μM, 10 μM, 100 μM, 1 mM, 2.5 mM, 5 mM) or $ZnCl_2$ (0 μM, 1 μM, 10 μM, 100 μM, 500 μM, 1 mM, 2.5 mM). The OD_{600} value was monitored with incubation using the plate reader after the addition of Lys-phiSA012.

2.6. MIC and MBC Assays

MIC and MBC assays were performed as described previously [45,52] with some modifications. The MIC values of oxacillin with or without Lys-phiSA012 towards SA003 were determined in 96-well plates. Each plate incubated serial 2-fold dilution of oxacillin and Lys-phiSA012 using LB medium overnight at 37 °C at concentrations ranging from 64 to 0 μg/mL and from 2.0 to 0 μg/mL, respectively. Overnight incubation was initiated by adding 10 μL SA003 to each well of the 96-well plate that also contained 100 μL LB medium. The MBC values of Lys-phiSA012 towards SA003 with 25% glycerol were determined using LB medium after overnight incubation at 37 °C. After the MIC assay of Lys-phiSA012 with 25% glycerol, 10 μL of liquid from each well in the 96-well plate was transferred to a fresh 96-well plate containing 100 μL antimicrobial agent free LB medium. The MIC and MBC values were evaluated by visual inspection after overnight incubation. MIC and MBC assays of glycerol were also performed using the same methods.

2.7. Bioinformatics Analysis

Amino acid sequences for multiple alignment and protein structure homology modeling were obtained from the National Center for Biotechnology Information (NCBI) database. Multiple alignment analysis between endolysin sequences was performed using GENETYX software v.10. The 3D protein structure models of the cysteine, histidine dependent amidohydrolases/peptidases (CHAP) and amidase (AMID) domain on Lys-phiSA012 were constructed and analyzed with modeling by homology to the existing crystal structure using the SWISS-MODEL server [53–56]. Homologous proteins and amino acid sequence alignments are summarized in Table 3 and Supplementary Materials Figure S1. A BLAST search was performed using the nucleotide sequence of Lys-phiK obtained from NCBI database as a query sequence. Endolysins which revealed over 90% query cover and identity are summarized in Table 4.

Table 3. Protein structure modeling information.

	Homologous Protein	Source Organism	Residues	Protein ID in PDBe	Seq. Identity	Ligands
Lys-phiSA012 CHAP	ORF30/31 CHAP domain	*Staphylococcus* virus K (Gene name: PhageK_071)	1–165	4ct3.1	99.39%	Ca^{2+} Cl^{-} Hg^{2+}
Lys-phiSA012 AMID	Endolysin / *N*-acetylmuramoyl-L-alanine amidase	*Staphylococcus* phage GH15 (Gene name: GH15_071)	165–403	4ols	100%	Zn^{2+} Mg^{2+} Fe^{3+}

Table 4. LysK-like endolysins.

Source of Endolysin	Query Cover (Nucleotide)	Identity (Nucleotide)	Accession	26	48	83	107	109	113	165	231	300	372	380	383	406	414	425	437	452	453	470	484	485	486	493	Identity (Amino Acid)
																											Residue at Position (Amino Asid)
Bacteriophage K	100%	100%	AY176327.1	V	G	S	F	S	E	A	N	A	D	V	D	Y	N	V	V	V	C	N	N	Q	I	V	100.00%
Bacteriophage JD007	100%	99%	JX878671.1	V	G	S	F	S	E	A	A	A	D	V	D	Y	N	V	V	V	C	N	N	Q	I	V	100.00%
Bacteriophage SA012	100%	99%	AB903967.1	V	G	N	F	S	E	A	N	A	D	V	D	Y	N	V	V	V	C	N	N	Q	I	V	99.80%
Bacteriophage vB_Sau_CG	100%	99%	KY794641.1	V	G	N	F	S	Q	A	T	A	D	V	D	Y	N	V	V	V	C	N	N	Q	I	V	99.39%
Bacteriophage S25-3	100%	99%	AB853330.1	V	G	N	F	S	E	E	N	T	D	V	D	Y	N	V	V	V	C	N	N	Q	I	V	99.39%
Bacteriophage S25-4	100%	99%	AB853331.1	V	G	N	F	S	E	E	N	T	D	V	D	Y	N	V	V	V	C	N	N	Q	I	V	99.39%
Bacteriophage SA3	100%	96%	MF001365.1	I	G	S	F	S	Q	A	N	A	D	V	D	Y	N	V	V	V	C	N	N	H	I	V	99.39%
Bacteriophage qdsa002	100%	96%	KY779849.1	I	G	S	F	S	Q	A	N	A	D	V	D	Y	N	V	V	V	C	N	N	H	I	V	99.39%
Bacteriophage GH15	100%	96%	JQ686190.1	I	G	S	F	S	Q	A	N	A	D	V	D	Y	N	V	V	V	C	D	N	H	I	V	99.19%
Bacteriophage vB_Sau_Clo6	100%	94%	KY794642.1	V	K	N	Y	E	E	A	K	A	N	K	K	Y	N	V	V	I	A	D	S	Y	T	I	97.98%
Bacteriophage vB_Sau_S24	100%	94%	KY794643.1	V	K	N	Y	E	E	A	K	A	N	V	K	Y	N	V	V	V	N	N	S	Q	V	T	97.37%
Bacteriophage MCE-2014	99%	99%	KJ888149.1	V	G	S	F	S	E	A	N	A	D	V	D	Y	N	V	I	V	C	N	N	H	V	V	99.39%
Bacteriophage IPLA-RODI	99%	95%	KP027446.1	I	G	S	F	S	Q	A	N	A	F	S	I	D	F	S	I	I	V	C	N	N	H	I	V	98.38%
						CHAP						Amidase							SH3b									

Amino acid changes compared to Lys-phiK are indicated in blue (Lys-phiSA012) or yellow (other).

2.8. Statistical Analysis

Statistical analysis was conducted using the Tukey-Kramer test based on one-way ANOVA from three independent experiments. Statistically significant differences are indicated by asterisks (*: $p < 0.05$, **: $p < 0.01$) or crosses (†: $p < 0.05$).

3. Results

3.1. Lytic Activity and the Antimicrobial Spectrum of Lys-phiSA012.

The endolysin of phiSA012, Lys-phiSA012, is encoded in ORF51 and is composed of 495 amino acids. The conserved domain of Lys-phiSA012 was shown by bioinformatics analysis to be a cysteine, histidine dependent amidohydrolase/peptidase (CHAP) domain at the N-terminus encompassing amino acid residues 29–160, an amidase (AMID) domain encompassing amino acid residues 188–385, and a SH3b cell wall binding domain at the C-terminus encompassing amino acid residues 409–481 (Figure 1).

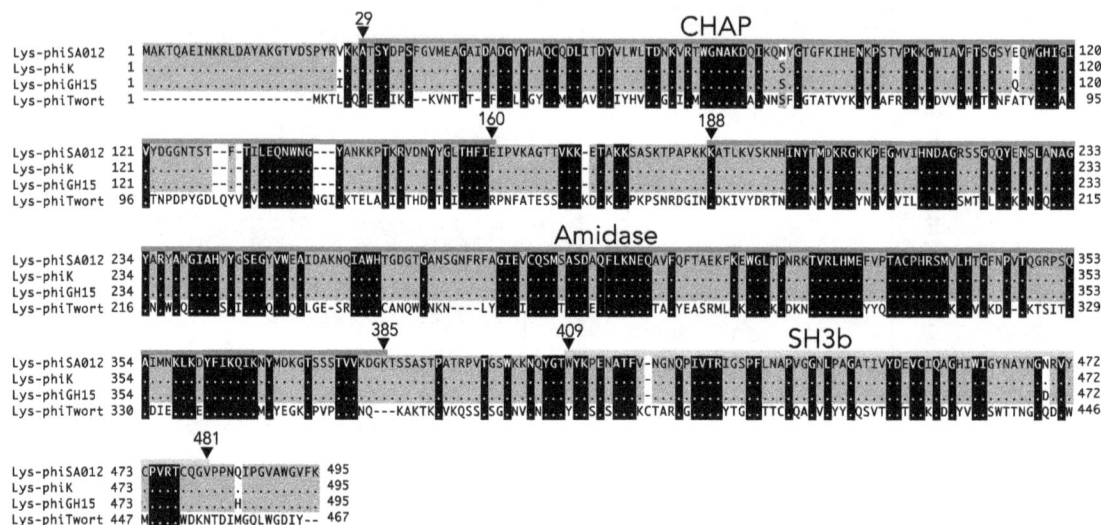

Figure 1. Prediction of the domain architecture and multiple alignment analysis of Lys-phiSA012. Lys-phiSA012 is composed of a CHAP, AMID, and SH3b domain. The amino acid sequence of Lys-phiSA012 was analyzed using InterPro. Blue and yellow lines indicate the domain structure of Lys-phiSA012. Multiple alignment analysis of the full length endolysins Lys-phiSA012, Lys-phiK, Lys-phiGH15, and Lys-phiTwort. Identical residues are shown as dots and amino acid residues conserved between the four endolysins are highlighted by a black (100%) or gray (80%) scale.

Comparison of the amino acid sequences of Lys-phiSA012 with the characterized *Staphylococcus* endolysins, Lys-phiK, Lys-phiGH15, and Lys-phiTwort, revealed that Lys-phiSA012 has high amino acid sequence similarity with Lys-phiK (99.80%) and Lys-phiGH15 (98.99%), but not with Lys-phiTwort (44.54%) (Figure 1). Furthermore, endolysins which have high nucleotide sequence similarity with Lys-phiK (LysK-like eondolysins) were found by a BLAST search, as summarized in Table 4; however, the lytic capabilities of LysK-like endolysins (with the exception of Lys-GH15) remain poorly characterized. Previous reports have focused on the lytic capabilities of the bacteriophages vB_Sau_CG, vB_Sau_Clo6, vB_Sau_S24 [57], S25-3 [58], MCE-2014 [59] and IPLA-RODI [60], from which the LysK-like endolysins are derived, or only genome sequences of bacteriophages JD007, S25-4, SA3 and qdsa002 have been registered. Therefore, we initially produced Lys-phiSA012WT and performed turbidity reduction assays to confirm the lytic activity of Lys-phiSA012. As shown in Figure 2A, Lys-phiSA012 showed high lytic activity towards SA003 (A schematic of the produced Lys-phiSA012WT protein and SDS-PAGE analysis of the purified protein are shown in Figure 3A,B).

Broad lytic activity of phiSA012 and Lys-phiK has been reported [28,40]. To determine whether Lys-phiSA012 similarly has lytic activity beyond *S. aureus*, we examined the antimicrobial spectrum of Lys-phiSA012 towards staphylococcal strains and *Streptococcus agalactiae*. Lys-phiSA012 showed high antimicrobial activity towards not only SA003, but also StaP001 and StaH001 as expected. In addition, the OD_{600} was reduced within a few minutes of adding Lys-phiSA012, with an initial OD_{600} of 0.4–0.6 being reduced to OD_{600} <0.2 over 10 min (Figure 2A–C).

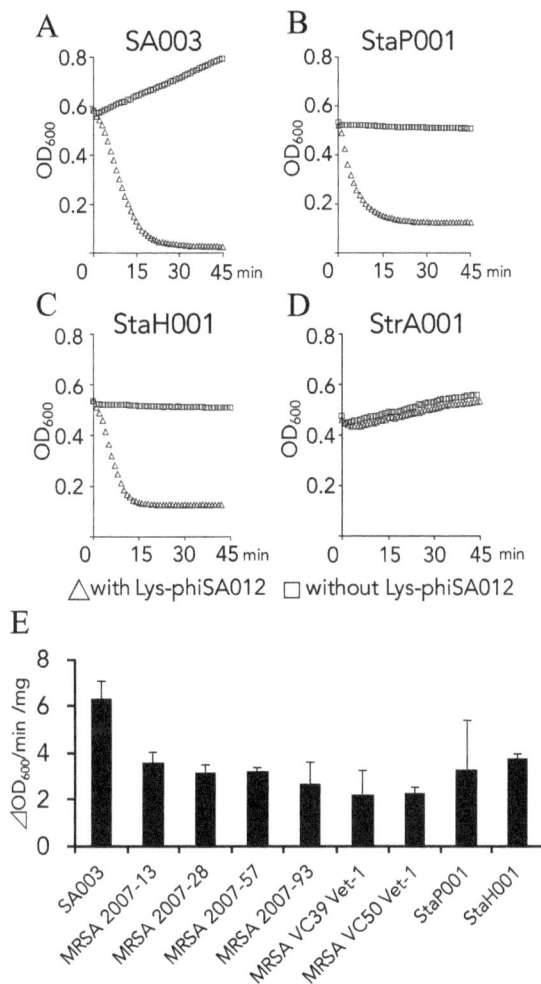

Figure 2. Antimicrobial spectrum of Lys-phiSA012. Lytic activities towards SA003, StaP, StaH, StrA and MRSA were examined using a turbidity reduction assay, as described in the materials and methods section. SA003 was isolated from bovine milk and has been reported to be susceptible to phiSA012 [28]. SA003 was also used in a mouse mastitis model [29]. MRSA strains were isolated from veterinarians and staff members of veterinary clinics [48,49]. Lys-phiSA012 (**A**) 109 μg/mL, (**B**) 132 μg/mL, (**C**) 132 μg/mL and (**D**) 106 μg/mL was added to the bacterial cultures. The values of OD_{600} were plotted each minute. (**E**) Lytic activities towards staphylococcal strains were examined. The maximum rate for each reaction is represented as ΔOD_{600} min^{-1} mg^{-1}, calculated as previously reported [61] and presented as means ± standard deviation (SD).

However, Lys-phiSA012 could not lyse StrA001, as shown by the turbidity reduction assay, and the initial OD_{600} increased with increasing incubation time (Figure 2D). We next assessed the antimicrobial activity of Lys-phiSA012 towards MRSA strains resistant against more than four antibiotics (Table 1). The turbidity reduction assay showed lytic activity of Lys-phiSA012 towards six MRSA strains (Figure 2E). The maximum rate for the lysis of SA003 (ΔOD_{600} min^{-1} mg^{-1}) was higher than that for the other strains.

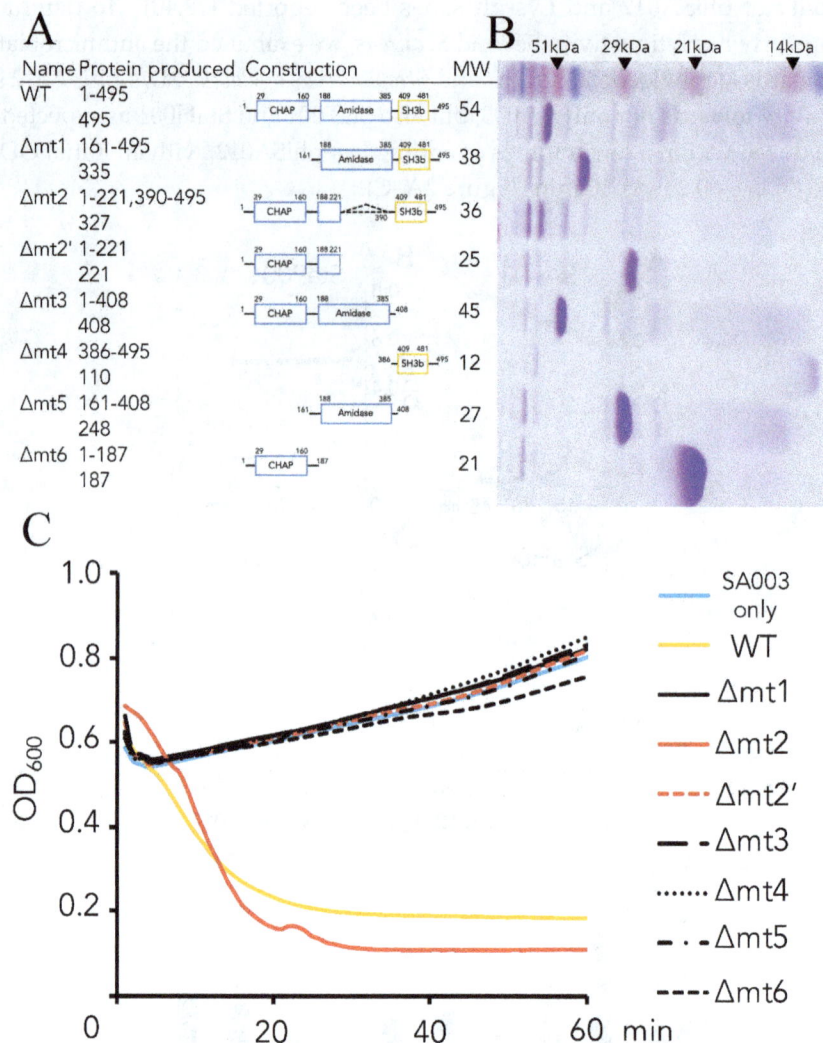

Figure 3. Schematic representation of Lys-phiSA012 and domain(s) deletion mutants and their lytic activities towards SA003. (**A**) Schematic representation of the Lys-phiSA012 protein construct. Amino acid residues 29–160: CHAP domain, 188–385: AMID domain, 409–481: SH3b domain. (**B**) SDS-PAGE of purified Lys-phiSA012 and each domain(s) deletion mutant, performed using 15% polyacrylamide gel. Upper lane; Standard molecular weight markers. (**C**) Lytic activities of Lys-phiSA012 and each domain(s) deletion mutant towards SA003. Except for Δmt2, 163.8 pmol of the endolysin was added to the culture medium. For Δmt2, 45.98 pmol was added.

3.2. Critical Region of the Lys-phiSA012 Protein Required for Lytic Activity

Next, we constructed plasmids encoding Lys-phiSA012 domain(s) deletion mutants to clarify the region of Lys-phiSA012 constructs critical for lytic activity towards SA003. The purified proteins were identified by SDS-PAGE analysis (Figure 3B). Turbidity reduction assays using the domain(s) deletion mutants clearly demonstrated that Lys-phiSA012Δmt2 showed high lytic activity similar to Lys-phiSA012WT (Figure 3C) whereas the other mutants showed no lytic activity towards SA003.

3.3. Optimal Ca^{2+} and Zn^{2+} Concentration for the Lytic Activity of Lys-phiSA012

Deletion analysis demonstrated that a CHAP domain and a SH3b domain play important roles for lytic activity. Enhancement of the lytic activity of endolysins by ions was previously reported [45,50]. Therefore, we next investigated the presence of an ion binding site in the Lys-phiSA012 catalytic domains. 3D models of the CHAP and AMID domain structures were constructed using the

SWISS-MODEL server. The homologous proteins used in structure modeling are summarized in Table 3 and the model-template alignment is shown in Figure A1.

The constructed model of the CHAP domain revealed that Ca^{2+} is bound in the N-terminal region and interacts with the side chains of Asp45, Asp47, Tyr49, His51 and Asp56 (Figure 4A). In addition, Cl^- and Hg^{2+} were indicated as bound ligands for the CHAP domain (Table 3). The constructed model of the AMID domain showed that Zn^{2+} is bound in the center of the domain and interacts with the side chains of His214, His324 and Cys332 (Figure 4B), and Mg^{2+} and Fe^{3+} were indicated as bound ligands for the AMID domain (Table 3). As shown in Figure 4C, no amino acid changes were observed in LysK-like endolysins at the Ca^{2+} and Zn^{2+}-binding site residues or at the CHAP active site residues of Lys-phiK [62].

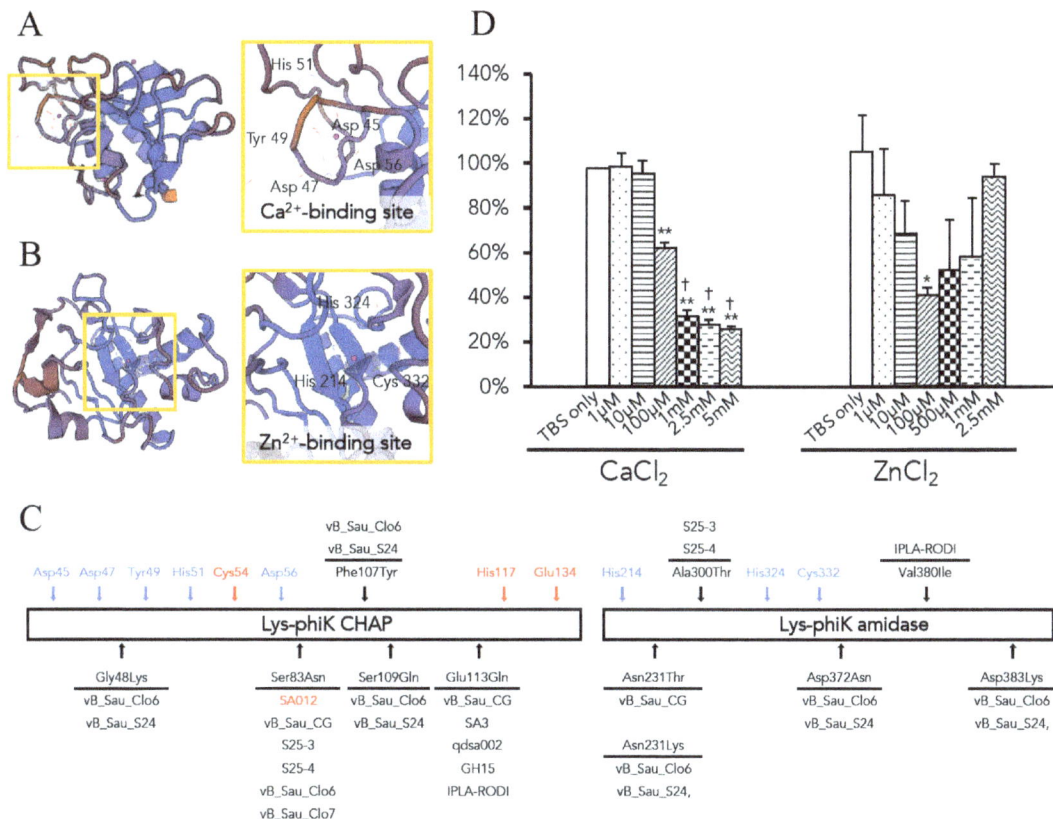

Figure 4. Protein structure modeling of the CHAP and AMID domains, and the effects of Ca^{2+} and Zn^{2+} on the lytic activity of Lys-phiSA012. Protein structure models of (**A**) the CHAP and (**B**) AMID domains in Lys-phiSA012. The models were constructed using the SWISS-MODEL server and the homologous proteins used for protein structure modeling are summarized in Table 3. Detailed views of the Ca^{2+} and Zn^{2+} coordination sites are framed in yellow. The Ca^{2+}-binding site is composed of Asp45, Asp47, Tyr49, His51 and Asp56. The Zn^{2+}-binding site is composed of His214, His324 and Cys332. Ions are shown as pink spheres. (**C**) Schematic image of the CHAP and AMID domain of Lys-phiK. Blue arrows indicate the amino acid residues which contacts with Ca^{2+} and Zn^{2+}. Red arrows indicate the active site residues of the CHAP domain. Black arrows indicate the amino acid changes in LysK-like endolysins summarized in Table 4. Bacteriophages whose endolysins are related to Lys-phiK are also indicated. Lys-phiSA012 differs by single amino acid residue from Lys-phiK, Ser83Asn on a CHAP domain. (**D**) The effects of Ca^{2+} and Zn^2 on the lytic activity of Lys-phiSA012 were analyzed using a turbidity reduction assay as described in the materials and methods section. Data are shown as relative OD_{600} reduction rate (initial OD600 divided by OD600 60 min after adding Lys-phiSA012). The values represent means ± SD. Significance was analyzed by the Tukey-Kramer test based on one-way ANOVA and is indicated by asterisks compared to TBS alone (*: $p < 0.05$, **: $p < 0.01$) or crosses against 100 μM Ca^{2+} (†: $p < 0.05$).

It was reported that Zn^{2+} inhibits the Lys-phiK activity and that Ca^{2+} enhances the stability of Lys-phiK but has no effect on lytic activity [63]. However, ions in the Lys-phiK buffer were not removed in those assays. Sanz-Gaitero et al. also commented on this point and suggested that Zn^{2+} might play a regulatory role [46]. Therefore, we examined the effects of Ca^{2+} and Zn^{2+} on the lytic activity of Lys-phiSA012 to determine the optimal Ca^{2+} and Zn^{2+} concentrations. Turbidity reduction assays were performed in the presence and absence of Ca^{2+} or Zn^{2+} in TBS buffer. The addition of Ca^{2+} significantly reduced the OD_{600} in a dose dependent manner. Notably, a high concentration of Ca^{2+} (above 1 mM) significantly increased Lys-phiSA012 activity compared to the addition of 100 µM Ca^{2+} (Figure 4C). Lys-phiSA012 exhibited no lytic activity in the absence of Ca^{2+} and the OD_{600} value did not change from the initial value of OD_{600} 0.6. The addition of 100 µM Zn^{2+} resulted in a significant decrease in OD_{600} compared to TBS alone; interestingly, however, the addition of 1 µM Zn^{2+} did not enhance the lytic activity of Lys-phiSA012 compared to TBS alone. We further examined whether divalent ions in LB medium affect lytic activity. Lys-phiSA012 in LB medium containing 10 µM EGTA did not inhibit the growth of SA003 (Figure A2).

3.4. MIC Assays of Oxacillin w/wo Lys-phiSA012

The MIC of oxacillin towards SA003 with or without (w/wo) Lys-phiSA012 was determined to confirm whether Lys-phiSA012 acts cooperatively with antibiotics due to the different mechanisms underlying the antimicrobial activities of endolysins and antibiotics. The oxacillin MIC without Lys-phiSA012 was ≥ 32 µg/mL, whereas the addition of 1.0 µg/mL or 2.0 µg/mL Lys-phiSA012 reduced the oxacillin MIC 16-fold (Figure 5A).

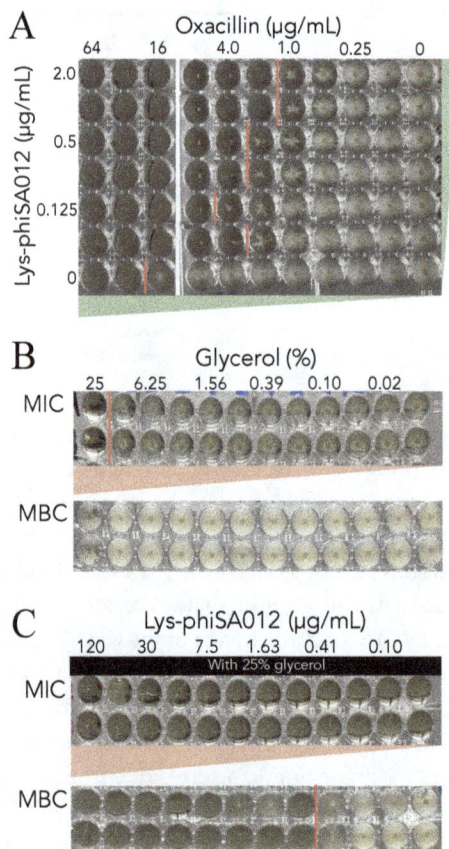

Figure 5. MIC and MBC assays. MIC and MBC assays were performed in 96-well plates. Red lines indicate the border of bacterial growth. (**A**) MIC assay of oxacillin towards SA003 with or without Lys-phiSA012. (**B**) MIC and MBC assays of glycerol towards SA003. (**C**) MIC and MBC assays of Lys-phiSA012 with 25% glycerol towards SA003.

Next, we examined suitable vehicles for endolysins. As shown in Figure 5B, 25% glycerol inhibited SA003 growth in MIC assays due to its bacteriostatic (and not bactericidal) activity, given that bacterial growth resumed after subculture, as confirmed by MBC assays (Figure 5B). An accurate MIC for Lys-phiSA012 could not be determined due to the initial high lytic activity of endolysins, as shown in Figure 2A–D and 3C, and their subsequent inactivation during overnight incubation. However, Lys-phiSA012 in 25% glycerol inhibited bacterial growth as shown by MIC assay after overnight incubation. Furthermore, the MBC of Lys-phiSA012 in 25% glycerol decreased at $\geq$0.815 µg/mL (Figure 5C).

4. Discussion

The discovery of penicillin by Alexander Fleming in 1928 lead to the purification and development of antibiotics in the 1940s, called the beginning of the era of antibiotics. The prevailing feeling during this era was that bacterial infectious diseases would be overcome by the development of various antibiotics. However, these antibiotics are no longer as effective as they were 70 years ago [5]. Furthermore, Gram-negative pathogens resistant to colistin, the last resort antibiotic against MDR, have been reported [64,65]. On the other hand, a personalized bacteriophage-based treatment approved by the Food and Drug Administration (FDA) of the United States as an emergency investigational new drug (eIND) was administered to a 68-year-old patient infected with multidrug-resistant *Acinetobacter baumannii* and resulted in dramatic improvement from a comatose state, despite the patient not responding to several antibiotics, including colistin [66]. In addition, the efficient lytic capability of endolysins towards MRSA in an in vivo assay has been reported [43,67,68]. These data suggested that the therapeutic use of bacteriophages could be applicable to similar cases, and endolysins might have the same potential as bacteriophages.

The present study has clearly demonstrated that Lys-phiSA012 shows high lytic activity towards *S. aureus,* including MRSA strains. The OD_{600} was reduced within a few minutes of adding Lys-phiSA012, and bacterial growth was clearly inhibited in the turbidity reduction assay, as it was previously shown for Lys-phiK [69]. Lys-phiSA012 also showed lytic activity towards *S. pseudintermidius* and *S. haemoliticus* (Figure 2A–C) but not towards *Streptococcus agalactiae* (Figure 2D), indicating that it has a specific antimicrobial spectrum limited to staphylococci, including MDR *S. aureus.* Specific host ranges of bacteriophages and endolysins could be advantageous for clinical applications as they would not disrupt our normal microbiota. Broad host ranges of bacteriophage SA012 [28], bacteriophage K [70] and bacteriophage Twort [71] towards *S. aureus* strains have been reported but the amino acid sequences of their endolysins showed incomplete identity. In particular, the sequence similarity between Lys-phiSA012 and Lys-phiTwort is less than 50% (Figure 1C), suggesting that endolysins have evolved to have highly diverse activities, allowing us to select the most effective and specific endolysin for combatting a specific bacterial strain. Further evaluation of Lys-phiSA012 efficacy in vivo is needed prior to its clinical application. In addition, Lys-phiSA012 showed high lytic activity within a few minutes, as shown in Figure 2A–C, which might lead to the rapid release of toxins from lysed bacterial cells. Therefore, it may be necessary to develop extended release Lys-phiSA012 that kill bacteria gradually in the body.

The recognition of peptidoglycans by endolysins determines their spectrum of activity and is regulated by a SH3b domain which binds a highly specific bacterial ligand [72]. In addition, the maximum lytic activities of several endolysins, such as Lys-phiK [45], LytA [73], and lysostaphin [74], depend on a SH3b domain. As shown in Figure 3C, Lys-phiSA012WT and Δmt2, both containing CHAP-SH3b, showed maximum lytic activity towards SA003, suggesting that the Lys-phiSA012 SH3b domain is required for catalytic activity of the CHAP domain and plays a critical role in cell lysis. In addition, Δmt3, which contains AMID-SH3b, showed no lytic activity, indicating that the AMID domain of Lys-phiSA012 may not play an essential role in lytic activity towards SA003 as assessed using turbidity reduction assays, or that deletion of this domain might cause conformational changes leading to defective lytic activity. These data are consistent with previous reports regarding various staphylococcal endolysins harboring a SH3b domain [73,75].

A Ca^{2+}-binding site in the CHAP domain and a Zn^{2+}-binding site in the AMID domain of Lys-phiSA012 were identified by bioinformatics analysis (Figure 4A,B). We estimated that the presence of Zn^{2+} might not effect lytic activity significantly because Δmt3 might not efficiently lyse bacterial cell wall peptidoglycan; however, high lytic activity was observed in the presence of 100 μM Zn^{2+} (Figure 4C). It was reported that the CHAP domain of Lys-phiK, which has 99.39% amino acid sequence identity (Table 3, Figure A1A) with that of Lys-phiSA012, also harbors a Zn^{2+}-binding site [64] based on structural analysis. We suggest that Zn^{2+} affects not only the AMID domain but also the CHAP domain, leading to potent lytic activity. Furthermore, Donovan et al. [73] and Becker et al. [50] provided clues for the relationship between the catalytic roles of the CHAP and AMID domains, suggesting that endolysins harboring dual lytic domains derived from staphylococcal phages might respond differently (i.e., either exolytic or endolytic) to bacterial peptidoglycan. Here, we demonstrated that divalent ions in the medium play a critical role in the lytic activity of Lys-phiSA012 (Figure A2), and maximum lytic activity was observed in the presence of at least 1 mM Ca^{2+}, consistent with the extracellular concentration of Ca^{2+} which is closely regulated at around 1.2 mM [76], and 100 μM Zn^{2+}, consistent with the intracellular concentration of Zn^{2+} [77]. Taken together, we suggest that Lys-phiSA012 is activated by divalent ions, especially Ca^{2+} and Zn^{2+}, at specific minimum concentrations, binding to a specific site in the catalytic domains. As we known, the present study is the first to characterize the optimal range of Ca^{2+} and Zn^{2+} concentrations for the lytic activity of Lys-phiK and LysK-like endolysins. Changes in the amino acid residues in the CHAP and AMID domain among Lys-phiK, Lys-phiSA012 and other LysK-like endolysins (Table 4) are not located at the Ca^{2+}-, Zn^{2+}-binding sites (Figure 4C), suggesting that at least 1 mM Ca^{2+} and 100 μM Zn^{2+} might be required for efficient Lys-phiK and LysK-like endolysin lytic activity. Further investigations are needed to clarify the relationship between amino acid change(s) and the lytic activity of LysK-like endolysins compared to the lytic activity of Lys-phiK. In particular, further studies of the role of Ser83Asn found in more than half of LysK-like endolysins, including Lys-phiSA012 (Table 4, Figure 3C), are required because it was previously reported that certain single amino acid changes in the CHAP domain of Lys-phiK enhance lytic activity toward *S. aureus* stains [78].

It was reported that the CHAP domain of Lys-phiK cleaves at the pentaglycine linkage between peptidoglycan chains and that the AMID domain of Lys-phiK cleaves between N-acetylmuramic acid and L-alanine [45,79]. The mechanism underlying cell wall peptidoglycan digestion is different between endolysins and other antibiotics, and thus we tested the efficacy of Lys-phiSA012 with oxacillin towards *S. aureus*. As shown in Figure 5A, endolysins have significant potential for reducing antibiotics use because Lys-phiSA012 decreased the MIC of oxacillin more than 16-fold. In addition, the bactericidal activity of Lys-phiSA012 was shown to be limited in the presence of 25% glycerol, which we used as a vehicle for Lys-phiSA012 (Figure 5C). Notably, it was previously reported that MIC of Lys-phiK towards *S. aureus* is 78 ± 20 μg/mL [45]. A large amount of Lys-phiK might be required to kill these bacteria completely due to the inactivation of endolysin during overnight incubation in MIC assays; however, Lys-phiSA012 ($\geq$0.815 μg/mL) with 25% glycerol clearly inhibited bacterial growth in the present study, suggesting that the combination of Lys-phiSA012 with bacteriostatic agents might enhance and prolong the lytic activity of endolysins.

Generally, endolysins can directly access and subsequently digest the cell wall peptidoglycans of Gram-positive bacteria, as shown in Figure 2A, but are largely ineffective towards Gram-negative bacteria due to the outer membrane barrier [25,34]. In addition, some bacteria, including *S. aureus*, can move into the intracellular spaces to escape the immune system, making antibiotics and endolysins ineffective because they cannot access the cytosol due to the cellular membrane [80]. However, endolysins can be engineered to overcome their limited activity towards Gram-negative and intracellular bacteria by being fused to outer membrane permeabilizing peptides, allowing their transfer across the membrane barrier [81–83]. Further investigations are needed to develop Lys-phiSA012 for use against intracellular *S. aureus*.

In conclusion, we purified a LysK-like endolysin, Lys-phiSA012, and demonstrated that its highly potent lytic activity towards staphylococci is not limited to *S. aureus*. Furthermore, our results suggest optimal conditions for Lys-phiK and LysK-like endolysins. Our results will contribute to the understanding of LysK-like endolysins and to promoting the development of alternatives for antibiotics, leading to the reduction of antibiotic-resistant bacteria and supporting the proper use of antibiotics.

Acknowledgments: This study was supported in part by the Japan Society for the Promotion of Science (JSPS) KAKENHI, Grant-in-Aid for Scientific Research (B) program (numbers 22380174, 25292182) and (A) program (number 17H01506), and the Ministry of Education, Culture, Sports, Science and Technology of Japan (MEXT)-Supported Program for the Strategic Research Foundation at Private Universities, 2013-2017.

Author Contributions: Hidetoshi Higuchi, Yasunori Tanji, Yutaka Tamura and Hidetomo Iwano conceived and designed the experiments; Masaru Usui contributed reagents, materials and analysis tools; Jumpei Fujiki, Tomohiro Nakamura, Takaaki Furusawa, Hazuki Ohno, Hiromichi Takahashi and Junya Kitana performed experiments and analyzed the data; and Jumpei Fujiki and Hidetomo Iwano wrote the paper.

Appendix A

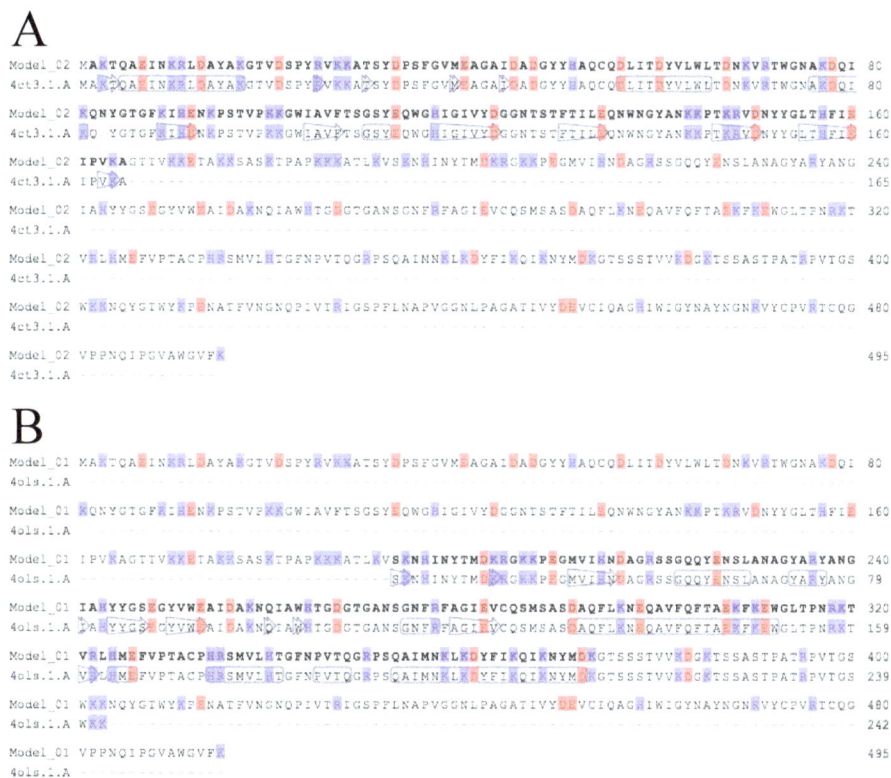

Figure A1. Model-template alignment in the protein structure model. Circles and arrows represent alpha-helices and beta-strands, respectively. Blue: positively charged amino acids, red: negatively charged amino acids. (**A**) Model-template alignment of the CHAP domain. Model_02; Lys-phiSA012 sequence. 4act. 1. A; Lys-phiK sequence. Lys-phiSA012 and Lys-phiK alignments of the other domains are described in Figure 1. (**B**) Model-template alignment of the AMID domain. Model_01; Lys-phiSA012 sequence. 4ols. 1. A; Lys-phiGH15 sequence. Lys-phiSA012 and Lys-phiGH15 alignments of the other domains are described in Figure 1. These data were analyzed using the SWISS-MODEL server.

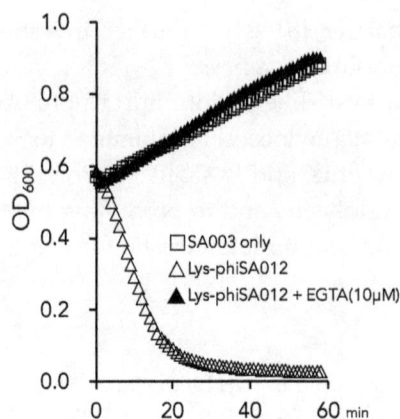

Figure A2. The effect of EGTA treatment on Lys-phiSA012 lytic activity. The lytic activity of Lys-phiSA012 w/wo EGTA was determined using the turbidity reduction assay. SA003 was grown in LB medium w/wo 10 mM EGTA and the assays were initiated by the addition of 64 µg/mL Lys-phiSA012.

References

1. Maragakis, L.L.; Perencevich, E.N.; Cosgrove, S.E. Clinical and economic burden of antimicrobial resistance. *Expert Rev. Anti-Infect. Ther.* **2008**, *6*, 751–763. [CrossRef] [PubMed]

2. De Kraker, M.E.; Wolkewitz, M.; Davey, P.G.; Koller, W.; Berger, J.; Nagler, J.; Icket, C.; Kalenic, S.; Horvatic, J.; Seifert, H.; et al. Clinical impact of antimicrobial resistance in European hospitals: Excess mortality and length of hospital stay related to methicillin-resistant *Staphylococcus aureus* bloodstream infections. *Antimicrob. Agents Chemother.* **2011**, *55*, 1598–1605. [CrossRef] [PubMed]

3. De Kraker, M.E.; Davey, P.G.; Grundmann, H.; Burden Study Group. Mortality and hospital stay associated with resistant *Staphylococcus aureus* and *Escherichia coli* bacteremia: Estimating the burden of antibiotic resistance in europe. *PLoS Med.* **2011**, *8*, e1001104. [CrossRef] [PubMed]

4. Asai, T.; Kojima, A.; Harada, K.; Ishihara, K.; Takahashi, T.; Tamura, Y. Correlation between the usage volume of veterinary therapeutic antimicrobials and resistance in *Escherichia coli* isolated from the feces of food-producing animals in japan. *Jpn. J. Infect. Dis.* **2005**, *58*, 369–372. [PubMed]

5. Golkar, Z.; Bagasra, O.; Pace, D.G. Bacteriophage therapy: A potential solution for the antibiotic resistance crisis. *J. Infect. Dev. Ctries.* **2014**, *8*, 129–136. [CrossRef] [PubMed]

6. Silbergeld, E.K.; Graham, J.; Price, L.B. Industrial food animal production, antimicrobial resistance, and human health. *Annu. Rev. Public Health* **2008**, *29*, 151–169. [CrossRef] [PubMed]

7. Sarmah, A.K.; Meyer, M.T.; Boxall, A.B. A global perspective on the use, sales, exposure pathways, occurrence, fate and effects of veterinary antibiotics (VAs) in the environment. *Chemosphere* **2006**, *65*, 725–759. [CrossRef] [PubMed]

8. Li, Y.X.; Zhang, X.L.; Li, W.; Lu, X.F.; Liu, B.; Wang, J. The residues and environmental risks of multiple veterinary antibiotics in animal faeces. *Environ. Monit. Assess* **2013**, *185*, 2211–2220. [CrossRef] [PubMed]

9. Smith, T.C.; Gebreyes, W.A.; Abley, M.J.; Harper, A.L.; Forshey, B.M.; Male, M.J.; Martin, H.W.; Molla, B.Z.; Sreevatsan, S.; Thakur, S.; et al. Methicillin-resistant *Staphylococcus aureus* in pigs and farm workers on conventional and antibiotic-free swine farms in the USA. *PLoS ONE* **2013**, *8*, e63704. [CrossRef] [PubMed]

10. Neyra, R.C.; Frisancho, J.A.; Rinsky, J.L.; Resnick, C.; Carroll, K.C.; Rule, A.M.; Ross, T.; You, Y.; Price, L.B.; Silbergeld, E.K. Multidrug-resistant and methicillin-resistant *Staphylococcus aureus* (MRSA) in hog slaughter and processing plant workers and their community in North Carolina (USA). *Environ. Health Perspect.* **2014**, *122*, 471–477. [PubMed]

11. Khanna, T.; Friendship, R.; Dewey, C.; Weese, J.S. Methicillin resistant *Staphylococcus aureus* colonization in pigs and pig farmers. *Vet. Microbiol.* **2008**, *128*, 298–303. [CrossRef] [PubMed]

12. Smith, T.C. Livestock-associated *Staphylococcus aureus*: The United States experience. *PLoS Pathog.* **2015**, *11*, e1004564. [CrossRef] [PubMed]

13. Geenen, P.L.; Graat, E.A.; Haenen, A.; Hengeveld, P.D.; Van Hoek, A.H.; Huijsdens, X.W.; Kappert, C.C.; Lammers, G.A.; Van Duijkeren, E.; Van De Giessen, A.W. Prevalence of livestock-associated MRSA on Dutch broiler farms and in people living and/or working on these farms. *Epidemiol. Infect.* **2013**, *141*, 1099–1108. [CrossRef] [PubMed]

14. Morcillo, A.; Castro, B.; Rodriguez-Alvarez, C.; Gonzalez, J.C.; Sierra, A.; Montesinos, M.I.; Abreu, R.; Arias, A. Prevalence and characteristics of methicillin-resistant *Staphylococcus aureus* in pigs and pig workers in Tenerife, Spain. *Foodborne Pathog. Dis.* **2012**, *9*, 207–210. [CrossRef] [PubMed]

15. Denis, O.; Suetens, C.; Hallin, M.; Catry, B.; Ramboer, I.; Dispas, M.; Willems, G.; Gordts, B.; Butaye, P.; Struelens, M.J. Methicillin-resistant *Staphylococcus aureus* st398 in swine farm personnel, Belgium. *Emerg. Infect. Dis.* **2009**, *15*, 1098–1101. [CrossRef] [PubMed]

16. Aubry-Damon, H.; Grenet, K.; Sall-Ndiaye, P.; Che, D.; Cordeiro, E.; Bougnoux, M.E.; Rigaud, E.; Le Strat, Y.; Lemanissier, V.; Armand-Lefevre, L.; et al. Antimicrobial resistance in commensal flora of pig farmers. *Emerg. Infect. Dis.* **2004**, *10*, 873–879. [CrossRef] [PubMed]

17. Sordillo, L.M.; Streicher, K.L. Mammary gland immunity and mastitis susceptibility. *J. Mammary Gland Biol. Neoplasia* **2002**, *7*, 135–146. [CrossRef] [PubMed]

18. Yamane, I. Epidemiological survey and economical evaluation of bovine mastitis in tie-stall dairy farms. *J. Jpn. Vet. Med. Assoc.* **2006**, *59*, 674–678. [CrossRef]

19. Costa, E.O.; Benites, N.R.; Guerra, J.L.; Melville, P.A. Antimicrobial susceptibility of *Staphylococcus* spp. isolated from mammary parenchymas of slaughtered dairy cows. *J. Vet. Med. B Infect. Dis. Vet. Public Health* **2000**, *47*, 99–103. [CrossRef] [PubMed]

20. Aires-de-Sousa, M. Methicillin-resistant *Staphylococcus aureus* among animals: Current overview. *Clin. Microbiol. Infect.* **2017**, *23*, 373–380. [CrossRef] [PubMed]

21. De Kraker, M.E.; Stewardson, A.J.; Harbarth, S. Will 10 million people die a year due to antimicrobial resistance by 2050? *PLoS Med.* **2016**, *13*, e1002184. [CrossRef] [PubMed]

22. O'Neill, L.J. Review on Antimicrobial Resistance Antimicrobial Resistance: Tackling a Crisis for the Health and Wealth of Nations. Available online: https://amr-review.org/sites/default/files/AMR%20Review% 20Paper%20-%20Tackling%20a%20crisis%20for%20the%20health%20and%20wealth%20of%20nations_1. pdf (accessed on 22 February 2018).

23. Haddad Kashani, H.; Schmelcher, M.; Sabzalipoor, H.; Seyed Hosseini, E.; Moniri, R. Recombinant endolysins as potential therapeutics against antibiotic-resistant *Staphylococcus aureus*: Current status of research and novel delivery strategies. *Clin. Microbiol. Rev.* **2018**, *31*. [CrossRef]

24. Cisek, A.A.; Dabrowska, I.; Gregorczyk, K.P.; Wyzewski, Z. Phage therapy in bacterial infections treatment: One hundred years after the discovery of bacteriophages. *Curr. Microbiol.* **2017**, *74*, 277–283. [CrossRef] [PubMed]

25. Doss, J.; Culbertson, K.; Hahn, D.; Camacho, J.; Barekzi, N. A review of phage therapy against bacterial pathogens of aquatic and terrestrial organisms. *Viruses* **2017**, *9*, 50. [CrossRef] [PubMed]

26. Furusawa, T.; Iwano, H.; Hiyashimizu, Y.; Matsubara, K.; Higuchi, H.; Nagahata, H.; Niwa, H.; Katayama, Y.; Kinoshita, Y.; Hagiwara, K.; et al. Phage therapy is effective in a mouse model of bacterial equine keratitis. *Appl. Environ. Microbiol.* **2016**, *82*, 5332–5339. [CrossRef] [PubMed]

27. Furusawa, T.; Iwano, H.; Higuchi, H.; Yokota, H.; Usui, M.; Iwasaki, T.; Tamura, Y. Bacteriophage can lyse antibiotic-resistant *Pseudomonas aeruginosa* isolated from canine diseases. *J. Vet. Med. Sci.* **2016**, *78*, 1035–1038. [CrossRef] [PubMed]

28. Synnott, A.J.; Kuang, Y.; Kurimoto, M.; Yamamichi, K.; Iwano, H.; Tanji, Y. Isolation from sewage influent and characterization of novel *Staphylococcus aureus* bacteriophages with wide host ranges and potent lytic capabilities. *Appl. Environ. Microbiol.* **2009**, *75*, 4483–4490. [CrossRef] [PubMed]

29. Iwano, H.; Inoue, Y.; Takasago, T.; Kobayashi, H.; Furusawa, T.; Taniguchi, K.; Fujiki, J.; Yokota, H.; Usui, M.; Tanji, Y.; et al. Bacteriophage ΦSA012 has a broad host range against *Staphylococcus aureus* and effective lytic capacity in a mouse mastitis model. *Biology* **2018**, *8*, 7.

30. Meaden, S.; Koskella, B. Exploring the risks of phage application in the environment. *Front. Microbiol.* **2013**, *4*, 358. [CrossRef] [PubMed]

31. Nobrega, F.L.; Costa, A.R.; Kluskens, L.D.; Azeredo, J. Revisiting phage therapy: New applications for old resources. *Trends Microbiol.* **2015**, *23*, 185–191. [CrossRef] [PubMed]

32. Guo, M.; Feng, C.; Ren, J.; Zhuang, X.; Zhang, Y.; Zhu, Y.; Dong, K.; He, P.; Guo, X.; Qin, J. A novel antimicrobial endolysin, lyspa26, against *Pseudomonas aeruginosa*. *Front. Microbiol.* **2017**, *8*, 293. [CrossRef] [PubMed]

33. Loeffler, J.M.; Nelson, D.; Fischetti, V.A. Rapid killing of *Streptococcus pneumoniae* with a bacteriophage cell wall hydrolase. *Science* **2001**, *294*, 2170–2172. [CrossRef] [PubMed]

34. Fischetti, V.A. Bacteriophage lytic enzymes: Novel anti-infectives. *Trends Microbiol.* **2005**, *13*, 491–496. [CrossRef] [PubMed]

35. Schuch, R.; Nelson, D.; Fischetti, V.A. A bacteriolytic agent that detects and kills bacillus anthracis. *Nature* **2002**, *418*, 884–889. [CrossRef] [PubMed]

36. Pastagia, M.; Euler, C.; Chahales, P.; Fuentes-Duculan, J.; Krueger, J.G.; Fischetti, V.A. A novel chimeric lysin shows superiority to mupirocin for skin decolonization of methicillin-resistant and -sensitive *Staphylococcus aureus* strains. *Antimicrob. Agents Chemother.* **2011**, *55*, 738–744. [CrossRef] [PubMed]

37. Rodriguez-Rubio, L.; Martinez, B.; Rodriguez, A.; Donovan, D.M.; Gotz, F.; Garcia, P. The phage lytic proteins from the *Staphylococcus aureus* bacteriophage vB_SauS-phiiPLA88 display multiple active catalytic domains and do not trigger staphylococcal resistance. *PLoS ONE* **2013**, *8*, e64671. [CrossRef] [PubMed]

38. Domenech, M.; Garcia, E.; Moscoso, M. In vitro destruction of *Streptococcus pneumoniae* biofilms with bacterial and phage peptidoglycan hydrolases. *Antimicrob. Agents Chemother.* **2011**, *55*, 4144–4148. [CrossRef] [PubMed]

39. Schuch, R.; Khan, B.K.; Raz, A.; Rotolo, J.A.; Wittekind, M. Bacteriophage lysin cf-301, a potent antistaphylococcal biofilm agent. *Antimicrob. Agents Chemother.* **2017**, *61*. [CrossRef] [PubMed]

40. O'Flaherty, S.; Coffey, A.; Meaney, W.; Fitzgerald, G.F.; Ross, R.P. The recombinant phage lysin lysk has a broad spectrum of lytic activity against clinically relevant staphylococci, including methicillin-resistant *Staphylococcus aureus*. *J. Bacteriol.* **2005**, *187*, 7161–7164. [CrossRef] [PubMed]

41. Gu, J.; Xu, W.; Lei, L.; Huang, J.; Feng, X.; Sun, C.; Du, C.; Zuo, J.; Li, Y.; Du, T.; et al. Lysgh15, a novel bacteriophage lysin, protects a murine bacteremia model efficiently against lethal methicillin-resistant *Staphylococcus aureus* infection. *J. Clin. Microbiol.* **2011**, *49*, 111–117. [CrossRef] [PubMed]

42. Loessner, M.J.; Gaeng, S.; Wendlinger, G.; Maier, S.K.; Scherer, S. The two-component lysis system of *Staphylococcus aureus* bacteriophage twort: A large TTG-start holin and an associated amidase endolysin. *FEMS Microbiol. Lett.* **1998**, *162*, 265–274. [CrossRef] [PubMed]

43. Zhang, L.; Li, D.; Li, X.; Hu, L.; Cheng, M.; Xia, F.; Gong, P.; Wang, B.; Ge, J.; Zhang, H.; et al. Lysgh15 kills *Staphylococcus aureus* without being affected by the humoral immune response or inducing inflammation. *Sci. Rep.* **2016**, *6*, 29344. [CrossRef] [PubMed]

44. Gu, J.; Feng, Y.; Feng, X.; Sun, C.; Lei, L.; Ding, W.; Niu, F.; Jiao, L.; Yang, M.; Li, Y.; et al. Structural and biochemical characterization reveals LysGH15 as an unprecedented "EF-Hand-Like" calcium-binding phage lysin. *PLoS Pathog.* **2014**, *10*, e1004109. [CrossRef] [PubMed]

45. Becker, S.C.; Dong, S.; Baker, J.R.; Foster-Frey, J.; Pritchard, D.G.; Donovan, D.M. Lysk chap endopeptidase domain is required for lysis of live staphylococcal cells. *FEMS Microbiol. Lett.* **2009**, *294*, 52–60. [CrossRef] [PubMed]

46. Sanz-Gaitero, M.; Keary, R.; Garcia-Doval, C.; Coffey, A.; van Raaij, M.J. Crystal structure of the lytic chap(k) domain of the endolysin Lysk from *Staphylococcus aureus* bacteriophage k. *Virol. J.* **2014**, *11*, 133. [CrossRef] [PubMed]

47. Ishihara, K.; Shimokubo, N.; Sakagami, A.; Ueno, H.; Muramatsu, Y.; Kadosawa, T.; Yanagisawa, C.; Hanaki, H.; Nakajima, C.; Suzuki, Y.; et al. Occurrence and molecular characteristics of methicillin-resistant *Staphylococcus aureus* and methicillin-resistant *Staphylococcus pseudintermedius* in an academic veterinary hospital. *Appl. Environ. Microbiol.* **2010**, *76*, 5165–5174. [CrossRef] [PubMed]

48. Ishihara, K.; Saito, M.; Shimokubo, N.; Muramatsu, Y.; Maetani, S.; Tamura, Y. Methicillin-resistant *Staphylococcus aureus* carriage among veterinary staff and dogs in private veterinary clinics in Hokkaido, Japan. *Microbiol. Immunol.* **2014**, *58*, 149–154. [CrossRef] [PubMed]

49. clinical and Laboratory standards Institute. Performance standards for antimicrobial susceptibility testing. *Twenty-First Inf. Suppl.* **2011**, *31*, 68–76.

50. Becker, S.C.; Swift, S.; Korobova, O.; Schischkova, N.; Kopylov, P.; Donovan, D.M.; Abaev, I. Lytic activity of the staphylolytic Twort phage endolysin CHAP domain is enhanced by the SH3b cell wall binding domain. *FEMS Microbiol. Lett.* **2015**, *362*, 1–8. [CrossRef] [PubMed]

51. Son, B.; Yun, J.; Lim, J.A.; Shin, H.; Heu, S.; Ryu, S. Characterization of lysb4, an endolysin from the *Bacillus cereus*-infecting bacteriophage b4. *BMC Microbiol.* **2012**, *12*, 33. [CrossRef] [PubMed]

52. Sader, H.S.; Flamm, R.K.; Jones, R.N. Antimicrobial activity of daptomycin tested against Gram-positive pathogens collected in Europe, Latin America, and selected countries in the Asia-Pacific region (2011). *Diagn. Microbiol. Infect. Dis.* **2013**, *75*, 417–422. [CrossRef] [PubMed]

53. Arnold, K.; Bordoli, L.; Kopp, J.; Schwede, T. The swiss-model workspace: A web-based environment for protein structure homology modelling. *Bioinformatics* **2006**, *22*, 195–201. [CrossRef] [PubMed]

54. Kiefer, F.; Arnold, K.; Kunzli, M.; Bordoli, L.; Schwede, T. The swiss-model repository and associated resources. *Nucleic Acids Res.* **2009**, *37*, D387–D392. [CrossRef] [PubMed]

55. Guex, N.; Peitsch, M.C.; Schwede, T. Automated comparative protein structure modeling with SWISS-MODEL and SWISS-PDBVIEWER: A historical perspective. *Electrophoresis* **2009**, *30*, S162–S173. [CrossRef] [PubMed]

56. Biasini, M.; Bienert, S.; Waterhouse, A.; Arnold, K.; Studer, G.; Schmidt, T.; Kiefer, F.; Gallo Cassarino, T.; Bertoni, M.; Bordoli, L.; et al. Swiss-Model: Modelling protein tertiary and quaternary structure using evolutionary information. *Nucleic Acids Res.* **2014**, *42*, W252–W258. [CrossRef] [PubMed]

57. Abatangelo, V.; Peressutti Bacci, N.; Boncompain, C.A.; Amadio, A.F.; Carrasco, S.; Suarez, C.A.; Morbidoni, H.R. Broad-range lytic bacteriophages that kill *Staphylococcus aureus* local field strains. *PLoS ONE* **2017**, *12*, e0181671. [CrossRef] [PubMed]

58. Takemura-Uchiyama, I.; Uchiyama, J.; Kato, S.; Inoue, T.; Ujihara, T.; Ohara, N.; Daibata, M.; Matsuzaki, S. Evaluating efficacy of bacteriophage therapy against *Staphylococcus aureus* infections using a silkworm larval infection model. *FEMS Microbiol. Lett.* **2013**, *347*, 52–60. [CrossRef] [PubMed]

59. Alves, D.R.; Gaudion, A.; Bean, J.E.; Perez Esteban, P.; Arnot, T.C.; Harper, D.R.; Kot, W.; Hansen, L.H.; Enright, M.C.; Jenkins, A.T. Combined use of bacteriophage k and a novel bacteriophage to reduce *Staphylococcus aureus* biofilm formation. *Appl. Environ. Microbiol.* **2014**, *80*, 6694–6703. [CrossRef] [PubMed]

60. Gutierrez, D.; Vandenheuvel, D.; Martinez, B.; Rodriguez, A.; Lavigne, R.; Garcia, P. Two phages, phiIPLA-RODI and phiIPLA-C1C, lyse mono- and dual-species staphylococcal biofilms. *Appl. Environ. Microbiol.* **2015**, *81*, 3336–3348. [CrossRef] [PubMed]

61. Dreher-Lesnick, S.M.; Schreier, J.E.; Stibitz, S. Development of phage lysin Lysa2 for use in improved purity assays for live biotherapeutic products. *Viruses* **2015**, *7*, 6675–6688. [CrossRef] [PubMed]

62. Fenton, M.; Cooney, J.C.; Ross, R.P.; Sleator, R.D.; McAuliffe, O.; O'Mahony, J.; Coffey, A. In silico modeling of the staphylococcal bacteriophage-derived peptidase chap(k). *Bacteriophage* **2011**, *1*, 198–206. [CrossRef] [PubMed]

63. Filatova, L.Y.; Donovan, D.M.; Becker, S.C.; Lebedev, D.N.; Priyma, A.D.; Koudriachova, H.V.; Kabanov, A.V.; Klyachko, N.L. Physicochemical characterization of the staphylolytic lysk enzyme in complexes with polycationic polymers as a potent antimicrobial. *Biochimie* **2013**, *95*, 1689–1696. [CrossRef] [PubMed]

64. Munoz-Price, L.S.; Poirel, L.; Bonomo, R.A.; Schwaber, M.J.; Daikos, G.L.; Cormican, M.; Cornaglia, G.; Garau, J.; Gniadkowski, M.; Hayden, M.K.; et al. Clinical epidemiology of the global expansion of *Klebsiella pneumoniae* carbapenemases. *Lancet Infect. Dis.* **2013**, *13*, 785–796. [CrossRef]

65. Zou, D.; Huang, S.; Lei, H.; Yang, Z.; Su, Y.; He, X.; Zhao, Q.; Wang, Y.; Liu, W.; Huang, L. Sensitive and rapid detection of the plasmid-encoded colistin-resistance gene *mcr-1* in enterobacteriaceae isolates by loop-mediated isothermal amplification. *Front. Microbiol.* **2017**, *8*, 2356. [CrossRef] [PubMed]

66. Schooley, R.T.; Biswas, B.; Gill, J.J.; Hernandez-Morales, A.; Lancaster, J.; Lessor, L.; Barr, J.J.; Reed, S.L.; Rohwer, F.; Benler, S.; et al. Development and use of personalized bacteriophage-based therapeutic cocktails to treat a patient with a disseminated resistant *Acinetobacter baumannii* infection. *Antimicrob. Agents Chemother.* **2017**. [CrossRef] [PubMed]

67. Daniel, A.; Euler, C.; Collin, M.; Chahales, P.; Gorelick, K.J.; Fischetti, V.A. Synergism between a novel chimeric lysin and oxacillin protects against infection by methicillin-resistant *Staphylococcus aureus*. *Antimicrob. Agents Chemother.* **2010**, *54*, 1603–1612. [CrossRef] [PubMed]

68. Rashel, M.; Uchiyama, J.; Ujihara, T.; Uehara, Y.; Kuramoto, S.; Sugihara, S.; Yagyu, K.; Muraoka, A.; Sugai, M.; Hiramatsu, K.; et al. Efficient elimination of multidrug-resistant *Staphylococcus aureus* by cloned lysin derived from bacteriophage ΦMR11. *J. Infect. Dis.* **2007**, *196*, 1237–1247. [CrossRef] [PubMed]

69. Becker, S.C.; Foster-Frey, J.; Donovan, D.M. The phage k lytic enzyme lysk and lysostaphin act synergistically to kill MRSA. *FEMS Microbiol. Lett.* **2008**, *287*, 185–191. [CrossRef] [PubMed]

70.   O'Flaherty, S.; Ross, R.P.; Meaney, W.; Fitzgerald, G.F.; Elbreki, M.F.; Coffey, A. Potential of the polyvalent anti-staphylococcus bacteriophage k for control of antibiotic-resistant staphylococci from hospitals. *Appl. Environ. Microbiol.* **2005**, *71*, 1836–1842. [CrossRef] [PubMed]

71.   Pantucek, R.; Rosypalova, A.; Doskar, J.; Kailerova, J.; Ruzickova, V.; Borecka, P.; Snopkova, S.; Horvath, R.; Gotz, F.; Rosypal, S. The polyvalent staphylococcal phage phi 812: Its host-range mutants and related phages. *Virology* **1998**, *246*, 241–252. [CrossRef] [PubMed]

72.   Schmelcher, M.; Shabarova, T.; Eugster, M.R.; Eichenseher, F.; Tchang, V.S.; Banz, M.; Loessner, M.J. Rapid multiplex detection and differentiation of listeria cells by use of fluorescent phage endolysin cell wall binding domains. *Appl. Environ. Microbiol.* **2010**, *76*, 5745–5756. [CrossRef] [PubMed]

73.   Donovan, D.M.; Lardeo, M.; Foster-Frey, J. Lysis of staphylococcal mastitis pathogens by bacteriophage phi11 endolysin. *FEMS Microbiol. Lett.* **2006**, *265*, 133–139. [CrossRef] [PubMed]

74.   Baba, T.; Schneewind, O. Target cell specificity of a bacteriocin molecule: A c-terminal signal directs lysostaphin to the cell wall of *Staphylococcus aureus*. *EMBO J.* **1996**, *15*, 4789–4797. [PubMed]

75.   Cheng, Q.; Fischetti, V.A. Mutagenesis of a bacteriophage lytic enzyme plygbs significantly increases its antibacterial activity against group b streptococci. *Appl. Microbiol. Biotechnol.* **2007**, *74*, 1284–1291. [CrossRef] [PubMed]

76.   Bronner, F. Extracellular and intracellular regulation of calcium homeostasis. *Sci. World J.* **2001**, *1*, 919–925. [CrossRef] [PubMed]

77.   Kambe, T.; Tsuji, T.; Hashimoto, A.; Itsumura, N. The physiological, biochemical, and molecular roles of zinc transporters in zinc homeostasis and metabolism. *Physiol. Rev.* **2015**, *95*, 749–784. [CrossRef] [PubMed]

78.   Jun, S.Y.; Jung, G.M.; Son, J.S.; Yoon, S.J.; Choi, Y.J.; Kang, S.H. Comparison of the antibacterial properties of phage endolysins sal-1 and lysk. *Antimicrob. Agents Chemother.* **2011**, *55*, 1764–1767. [CrossRef] [PubMed]

79.   Lu, J.Z.; Fujiwara, T.; Komatsuzawa, H.; Sugai, M.; Sakon, J. Cell wall-targeting domain of glycylglycine endopeptidase distinguishes among peptidoglycan cross-bridges. *J. Biol. Chem.* **2006**, *281*, 549–558. [CrossRef] [PubMed]

80.   Loffler, B.; Tuchscherr, L.; Niemann, S.; Peters, G. *Staphylococcus aureus* persistence in non-professional phagocytes. *Int. J. Med. Microbiol.* **2014**, *304*, 170–176. [CrossRef] [PubMed]

81.   Briers, Y.; Walmagh, M.; Van Puyenbroeck, V.; Cornelissen, A.; Cenens, W.; Aertsen, A.; Oliveira, H.; Azeredo, J.; Verween, G.; Pirnay, J.P.; et al. Engineered endolysin-based "artilysins" to combat multidrug-resistant Gram-negative pathogens. *Am. Soc. Microbiol.* **2014**, *5*, e01379-14. [CrossRef] [PubMed]

82.   Rodriguez-Rubio, L.; Chang, W.L.; Gutierrez, D.; Lavigne, R.; Martinez, B.; Rodriguez, A.; Govers, S.K.; Aertsen, A.; Hirl, C.; Biebl, M.; et al. 'Artilysation' of endolysin lambdasa2lys strongly improves its enzymatic and antibacterial activity against streptococci. *Sci. Rep.* **2016**, *6*, 35382. [CrossRef] [PubMed]

83.   Becker, S.C.; Roach, D.R.; Chauhan, V.S.; Shen, Y.; Foster-Frey, J.; Powell, A.M.; Bauchan, G.; Lease, R.A.; Mohammadi, H.; Harty, W.J.; et al. Triple-acting lytic enzyme treatment of drug-resistant and intracellular *Staphylococcus aureus*. *Sci. Rep.* **2016**, *6*, 25063. [CrossRef] [PubMed]

Permissions

All chapters in this book were first published in PHARMACEUTICALS, by MDPI; hereby published with permission under the Creative Commons Attribution License or equivalent. Every chapter published in this book has been scrutinized by our experts. Their significance has been extensively debated. The topics covered herein carry significant findings which will fuel the growth of the discipline. They may even be implemented as practical applications or may be referred to as a beginning point for another development.

The contributors of this book come from diverse backgrounds, making this book a truly international effort. This book will bring forth new frontiers with its revolutionizing research information and detailed analysis of the nascent developments around the world.

We would like to thank all the contributing authors for lending their expertise to make the book truly unique. They have played a crucial role in the development of this book. Without their invaluable contributions this book wouldn't have been possible. They have made vital efforts to compile up to date information on the varied aspects of this subject to make this book a valuable addition to the collection of many professionals and students.

This book was conceptualized with the vision of imparting up-to-date information and advanced data in this field. To ensure the same, a matchless editorial board was set up. Every individual on the board went through rigorous rounds of assessment to prove their worth. After which they invested a large part of their time researching and compiling the most relevant data for our readers.

The editorial board has been involved in producing this book since its inception. They have spent rigorous hours researching and exploring the diverse topics which have resulted in the successful publishing of this book. They have passed on their knowledge of decades through this book. To expedite this challenging task, the publisher supported the team at every step. A small team of assistant editors was also appointed to further simplify the editing procedure and attain best results for the readers.

Apart from the editorial board, the designing team has also invested a significant amount of their time in understanding the subject and creating the most relevant covers. They scrutinized every image to scout for the most suitable representation of the subject and create an appropriate cover for the book.

The publishing team has been an ardent support to the editorial, designing and production team. Their endless efforts to recruit the best for this project, has resulted in the accomplishment of this book. They are a veteran in the field of academics and their pool of knowledge is as vast as their experience in printing. Their expertise and guidance has proved useful at every step. Their uncompromising quality standards have made this book an exceptional effort. Their encouragement from time to time has been an inspiration for everyone.

The publisher and the editorial board hope that this book will prove to be a valuable piece of knowledge for researchers, students, practitioners and scholars across the globe.

List of Contributors

Ammar Almaaytah, Mohammed T. Qaoud and Gubran Khalil Mohammed
Department of Pharmaceutical Technology, Faculty of Pharmacy, Jordan University of Science and Technology, Irbid 22110, Jordan

Ahmad Abualhaijaa
Department of Applied Biological Sciences, Faculty of Science and Arts, Jordan University of Science and Technology, Irbid 22110 Jordan

Daniel Knappe and Ralf Hoffmann
Institute of Bioanalytical Chemistry, Faculty of Chemistry and Mineralogy and Center for Biotechnology and Biomedicine, Universität Leipzig, Deutscher Platz 5, 04103 Leipzig, Germany

Qosay Al-Balas
Department of Medicinal Chemistry, Faculty of Pharmacy, Jordan University of Science and Technology, Irbid 22110, Jordan

Tetiana Marchyshak, Tetiana Yakovenko and Zenoviy Tkachuk
Institute of Molecular Biology and Genetics, National Academy of Sciences of Ukraine, 03680 Kyiv, Ukraine

Igor Shmarakov
Department of Biochemistry and Biotechnology, Yurii Fedkovych Chernivtsi National University, 58012 Chernivtsi, Ukraine

Malose J. Mphahlele
Department of Chemistry, College of Science, Engineering and Technology, University of South Africa, Private Bag X06, Florida 1710, South Africa

Nishal Parbhoo
Department of Life & Consumer Sciences, College of Agriculture and Environmental Sciences, University of South Africa, Private Bag X06, Florida 1710, South Africa

Sorah Yoon
Department of Molecular and Cellular Biology, Beckman Research Institute of City of Hope, Duarte, CA 91010, USA

John J. Rossi
Department of Molecular and Cellular Biology, Beckman Research Institute of City of Hope, Duarte, CA 91010, USA

Irell and Manella Graduate School of Biological Sciences, Beckman Research Institute of City of Hope, Duarte, CA 91010, USA

Zaril H. Zakaria
Ministry of Health Malaysia, Block E1, E3, E6, E7 & E10, Parcel E, Federal Government Administration Centre, Putrajaya 62590, Malaysia
Applied Health Research Group, School of Life and Health Sciences, Aston University, Birmingham B4 7ET, UK

Alan Y. Y. Fong
Ministry of Health Malaysia, Block E1, E3, E6, E7 & E10, Parcel E, Federal Government Administration Centre, Putrajaya 62590, Malaysia
Sarawak Heart Centre, Kota Samarahan 94300, Malaysia
Clinical Research Centre, Sarawak General Hospital, Kuching 93586, Malaysia

Raj K. S. Badhan
Applied Health Research Group, School of Life and Health Sciences, Aston University, Birmingham B4 7ET, UK
Aston Pharmacy School, Aston University, Birmingham B4 7ET, UK

Daniela Almeida, Rita Pinho, Verónica Correia, Jorge Soares, Maria de Lourdes Bastos, Félix Carvalho and Vera Marisa Costa
UCIBIO, REQUIMTE, Laboratory of Toxicology, Faculty of Pharmacy, University of Porto, Rua de Jorge Viterbo Ferreira, 228, 4050-313 Porto, Portugal

João Paulo Capela
UCIBIO, REQUIMTE, Laboratory of Toxicology, Faculty of Pharmacy, University of Porto, Rua de Jorge Viterbo Ferreira, 228, 4050-313 Porto, Portugal
FP-ENAS (Unidade de Investigação UFP em Energia, Ambiente e Saúde), CEBIMED (Centro de Estudos em Biomedicina), Faculdade de Ciências da Saúde, Universidade Fernando Pessoa, 4249-004 Porto, Portugal

Rafael Sebastián Fort
Laboratorio de Interacciones Moleculares, Facultad de Ciencias, Universidad de la República, Montevideo, C.P.11400, Uruguay

Juan M. Trinidad Barnech
Laboratorio de Interacciones Moleculares, Facultad de Ciencias, Universidad de la República, Montevideo, C.P.11400, Uruguay
Laboratorio de Moléculas Bioactivas, CENUR Litoral Norte, Universidad de la República, Ruta 3 (km 363), Paysandú, C.P. 60000, Uruguay

María Ana Duhagon
Laboratorio de Interacciones Moleculares, Facultad de Ciencias, Universidad de la República, Montevideo, C.P.11400, Uruguay
Departamento de Genética, Facultad de Medicina, Universidad de la República, Montevideo, C.P. 11800, Uruguay

Juliette Dourron and and Guzmán Álvarez
Laboratorio de Moléculas Bioactivas, CENUR Litoral Norte, Universidad de la República, Ruta 3 (km 363), Paysandú, C.P.60000, Uruguay

Marcos Colazzo
Departamento de Química del Litoral, CENUR Litoral Norte, Universidad de la República, Paysandú, C.P.60000, Uruguay

Francisco J. Aguirre-Crespo
Facultad de Ciencias Químico Biológicas, Universidad Autónoma de Campeche, Campeche, C.P. 24039, Mexico

Elenilze Figueiredo Batista Ferreira
Posgraduate Program of Pharmaceutical Innovation, Federal University of Amapá, 68902-280 Macapá, AP,Brazil
Laboratory of Modeling and Computational Chemistry, Department of Biological and Health Sciences, Federal University of Amapá, 68902-280 Macapá, AP, Brazil

Mayara Amoras Teles Fujishima
Posgraduate Program of Pharmaceutical Innovation, Federal University of Amapá, 68902-280 Macapá, AP,Brazil
Laboratory of Modeling and Computational Chemistry, Department of Biological and Health Sciences, Federal University of Amapá, 68902-280 Macapá, AP, Brazil
Laboratory of Toxicology, Department of Biological and Health Sciences, Federal University of Amapá, 68902-280 Macapá, AP, Brazil

Cleydson Breno Rodrigues dos Santos
Posgraduate Program of Pharmaceutical Innovation, Federal University of Amapá, 68902-280 Macapá, AP,Brazil
Laboratory of Modeling and Computational Chemistry, Department of Biological and Health Sciences, Federal University of Amapá, 68902-280 Macapá, AP, Brazil

Department of Pharmaceutical Organic Chemistry, University of Granada, 18071 Granada, Spain

Jocivania Oliveira da Silva
Posgraduate Program of Pharmaceutical Innovation, Federal University of Amapá, 68902-280 Macapá, AP,Brazil
Laboratory of Toxicology, Department of Biological and Health Sciences, Federal University of Amapá, 68902-280 Macapá, AP, Brazil

Nayara dos Santos Raulino da Silva, Ryan da Silva Ramos and Kelton Luís Belém dos Santos
Laboratory of Modeling and Computational Chemistry, Department of Biological and Health Sciences, Federal University of Amapá, 68902-280 Macapá, AP, Brazil

Carlos Henrique Tomich de Paula da Silva
Computational Laboratory of Pharmaceutical Chemistry, Faculty of Pharmaceutical Sciences of Ribeirão Preto, 14040-903 São Paulo, Brazil

Joaquín Maria Campos Rosa
Department of Pharmaceutical Organic Chemistry, University of Granada, 18071 Granada, Spain

Aymeric Ousset and Kalliopi Dodou
School of Pharmacy and Pharmaceutical Sciences, Faculty of Health Sciences and Wellbeing, University of Sunderland, Sunderland SR13SD, UK

Rosanna Chirico, Florent Robin, Martin Alexander Schubert and Pascal Somville
UCB Pharma S.A.,Product Development, B-1420 Braine l'Alleud, Belgium

Elvis Legala Ongey and Peter Neubauer
Department of Biotechnology, Technische Universität Berlin, Ackerstraße 76, ACK24, D-13355 Berlin, Germany

Stephan Pflugmacher
Aquatic Ecotoxicology in an Urban Environment, Ecosystems and Environment Research Program, Faculty of Biological and Environmental Sciences, University of Helsinki, Niemenkatu 73, FI-15140 Lahti 2, 00100 Helsinki, Finland
Korean Institute of Science & Technology Europe, Joint Laboratory of Applied Ecotoxicology, Campus E7 1, 66123 Saarbrücken, Germany

Jumpei Fujiki, Tomohiro Nakamura, Takaaki Furusawa, Hazuki Ohno, Hiromichi Takahashi, Junya Kitana and Hidetomo Iwano
Laboratory of Biochemistry, School of Veterinary Medicine, Rakuno Gakuen University, Ebetsu 069-8501

Masaru Usui
Laboratory of Food Microbiology and Food Safety, School of Veterinary Medicine, Rakuno Gakuen University, Ebetsu 069-8501, Japan

Yutaka Tamura
Laboratory of Food Microbiology and Food Safety, School of Veterinary Medicine, Rakuno Gakuen University, Ebetsu 069-8501, Japan
Center for Veterinary Drug Development, Rakuno Gakuen University, Ebetsu 069-8501, Japan

Hidetoshi Higuchi
Laboratory of Veterinary Hygiene, School of Veterinary Medicine, Rakuno Gakuen University, Ebetsu 069-8501, Japan

Yasunori Tanji
Department of Bioengineering, Tokyo Institute of Technology, Yokohama 226-8502, Japan

Index